CASE REVIEW

Brain
Imaging

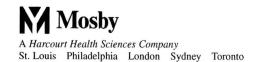

A Harcourt Health Sciences Company
St. Louis Philadelphia London Sydney Toronto

Laurie A. Loevner, MD
Assistant Professor
Department of Radiology
University of Pennsylvania Medical Center
Philadelphia, Pennsylvania

WITH 426 ILLUSTRATIONS

CASE REVIEW

Brain
Imaging

CASE REVIEW SERIES

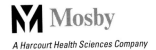

Mosby

A Harcourt Health Sciences Company

Publisher: Geoff Greenwood
Editor: Liz Corra
Associate Developmental Editor: Marla Sussman
Project Manager: Carol Sullivan Weis
Senior Production Editor: Rick Dudley
Designer: Jen Marmarinos

Printed in the United States of America

Mosby, Inc.
11830 Westline Industrial Drive
St. Louis, Missouri 63146

Library of Congress Cataloging-in-Publication Data

Loevner, Laurie A.
    Case review : brain imaging / Laurie A. Loevner.
      p.   cm. — (Case review series)
    Includes bibliographical references and index.
    ISBN 0-323-00430-X
    1. Brain—Imaging—Case studies. I. Title. II. Title: Brain imaging. III. Series.
    [DNLM: 1. Brain—radiography examination questions.
2. Brain—radiography case studies.   WL 18.2 L826c 1999]
    RC386.6.D52L64 1999
    616.8'04752'076—dc21
    DNLM/DLC   99-10768

00 01 02 03 / 9 8 7 6 5 4 3 2

To my loving and devoted husband Steven and
our beautiful son Benjamin,
You are my sunshine.

To my parents,
For your unconditional love and support.

My experience in teaching medical students, residents, fellows, practicing radiologists, and clinicians has been that they love the case conference format more than any other approach. I hope that the reason for this is not a reflection on my lecturing ability, but rather that people stay awake, alert, and on their toes more when they are in the hot seat (or may be the next person to assume the hot seat). In the dozens of continuing medical education courses I have directed, the case review sessions are almost always the most popular parts of the courses.

The idea of this Case Review series grew out of a need for books designed as exam preparation tools for the resident, fellow, or practicing radiologist about to take the boards or the certificate of additional qualification (CAQ) exams. Anxiety runs extremely high concerning the content of these exams, administered as unknown cases. Residents, fellows, and practicing radiologists are very hungry for formats that mimic this exam setting and that cover the types of cases they will encounter and have to accurately describe. In addition, books of this ilk serve as excellent practical reviews of a field and can help a practicing board-certified radiologist keep his or her skills sharpened. Thus heads banged together, and Mosby and I arrived at the format of the volume herein, which is applied consistently to each volume in the series. We believe that these volumes will strengthen the ability of the reader to interpret studies. By formatting the individual cases so that they can "stand alone," these case review books can be read in a leisurely fashion, a case at a time, on the whim of the reader.

The content of each volume is organized into three sections based on difficulty of interpretation and/or the rarity of the lesion presented. There are the Opening Round cases, which graduating radiology residents should have relatively little difficulty mastering. The Fair Game section consists of cases that require more study, but most people should get into the ballpark with their differential diagnoses. Finally, there is the Challenge section. Most fellows or fellowship-trained practicing radiologists will be able to mention entities in the differential diagnoses of these challenging cases, but one shouldn't expect to consistently "hit home runs" a la Mark McGwire. The Challenge cases are really designed to whet one's appetite for further reading on these entities and to test one's wits. Within each of these sections, the selection of cases is entirely random, as one would expect at the boards (in your office or in Louisville).

For many cases in this series, a specific diagnosis may not be what is expected—the quality of the differential diagnosis and the inclusion of appropriate options are most important. Teaching how to distinguish between the diagnostic options (taught in the question and answer and comment sections) will be the goal of the authors of each Case Review volume.

The best way to go through these books is to look at the images, guess the diagnosis, answer the questions, and then turn the page for the answers. If there are two cases on a page, do them two at a time. No peeking!

Mosby (through the strong work of Liz Corra) and I have recruited most of the authors of THE REQUISITES series (editor, James Thrall, MD) to create Case Review books for their subspecialties. To meet the needs of certain subspecialties and to keep each of the volumes to a consistent, practical size, some specialties will have more than one volume (e.g., ultrasound, interventional and vascular radiology, and neuroradiology). Nonetheless, the pleasing tone of THE REQUISITES series and its emphasis on condensing the fields of radiology into its foundations will be inculcated into the Case Review volumes. In many situations, THE REQUISITES authors have enlisted new coauthors to breathe a novel approach and excitement into the cases submitted. I think the fact that so many of THE REQUISITES authors are "on board" for this new series is a testament to their dedication to teaching. I hope that the success of THE REQUISITES is duplicated with the new Case Review series. Just as THE REQUISITES series provides coverage of the essentials in each subspecialty and successfully meets that overwhelming need in the market, I hope that the

Case Review series successfully meets the overwhelming need in the market for practical, focused case reviews.

In this volume on brain imaging authored by Dr. Laurie A. Loevner, you gain the perspective of one of the young bright academicians in neuroradiology. Dr. Loevner has one of the sharpest eyes in the business, and her ability to consistently arrive at the correct diagnosis has impressed all the members of the Neuroradiology Section of the University of Pennsylvania Medical Center. She was the unanimous choice of Bob Grossman and myself to author the Brain version of the Case Review Series, which has cross-references to our REQUISITES volume (*Neuroradiology: THE REQUISITES,* Mosby, 1994). I am certain that the reader will benefit immensely as Dr. Loevner imparts her uncanny acumen in reading cases. I hope you have fun learning neuroradiology via the case study approach. We'd all love your feedback!

David M. Yousem, MD

I was delighted when I was asked to prepare the foreword for the new book authored by my friend and colleague, Dr. Laurie Loevner. I have watched Dr. Loevner's career since she was a resident. She has rapidly matured from resident, through attending, lecturer, and researcher, and has now become author of a wonderful new book. This volume is the second in a series of Case Review books and covers Brain Imaging. The Case Review series consists of well-priced books that focus, volume by volume, on the individual radiology subspecialties. These books can be used independently or in tandem with the immensely popular series from Mosby— THE REQUISITES.

Dr. Loevner's book contains 200 well-chosen cases. Each of them models a typical clinical radiologic diagnostic problem. Each of the 200 cases is illustrated with one to four figures, for a total of over 400 MR, CT, and angiographic images. These cases are presented in a randomized manner. One case may be metastatic disease and the very next could be a vascular process. This creates novelty for the reader. Each case includes four key questions. The reader then turns the page to reveal the actual case diagnosis, the answers to the four key questions, a small number of key references, and a cross-reference to the *Neuroradiology: THE REQUISITES* textbook. Reviewing these cases simulates the real world of radiologic diagnosis, but it also serves as practice and review for those pesky examinations.

Teaching, especially at the resident level, has been both my vocation and my avocation for the past 19 years. During that time, I have observed that everyone learns differently. Some prefer to follow a linear course, with new incremental knowledge being added to what has already been learned. This is the traditional method used in most textbooks and in most didactic lecture series. Some of us prefer to learn by analysis, by breaking down a problem—a case—and then learning through understanding how our analysis worked, or how our thought process failed. Most of us prefer some combination of these two extremes. Thus it is marvelous when a set of integrated teaching tools is developed that allows us to choose how we learn. The combination of THE REQUISITES textbooks with the Case Review series is an excellent example of providing coordination between didactic and problem-based learning. The detailed didactic material is presented sequentially through the textbook approach of THE REQUISITES, whereas the Case Reviews allow a simulation of the "real world" environment—where every case is first seen as an "unknown." These books fit hand-in-glove.

I think that anyone who successfully navigates through these carefully selected cases will be much better prepared and will enjoy greater self-confidence as they face the real examiners.

James G. Smirniotopoulos, MD
Professor of Radiology and Neurology
Chairman, Department of Radiology and Nuclear Medicine
Uniformed Services University of the Health Sciences

Having finished this book, I look back with a sense of amazement, wonder, and ecstasy. It has been the highlight thus far of my academic career. Writing this book has given me the opportunity to fulfill what I consider to be the most substantial role as an academician, that of an educator. I hope that you will find the pages that follow as informative and educational as I believe them to be.

The book is intended to provide insight into the interpretation of brain imaging studies, with particular attention to imaging features that allow one to distinguish one entity from among the other possible diagnoses. Hundreds of hours alone have been poured into the preparation of the images, hoping to provide superb quality for educational purposes. The book is a radiologic presentation of a spectrum of disease entities in a case-by-case format. The questions and answers that accompany each case are designed to provide insight into the significance of specific imaging findings, as well as to provide "pearls" and factual data regarding the clinical, pathologic, and demographic aspects of the diseases covered herein. Because the book is organized in a case-by-case format, you can sit down and read it for hours on end if you chose (and I hope you do), or you may pick it up and read when you find a few free moments here and there (without losing your place). Following the questions and answers for each entity covered, there is a discussion providing pertinent imaging, clinical, and factual information. For each case, a cross-reference in *Neuroradiology: THE REQUISITES* is provided, and in some instances, you are referred to pages in that text that cover some aspect of the anatomy, physiology, or other disease processes that involve that region. In addition, reference(s) is provided for each case. When appropriate, I have tried to cite the "classic" article for a particular entity. In other cases, I have tried to emphasize more current literature that provides new imaging pearls or future directions in the development of imaging techniques to improve our ability to perform our job as radiologists.

The energy and enthusiasm required to prepare this book was fueled by the curious and inquisitive radiology fellows, residents, and medical students with whom I work so closely everyday. Without your enthusiasm, support, and desire to be educated, I could not have completed it. In addition, David Yousem's enthusiasm for neuroradiology and his strong work ethic (which is unparalleled) recharged my battery in those wee hours of the night when I thought the lights would go out. With this book, I have tried to emphasize our role as radiologists. This book is intended as an educational tool for a wide spectrum of readers, including medical students, radiology residents (especially for preparation of exams), neuro-radiology fellows, practicing general radiologists, and neuroradiologists.

I hope that you find this Case Review fun and educational!

Laurie A. Loevner, MD

I could not have completed this book without the support of so many people who deserve credit in helping me with this arduous project.

I should probably start with my husband Steven. Marrying him was clearly my most ingenious accomplishment to date! I couldn't have picked anyone more supportive. Not only has he endured my incredible work schedule, which begins before the sun rises and typically ends long after it sets, he also has endured my travel schedule, which frequently takes me cross-country or overseas. I must reluctantly admit that he has also endured numerous nights with no dinner on the table. Before this project, the house was perfect and if you opened a kitchen cupboard, all the cans were neatly stacked and organized based on their contents. Furthermore, the kitchen counters and tabletops throughout the house were naked, spanking clean, frankly bare! This has all changed in the last few years. Quite simply, the book took over our house. In addition to taking over my computer, the book took over my husband's computer as well. Reluctantly, I think my husband would admit that he has become accustomed to my "organized chaos" and more relaxed about coming home to a house that looks lived in. I am fortunate to have married a man who finds my enthusiasm for my work infectious and my commitment to my work enticing. He balances the rest of my life.

On May 7, 1998, I gave birth to twins—my son Benjamin David and the first draft of this book! I must thank my beautiful son—little does he know that without him I could not have completed this book. At about the same time I started preparing this book, I happily found out that I was pregnant. During his months of in utero development, Ben has endured numerous business trips, has spent hours in the library with me retrieving journal articles, and was with me during the entire first draft of this book that was dictated. If talking to your children while they are in utero really works, my son's first words will probably be "MR imaging" or "signal intensity." It is said that being pregnant is intended to prepare you for those sleepless nights after the baby is born; however, nothing prepared me better than the preparation of this manuscript. On those nights that I was burning the midnight oil, I relished the moments when Benjamin would awaken. His big blue eyes and sparkling smile no matter what hour of the day make the sun shine.

I want to thank all of the fellows, residents, and medical students over the last 3 years who have fueled the foundation of my career. Their desire to learn makes work each day rewarding. In particular, I want to thank the fourth-year residents who were preparing for their oral boards at the time I was buried in the preparation of this book. Maj Wickstrom, David Roberts, Linda Kloss, Kathleen Dougherty, Lisa Collazzo, Sam Wu, and I spent countless hours reviewing cases. They were instrumental in providing insight not only into what cases to include in the book but also in directing the appropriate questions that accompany many of the cases. I had no doubt that they would all pass their oral boards with flying colors, and they did. I would like to thank two medical students in particular, Andrew Mong and Wendy Hsu, with whom I work closely. They have been a tremendous motivational force. Thanks to Sid Roychowdhury, Linda Kloss, Rita Patel, Ronald Wolf, Jill Langer, and the neuroradiology faculty at the Children's Hospital of Philadelphia for providing some of the interesting and challenging cases in the book. I am also indebted to many people who read portions of my book and provided useful feedback. In particular, I want to thank David Yousem, Azita Khorsandi, and Chad Holder, who each spent long hours reviewing the entire manuscript and providing thoughtful criticism that enhanced the final product.

To my friends and colleagues in the Neuroradiology Section at the University of Pennsylvania—David Hackney, Bob Hurst, Linda Bagley, Joseph Maldjian, Herb Goldberg, and Steve Imbesi—thanks for your support and encouragement. To Bob Grossman—my boss, a mentor, and friend—thanks for reminding me that you can't please everybody all the time and to be true to yourself. If nothing else, I have completed a project that I am proud of. To David Yousem, my partner, close friend, and mentor, I express deep gratitude for giving me the opportunity to write this book. I hope I have done you proud! Thank you for your support, encouragement, and insight. You have shown me that it is not necessarily the final destination that provides the greatest satisfaction but rather all the stops we make along the way. Corona and Carol—I couldn't have done it without you. A very special thank you to Corona, who transcribed the entire first draft of this book. With my "3-finger" typing technique, I might still be on the first draft without your help.

I want to thank the Mosby staff, in particular Liz Corra and Marla Sussman. Writing this book gave me the opportunity to meet some very special, hard-working, creative people. Thanks for your enthusiastic support. In addition, I would like to thank the Media Services at the University of Pennsylvania, who spent countless hours helping me to prepare the images.

Last but not least, I want to thank my family and friends. To my parents and the rest of the Loevner clan, thanks for years of support. I personally think all of you deserve your own MD degrees as you have journeyed with me each step of the way in my medical career. To the Berger family—thanks for your interest and support (and for providing my husband and me with dinner on occasions and holidays). To Judy and Jon Goodman, and Sandy and Arnie Galman—the summer barbecues were great (I believe they were my salvation to the outside world!). "Rosabear"—thanks for taking such good care of Ben! To Cindy Urbach, Natalie Carlson, Lynne Secatore, Lois Mannon, and Janice Ford—you've kept me focused and energized for so many years! To Ella Kazerooni my dear friend—it's been a grand decade knowing you! Thank you for your friendship, support, inspiration, and your confidence in me as a friend and physician. Thanks to my loving and devoted husband Steven, and our darling son Benjamin; where would I be without you?

To the readership, a very special thanks. I hope you enjoy this Case Review!

Opening Round

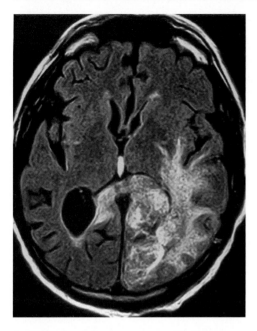 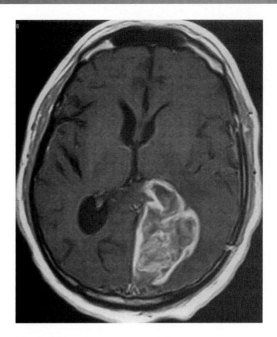

1. What neoplasms are most likely to present with this imaging appearance?
2. What radiologic feature favors a primary central nervous system (CNS) tumor over metastatic disease in this case?
3. Of the various histologic types of gliomas, which is most common?
4. According to the World Health Organization (WHO) classification of brain tumors, what are the three types of diffuse astrocytic brain tumors?

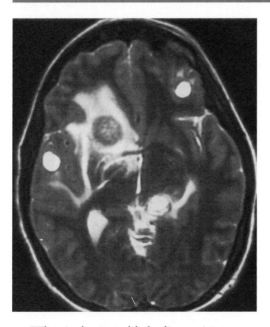 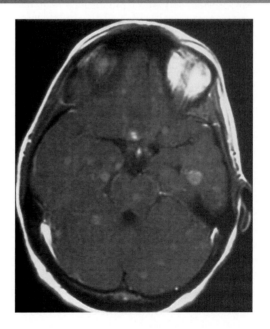

1. What is the most likely diagnosis?
2. What factors may contribute to a metastasis appearing hyperdense on an unenhanced CT and hypointense on a T2W MRI?
3. How often do solitary metastases to the brain occur?
4. What site of metastases may be associated with minimal or no edema such that they are frequently missed on T2W imaging and necessitate the administration of intravenous contrast for their detection?

Infiltrating Astrocytoma—Glioblastoma Multiforme

1. Primary glial neoplasm, lymphoma, and metastatic disease.

2. The enhancing portion of the mass extends directly into the splenium of the corpus callosum, which is expanded. Abnormal signal intensity on the fluid-attenuation inversion recovery (FLAIR) image extends across the corpus callosum to the right peritrigonal white matter.

3. Glioblastoma multiforme (GBM); represents at least 50% of all glial neoplasms.

4. Astrocytoma, anaplastic astrocytoma, and GBM.

Reference

Bagley LJ, Grossman RI, Judy KD, Curtis M, Loevner LA, Polansky M, Detre J: Gliomas: correlation of magnetic susceptibility artifact with histologic grade, *Radiology* 202: 511-516, 1997.

Cross-Reference

Neuroradiology: THE REQUISITES, pp 87-90.

Comment

According to the WHO classification, infiltrating astrocytic tumors may be divided into three subtypes: astrocytoma, anaplastic astrocytoma, and GBM. The histologic criteria for these subdivisions depend on many factors, including cellular density, number of mitoses, presence of necrosis, nuclear/cytoplasmic pleomorphism, and vascular endothelial proliferation. GBM typically has all of these histologic features, whereas the lower grade astrocytomas may only demonstrate minimal increased cellularity and cellular pleomorphism. The presence of necrosis and vascular endothelial proliferation in particular favor GBM, the most malignant of the glial neoplasms.

Glioblastomas are the most common supratentorial neoplasms in adults. The peak incidence is in the sixth decade of life. As with most types of gliomas, there is an increased incidence in men compared with women. Clinical presentation may include signs of increased intracranial pressure and/or focal neurologic symptoms. Prognosis is poor, with average survival at approximately 1 year. MRI is the most sensitive imaging modality for demarcating the extent of abnormality; however, on pathologic examination of resected neoplasms, tumor infiltration may be seen in areas of the brain that appear normal on MRI. Therefore MRI is not always accurate in defining the entire extent of a neoplasm. However, it does reflect many of the pathologic findings, including necrosis, hemorrhage, and hypercellularity (regions of T2W hypointensity). Flow voids representing vascular proliferation may be identified. Most GBMs enhance. Enhancement may be heterogeneous and ring-like around regions of necrosis. This enhancement pattern may also be seen in metastases and radiation necrosis.

Notes

Multiple Brain Metastases—Breast Carcinoma

1. Metastatic disease.

2. Acute hemorrhage, dense cellularity, high protein concentration, and metastases with calcification.

3. Approximately 30% to 50% of patients with parenchymal brain metastases have isolated lesions on imaging.

4. Cortical metastases.

Reference

Healy ME, Hesselink JR, Press GA, Middleton MS: Increased detection of intracranial metastases with intravenous Gd-DTPA, *Radiology* 165:619-624, 1987.

Cross-Reference

Neuroradiology: THE REQUISITES, pp 79-81, 87.

Comment

Metastatic disease is among the most common causes of intracranial masses in adults. More often than not metastases are multiple; however, in 30% to 50% of cases they may present as isolated lesions on imaging. The common systemic tumors associated with brain metastases include lung and breast carcinomas, melanoma, and vascular tumors such as renal and thyroid carcinoma. Enhanced MRI is clearly more sensitive than CT in detecting cerebral metastases. Metastases are typically rounded, circumscribed masses that demonstrate enhancement; however, the enhancement pattern may vary (solid, peripheral, or heterogeneous). In addition, metastatic lesions are often associated with a disproportionate amount of surrounding edema, which is manifested on T2W images as increased signal intensity (such is the case of the lesion in the inferior right frontal lobe in this patient).

Metastases typically occur at the gray-white matter interface because tumor cells lodge in the small caliber vessels in this location. Metastatic deposits may also involve the cortex. With cortical metastases in particular, edema may be absent such that metastatic lesions could be missed on T2W imaging. Therefore it is essential to give intravenous contrast in all patients with suspected brain metastases. Studies examining the role of double- and triple-dose gadolinium have shown that although higher doses of contrast reveal more metastases than does a single dose, this often occurs in patients whose standard dose study already shows more than one metastasis. Therefore management in these patients is not affected. In patients with no or a single metastasis on single-dose gadolinium, higher doses of contrast material yield additional metastases in less than 10% of cases.

Notes

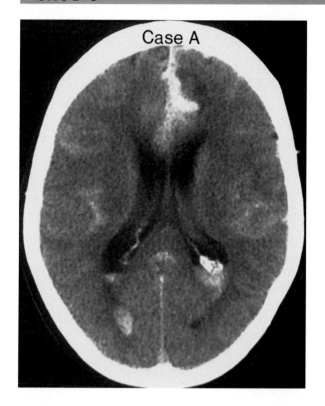

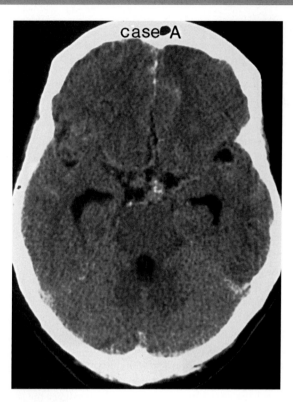

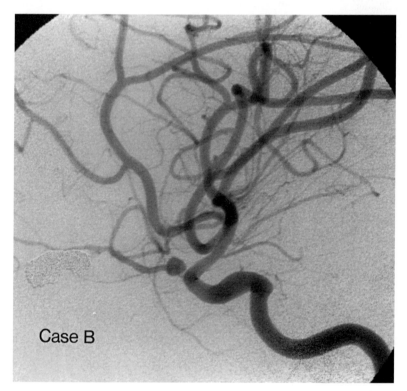

1. What are the major CT findings?
2. What was the clinical presentation of the patient in case A?
3. Given the CT findings, what imaging study should be performed next?
4. What type of aneurysms typically arises from the distal cerebral arteries?

Traumatic Pseudoaneurysm

1. Acute subarachnoid hemorrhage, intraventricular hemorrhage, and early hydrocephalus.

2. Worst headache of life.

3. Cerebral angiography.

4. Mycotic aneurysms, traumatic aneurysms, and aneurysms arising from invasion of the arterial wall by tumor emboli (atrial myxoma).

Reference

Loevner LA, Ting TY, Hurst RW, Goldberg H, Schut L: Spontaneous thrombosis of a basilar artery traumatic aneurysm in a child, *AJNR Am J Neuroradiol* 19:386-388, 1998.

Cross-Reference

Neuroradiology: THE REQUISITES, pp 136-139.

Comment

Prompt catheter angiography with meticulous technique is necessary in the evaluation of subarachnoid hemorrhage because this type of hemorrhage is associated with significant morbidity and mortality. Up to 15% of patients with acute subarachnoid hemorrhage die before reaching the hospital. The incidence of aneurysmal rebleeding occurs at a rate of approximately 2% per day in the first 2 weeks following the initial hemorrhage. With diagnostic angiography, there are several issues that the radiologist must address. These include identifying the vessel from which the aneurysm arises, aneurysm size, the presence or absence of an aneurysm neck, the orientation of the aneurysm, and the anatomy of the circle of Willis. A search to exclude multiple aneurysms is necessary. If there is more than one aneurysm, it is necessary to try to address which aneurysm bled.

In addition to subarachnoid and intraventricular hemorrhage with hydrocephalus, the first CT image also shows an intraparenchymal hematoma in the medial left frontal lobe caused by rupture of an aneurysm arising along the pericallosal artery. The aneurysm is most likely traumatic in this patient who had prior severe head injury. Case B shows a traumatic aneurysm of the ophthalmic artery caused by a gunshot wound to the head.

Traumatic aneurysms are rare, comprising less than 1% of all intracranial aneurysms. The majority involve branches of the middle and anterior cerebral arteries, or the internal carotid artery at the skull base. Traumatic aneurysms may result from penetrating injuries (e.g., direct arterial injury from projectiles, bone fragments from skull fractures) or blunt trauma. In closed head injuries, the mechanism of arterial injury may involve vessel stretching and torsion, or compression against the dura or bony prominences at the skull base. Rupture of traumatic pseudoaneurysms occurs in up to 33% of reported cases. (Did you notice the hyperdense mass in the suprasellar cistern corresponding to an incidental distal internal carotid artery aneurysm?)

Notes

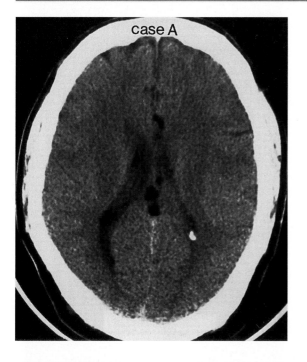

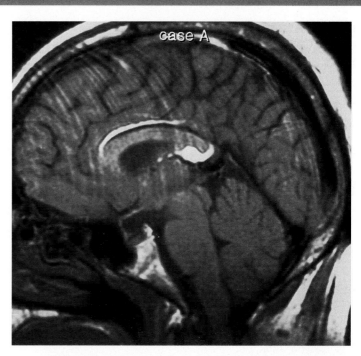

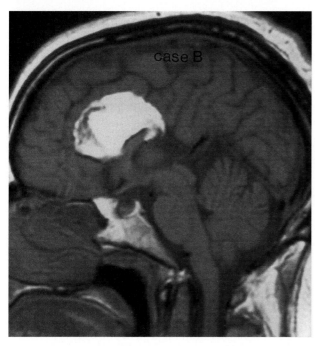

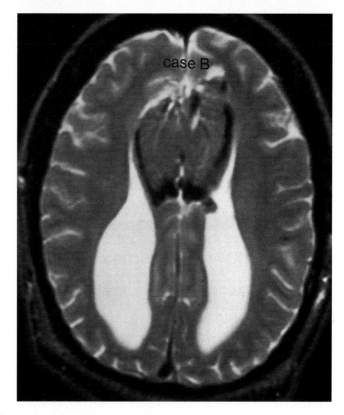

1. What structures may be responsible for the presence of signal voids in these masses?

2. What are the characteristic signal intensities of these lesions on spin-echo MRI sequences?

3. What are the most common locations of these lesions?

4. One can confirm that an intracranial mass is composed of fat by identifying what other MRI findings?

Lipoma Associated With Dysgenesis of the Corpus Callosum

1. Vessels or calcifications.

2. Hyperintense on T1W, intermediate-weighted, FLAIR, and fast spin-echo T2W sequences. On conventional spin-echo T2W imaging fat is hypointense (isointense to the brain).

3. The pericallosal region (interhemispheric fissure), cerebellopontine angle, suprasellar and quadrigeminal cisterns.

4. Chemical shift artifact on T2W images (which results in hypointensity at the periphery of the lesion along the frequency encoded axis while the contralateral edge is hyperintense) and loss of signal with the application of fat-suppression pulse.

References

Demaerel P, Van de Gaer P, Wilms G, et al: Interhemispheric lipoma with variable callosal dysgenesis: relationship between embryology, morphology, and symptomatology, *Eur Radiol* 6:904-909, 1996.

Dean B, Drayer BP, Berisini DC, Bird CR: MR imaging of pericallosal lipoma, *AJNR Am J Neuroradiol* 9:929-931, 1988.

Cross-Reference

Neuroradiology: THE REQUISITES, pp 77-78, 259, 320.

Comment

A widely accepted theory for the development of intracranial lipomas is they arise from abnormal differentiation of embryologic meninx primitiva (a mesodermal derivative of the neural crest). The meninx primitiva encases the CNS, and its inner lining is resorbed to allow formation of the subarachnoid spaces. Intracranial lipomas are not neoplasms but rather disorders of the development of subarachnoid spaces. Because lipomas are believed to develop from the inner layer of the meninx primitiva that forms the subarachnoid space, pericallosal arteries in interhemispheric lipomas and cranial nerves in cerebellopontine angle lipomas, respectively, often course through the lesions.

Intracranial lipomas most often occur in the interhemispheric fissure (up to 50%), followed by the quadrigeminal cistern (25%), the suprasellar cistern (15%), and the cerebellopontine cistern (10%). They are frequently associated with underdevelopment or dysgenesis of adjacent brain tissue. Lesions occurring around the posterior corpus callosum, especially the splenial region (case A), are "ribbon-like" in appearance. In these cases the corpus callosum is relatively normally developed. Lipomas along the anterior corpus callosum within the interhemispheric fissure (case B) are often "tumefactive" (mass-like in configuration) and are associated with partial agenesis of the corpus callosum. Lipomas in the quadrigeminal cistern may be associated with underdevelopment of the inferior colliculus.

Notes

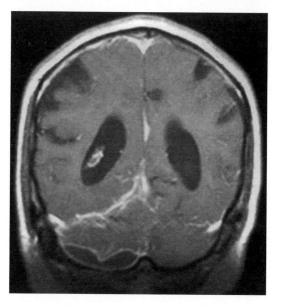
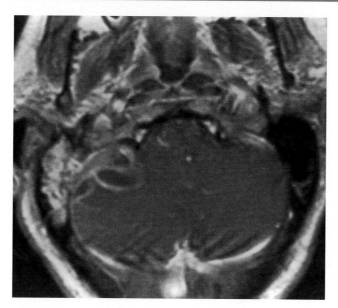

1. Direct extension from what areas is the most common cause of this entity?

2. Which paranasal sinuses are most commonly implicated in this disorder?

3. Which are more commonly complicated by brain abscess and/or venous thrombosis, epidural abscesses or subdural empyemas?

4. What is the standard treatment for subdural empyemas?

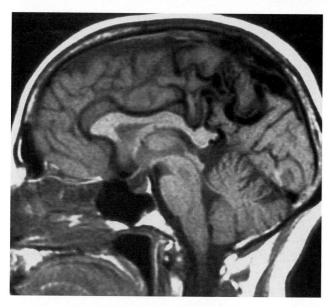
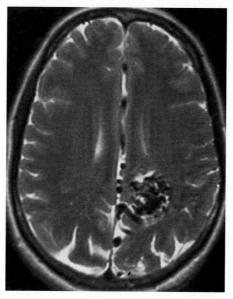

1. What is the estimated annual hemorrhage rate of these lesions?

2. What pathophysiology explains why brain tissue around these lesions may be atrophied?

3. What are causes of false negative angiograms in patients with surgically proven arteriovenous malformations (AVMs)?

4. What is the major vascular supply to the lesion in this case?

Epidural Abscess

1. The paranasal sinuses and mastoid air cells.

2. The frontal sinuses.

3. Subdural empyemas.

4. Surgical drainage and antibiotic therapy.

Reference

Tsuchiya K, Makita K, Furui F, Kusano S, Inoue Y: Contrast-enhanced magnetic resonance imaging of sub- and epidural empyemas, *Neuroradiology* 34:494-496, 1992.

Cross-Reference

Neuroradiology: THE REQUISITES, pp 172-173.

Comment

Epidural abscesses are most frequently caused by direct extension of infection from the paranasal sinuses or mastoid air cells. Of the paranasal sinuses, frontal sinusitis is probably the most common cause of intracranial epidural and subdural abscesses. These serious infections may also occur as a complication following craniotomy and meningitis. On imaging, these lesions share the common appearance of other extracerebral abnormalities. Epidural abscesses (like hematomas) are contained by the cranial sutures and may cross the midline. In contrast, subdural hematomas do not spread across the midline because they are confined by the falx, allowing differentiation from epidural collections. On CT epidural abscesses are usually hypodense relative to the brain parenchyma. On MRI they are usually hypointense to isointense on T1W imaging (depending on the protein concentration and the cellular content) and hyperintense relative to the brain on T2W imaging. After the administration of contrast, there is usually prominent enhancement of a thickened dura or dural membrane. Epidural and subdural empyemas may be complicated by cerebritis and intraparenchymal abscess formation. In addition, dural venous and/or cortical vein thrombosis with venous infarction may occur. In the presence of suspected epidural or subdural empyema on imaging, the radiologist (in addition to the clinician) should search for a site of origin of the infection, as well as its contiguous spread into the intracranial compartment.

Notes

Cerebral Arteriovenous Malformation

1. Two percent to 4%. The mean interval between hemorrhagic events is approximately 7 to 8 years.

2. The "steal" phenomenon in which there is parasitization of the blood supply from the normal brain preferentially to the AVM. Gliosis in the affected brain may result in focal neurologic symptoms or seizures.

3. Lack of angiographic visualization of a surgically proven AVM may be due to a very small AVM, thrombosis of the AVM, and mass effect usually related to an associated parenchymal hemorrhage that compresses the AVM and prevents its filling.

4. The pericallosal artery from the anterior cerebral circulation.

References

Nussel F, Wegmuller H, Huber P: Comparison of magnetic resonance angiography, magnetic resonance imaging, and conventional angiography in cerebral arteriovenous malformations, *Neuroradiology* 33:56-61, 1991.

Spetzler RF, Martin NA: A proposed grading system for arteriovenous malformations, *J Neurosurg* 65:476-483, 1986.

Cross-Reference

Neuroradiology: THE REQUISITES, pp 142-145.

Comment

Arteriovenous malformations represent a vascular nidus made up of a core of entangled vessels fed by one or more enlarged feeding arteries. Blood is shunted from the nidus to enlarged draining vein(s), which terminate in the deep and/or superficial venous system.

Spetzler and Martin have proposed a grading scheme for AVMs that is aimed at predicting the risk of operative morbidity and mortality. AVMs are graded on a scale of I to VI, determined by size (<3 cm, 3 to 6 cm, >6 cm), pattern of drainage (superficial or deep), and involvement of the cortex (noneloquent or eloquent). Grade I lesions are small, superficial, and do not involve eloquent cortex. On the opposite end of the spectrum, grade VI lesions are usually inoperable.

On CT the vascular nidus of an AVM and enlarged draining veins are usually isodense or hyperdense to gray matter on unenhanced images as a result of pooling of blood. Calcification may be present. Arteriovenous malformations enhance and have characteristic serpentine flow voids on MRI related to fast flow in dilated arteries. In lesions associated with an acute parenchymal hemorrhage, phase-contrast magnetic resonance angiography (MRA) best demonstrates the AVM (it subtracts out the signal intensity of the blood products in the hematoma, in contrast to time-of-flight MRA). Cerebral angiography shows enlarged feeding arteries, the vascular nidus, and early draining veins. In cases of very small AVMs, early venous filling should be sought on careful evaluation of the angiographic images.

Notes

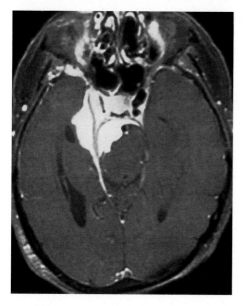

1. What is the most likely diagnosis?

2. What is the most common T2W appearance of hypercellular neoplasms?

3. What finding is highly suggestive of the diagnosis of meningioma?

4. By what mechanism do head and neck cancers extend to the cavernous sinus?

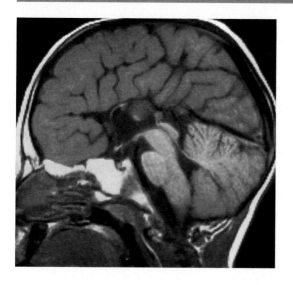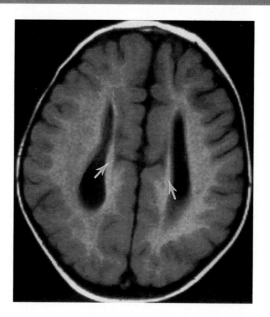

1. What are the names of these structures *(arrows)*?

2. In this entity, the mesial hemispheric sulci course uninterrupted in a radial manner all the way to the third ventricle because of the absence of what structure?

3. What congenital anomalies are associated with this entity?

4. In partial dysgenesis of the corpus callosum, which portions of the corpus callosum are typically spared?

Meningioma Involving the Right Cavernous Sinus

1. Meningioma invading the cavernous sinus.

2. They are frequently hypointense to cerebrospinal fluid (CSF; isointense to brain tissue).

3. Encasement and narrowing of the cavernous internal carotid artery.

4. Perineural spread through the skull base foramina.

References

O'Sullivan MG, van Loveren HR, Tew JM Jr: The surgical resectability of meningiomas of the cavernous sinus, *Neurosurgery* 40:238-244, 1997.

De Jesus O, Sekhar LN, Parikh HK, Wright DC, Wagner DP: Long-term follow-up of patients with meningiomas involving the cavernous sinus: recurrence, progression, and quality of life, *Neurosurgery* 39:915-919, 1996.

Cross-Reference

Neuroradiology: THE REQUISITES, p 327.

Comment

Lesions arising within the cavernous sinus tend to enlarge the sinus, resulting in outward convexity of its lateral dural margin. This lateral bulging may be focal (such as with a cavernous carotid aneurysm) or more diffuse (as is the case with meningiomas and schwannomas). Meningiomas of the cavernous sinus have a somewhat characteristic appearance, tending to grow along the lateral dural surface. As in this case, growth along the dura may extend anteriorly around the tip of the temporal lobe and posteriorly along the tentorium. Another finding of meningiomas involving the cavernous sinus that may help to differentiate them from other solid enhancing masses that occur in this location is that 66% partially or totally encase the cavernous internal carotid artery and 33% narrow the artery, as is shown in this patient. Occlusion of a vessel is unusual. Rarely, meningiomas may extend through the skull base foramina. Otherwise, the density on CT, intensity on MRI, and enhancement characteristics of meningiomas in this location are similar to those of meningiomas occurring in other locations. Besides meningioma, the differential diagnosis of solid, expansile masses in the cavernous sinus includes a schwannoma of cranial nerves III through VI; metastatic disease, including perineural spread of tumor; lymphoma; and infection.

Management of cavernous sinus meningiomas includes radiation therapy, surgical resection, gamma-knife radiosurgery, or a combination of these treatment modalities. Resectability is dependent on the degree of encasement of the internal carotid artery and the extent of cavernous sinus involvement. The primary cause of operative morbidity is cranial neuropathies, which affect eye motion and facial sensation.

Notes

Agenesis of the Corpus Callosum

1. The Probst bundles are the white matter tracts that were destined to cross the corpus callosum. The axons that would usually cross from right to left in the corpus callosum instead form tracts that run anterior to posterior along the medial walls of the lateral ventricles parallel to the interhemispheric fissure.

2. The cingulate gyrus.

3. Lipomas, migrational abnormalities, Dandy-Walker syndrome, Chiari malformations, and holoprosencephaly, to name just a few!

4. The anterior portions (except the rostrum).

Reference

Atlas SW, Zimmerman RA, Bilaniuk LT, et al: Corpus callosum and limbic system: neuroanatomic MR evaluation of developmental anomalies, *Radiology* 160:355-362, 1986.

Cross-Reference

Neuroradiology: THE REQUISITES, pp 254-256.

Comment

Axons arising from the right and left cerebral hemispheres grow into the lamina reuniens (the dorsal aspect of the lamina terminalis), giving rise to the corpus callosum (and also the hippocampal commissures). The corpus callosum develops between the eleventh and twentieth gestational weeks in an organized manner, with formation of the anterior genu first followed in order by the anterior body, posterior body, splenium, and rostrum. Given this pattern of development, in partial dysgenesis of the corpus callosum the anterior portion is formed and partial dysgenesis affects the posterior portions (posterior body, splenium) and rostrum. In cases in which the splenium is very small or not visualized, partial dysgenesis of the corpus callosum can be readily distinguished from an insult to a previously fully developed splenium by checking for the presence of the rostrum. If the rostrum is absent, the splenial abnormality corresponds to partial dysgenesis. However, if the rostrum is present given that it forms after the splenium, a splenial abnormality must have occurred on the basis of an insult resulting in secondary atrophy/volume loss.

Imaging findings in complete agenesis of the corpus callosum include lack of convergence of the lateral ventricles, which are displaced laterally and oriented in a vertical fashion; a high riding third ventricle (which may form an interhemispheric cyst); and ex-vacuo enlargement of the occipital and temporal horns (colpocephaly) related to deficient white matter.

Notes

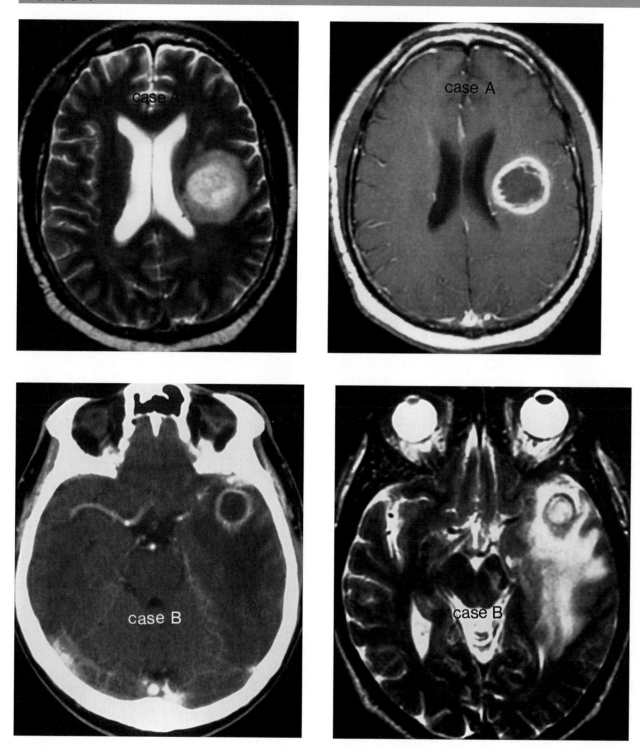

1. What is the differential diagnosis of a ring enhancing mass?

2. Regarding necrotic metastases, what is the most common cell type to result in this appearance?

3. Cerebritis and/or pyogenic brain abscesses are most commonly acquired through what routes of transmission?

4. What MRI findings regarding the rim of a mass favor the diagnosis of infection over other causes of a ring enhancing lesion?

Pyogenic Brain Abscess

1. Primary brain tumor, metastatic disease, pyogenic brain abscess, demyelinating disease, granuloma, other infectious processes, radiation necrosis, and a maturing hematoma.

2. Metastatic adenocarcinoma.

3. Either by direct spread from otorhinologic infections or by hematogenous spread.

4. A circumferential rim that is isointense to slightly hyperintense to white matter on unenhanced T1W images and hypointense on T2W images may be present around a brain abscess. This appearance is believed to be related to the presence of collagen, free radicals within macrophages, and/or small areas of hemorrhage.

References

Kim SH, Chang KH, Song IC, et al: Brain abscess and brain tumor: discrimination with in vivo H-1 MR spectroscopy, *Radiology* 204:239-245, 1997.

Haimes AB, Zimmerman RD, Morgello S, et al: MR imaging of brain abscesses, *AJR Am J Roentgenol* 152:1073-1085, 1989.

Cross-Reference

Neuroradiology: THE REQUISITES, pp 176-180.

Comment

The development of a pyogenic brain abscess may be divided into four stages: early cerebritis, late cerebritis, early capsule formation, and late capsule formation. The length of time required to form a mature abscess varies from approximately 2 weeks to months. In the mature abscess there is a collagen capsule that is slightly thinner on the ventricular side than on the cortical margin (this may be related to differences in perfusion). The presence of a dimple or small evagination pointing toward the ventricular margin from a ring enhancing lesion should raise suspicion for an abscess. This is also important because intraventricular rupture and ependymitis may occur and are associated with a very poor prognosis. In the presence of a mature abscess, there is relatively little surrounding cerebritis and edema (case A) compared with the early stages of abscess formation (case B). In case A the patient was treated with antibiotics for 10 days before the images were obtained.

The typical treatment for a mature brain abscess is surgical drainage and antibiotic therapy. Cerebritis and early abscesses may be managed with antibiotics and should be followed closely both with MRI, as well as clinically for signs of improvement. Successful management monitored with serial MRI examinations will reveal a decrease in the surrounding edema, mass effect, and associated enhancement. It is important to remember that the radiologic findings lag behind clinical improvement, and enhancement may persist for months. Resolution of an abscess may result in an area of gliosis with small calcifications.

Notes

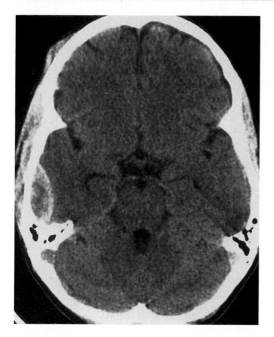 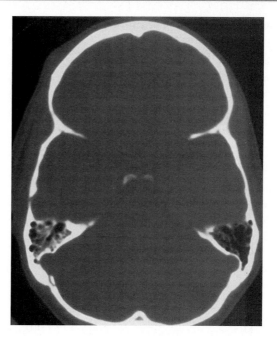

1. What is the most common cause of this extraaxial mass?

2. What arterial and venous complications may occasionally occur with calvarial fractures through the meningeal groove?

3. What are possible causes for the region of hypodensity within this hyperdense extraaxial mass?

4. How are venous epidural hematomas caused, and where do they occur?

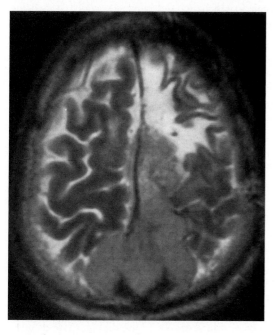 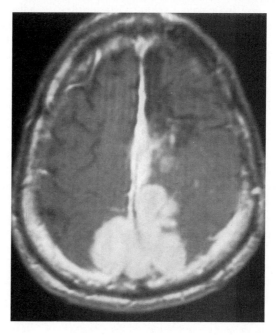

1. Is the mass intraaxial or extraaxial in origin, and from what structure does it arise?

2. What is the differential diagnosis?

3. What vascular structure is involved?

4. What clinical and imaging findings may occur with venous ischemia/congestion?

Acute Epidural Hematoma With a Small Nondisplaced Temporal Bone Fracture

1. Direct laceration of the middle meningeal artery related to a skull fracture (present in 80% to 90% of cases).

2. Pseudoaneurysms of the meningeal artery (most commonly the middle meningeal artery) and arteriovenous fistulas if a fracture lacerates both the middle meningeal artery and vein.

3. Leakage of serum from the epidural clot or active bleeding.

4. Laceration of a dural venous sinus by an underlying skull fracture. The most common location of venous epidural hematomas is the posterior fossa as a result of injury of the transverse or sigmoid sinus. These may also occur in the paramedian location over the cerebral convexities or in the middle cranial fossa related to a tear in the superior sagittal or sphenoparietal sinus, respectively.

Reference
Hamilton M, Wallace C: Nonoperative management of acute epidural hematoma diagnosed by CT: the neuroradiologist's role, *AJNR Am J Neuroradiol* 13:853-859, 1993.

Cross-Reference
Neuroradiology: THE REQUISITES, pp 151-152.

Comment
In the vast majority of cases, epidural hematomas are secondary to laceration of the meningeal arteries (most commonly the middle meningeal artery) by a skull fracture. Occasionally (10%) epidural hematomas occur as a result of tearing of meningeal arteries in the absence of a fracture. This is most common in children and may be related to transient depression of the soft calvaria on these arteries. Most arterial epidural hematomas occur in the temporoparietal region.

On CT acute epidural hematomas are hyperdense extraaxial masses that can usually be distinguished from acute subdural hematomas based on their shape. Epidural hematomas tend to be biconvex compared with subdural hematomas, which are usually lenticular in configuration. Another finding that may be useful is that epidural hematomas are usually confined by the cranial sutures because in these regions the dura is adherent to the periosteum of the inner calvaria. In comparison, subdural hematomas cross sutural boundaries because they occur deep to the dura.

Venous epidural hematomas are much less common than are arterial epidural hematomas. Venous epidural hematomas are usually related to laceration or tearing of a dural venous sinus. They are most common in the posterior fossa and are most frequently seen in the pediatric population. Unlike arterial epidural hematomas and subdural hematomas, venous epidural hematomas may extend across the tentorium involving both the supratentorial and the infratentorial compartments.

Notes

Falx Meningioma Invading the Superior Sagittal Sinus

1. Extraaxial, from the falx.

2. Meningioma is most likely; however, other neoplastic processes must be considered, including dural metastases and hemangiopericytomas.

3. There is invasion of the superior sagittal sinus.

4. Headache, papilledema, and focal neurologic deficits. Imaging findings suggesting venous infarction include subcortical high signal intensity, bilateral parenchymal hemorrhages (particularly in cases of superior sagittal sinus thrombosis), and hemorrhagic infarctions that are not in arterial distributions.

Reference
Hutzelmann A, Palmie S, Buhl R, Freund M, Heller M: Dural invasion of meningiomas adjacent to the tumor margin on Gd-DTPA-enhanced MR images: histopathologic correlation, *Eur Radiol* 8:746-748, 1998.

Cross-Reference
Neuroradiology: THE REQUISITES, pp 68-73, 131-132, 509-510.

Comment
These images demonstrate a poorly demarcated extraaxial mass in the interhemispheric fissure along the falx cerebri. The mass is only mildly hyperintense (because of its cellularity) to the adjacent brain parenchyma and enhances avidly. Enhancing tumor is noted obliterating the superior sagittal sinus. High signal intensity in the white matter of the posterior left frontal lobe with associated cortical atrophy is related to prior surgery. High signal intensity in the frontal white matter bilaterally may be the result of prior radiation therapy for residual tumor.

In trying to determine the cause of this lesion, it is important to view the remainder of the brain as well as the calvaria for other abnormalities. This is because the vast majority of malignant extraaxial neoplasms are caused by bone metastases. Destructive or infiltrative lesions within the calvaria that may affect the inner and outer cortical tables should be sought. In addition, metastases may be associated with extraosseous soft tissue masses within the scalp. Multiple lesions within the calvaria favor metastatic disease. Additional malignant extraaxial masses include metastases and lymphoma (which may involve the leptomeninges, dura, or bone). The most common cause of an extraaxial neoplasm in adults is meningioma. Although meningiomas may demonstrate changes along the inner table of the skull (hyperostosis and less commonly lysis), a dural-based mass in the absence of disease involving the diploic space or outer table of the skull still favors meningioma (as do statistics!)

Notes

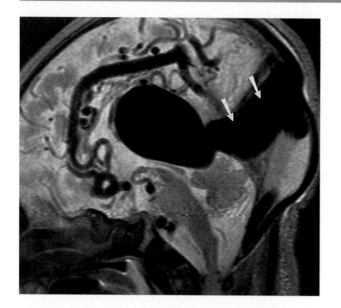

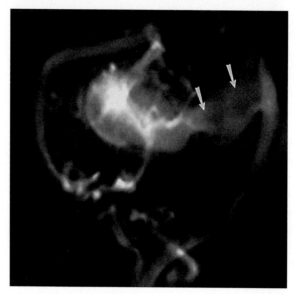

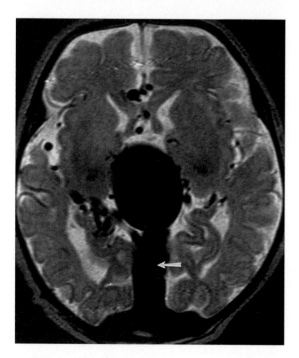

1. What is the diagnosis?

2. What are common clinical presentations of this abnormality in newborns?

3. What is the underlying pathology in this entity?

4. What sinus *(arrows)* is frequently present when the straight sinus is absent or thrombosed?

Vein of Galen Aneurysm

1. Vein of Galen aneurysm.

2. High-output congestive heart failure, hydrocephalus, and/or macrocephaly.

3. These malformations represent a spectrum of vascular malformations. The two major types of vascular abnormalities are true AVMs or direct arteriovenous fistulas (between choroidal arteries and vein of Galen).

4. The falcine sinus.

Reference

Raybaud CA, Strother CM, Hald JK: Aneurysms of the vein of Galen: embryonic considerations and anatomical features related to the pathogenesis of the malformation, *Neuroradiology* 31:109-128, 1989.

Cross-Reference

Neuroradiology: THE REQUISITES, pp 63, 239.

Comment

The CT appearance of a vein of Galen aneurysm in an infant is characteristic. On unenhanced images, the vein of Galen appears as a hyperdense, demarcated mass at the level of the posterior third ventricle and diencephalon. Following intravenous contrast administration, there is marked homogeneous enhancement of the malformation. MRI not only confirms the presence of flow within this abnormality, but it also better delineates both the arterial and venous anatomy. In combination with MRA, MRI may show large choroidal artery–venous fistulas and/or the presence of a parenchymal AVM. In this case, a vein of Galen aneurysm is associated with a large AVM confirmed by MRA. Because many women undergo obstetric ultrasound as part of their prenatal care, many of these malformations are detected in utero with color flow Doppler/sonography.

Early in embryologic development, the deep brain structures/diencephalon are drained by the median prosencephalic vein. As the internal cerebral veins begin to develop, this vein slowly regresses. A caudal remnant of the median prosencephalic vein will become the normal vein of Galen. In patients with vein of Galen aneurysms related to either a parenchymal AVM or a direct arteriovenous fistula between the choroidal vessels, a persistent median prosencephalic vein may occur. In that this provides diencephalic venous drainage, the straight sinus may not form. Instead, a falcine sinus is frequently noted (as in this case; *arrows*). Vein of Galen malformations resulting from direct arteriovenous fistulas are frequently associated with venous obstruction and venous hypertension.

Notes

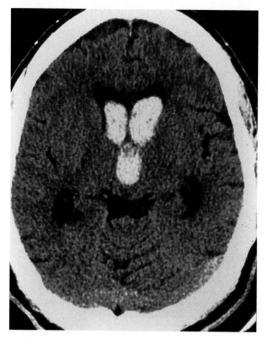
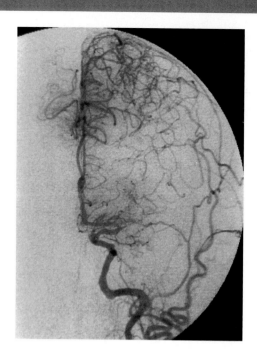

1. What are the major imaging findings?
2. What is the major risk factor for intraventricular hemorrhage related to germinal matrix bleeds in newborns?
3. In the setting of trauma, intraventricular hemorrhage is commonly associated with what other traumatic brain injury?
4. In adults, what conditions may present with spontaneous intraventricular hemorrhage in the absence of trauma?

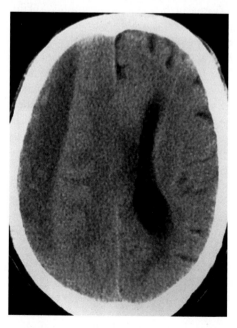
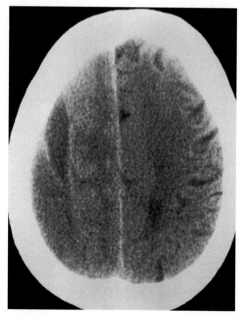

1. Which type of extracerebral hematoma is usually related to an arterial injury?
2. What factors may contribute to the development of an isodense to hypodense acute subdural hematoma?
3. Which type of extraaxial hematoma is confined by the cranial sutures?
4. What are causes of subacute and chronic subdural hematomas in infants?

Intraventricular Hemorrhage

1. Diffuse intraventricular hemorrhage with acute hydro-cephalus.

2. Prematurity/low birth weight.

3. Diffuse axonal injury of the corpus callosum.

4. A vascular malformation (e.g., choroidal AVM), rupture of a cerebral hematoma into the ventricular system (as might be seen with a deep gray matter bleed in hypertension), and rupture of an aneurysm of the posterior inferior cerebellar artery.

Reference

Gentry LR, Thompson B, Godersky JC: Trauma to the corpus callosum: MR features, *AJNR Am J Neuroradiol* 9:1129-1138, 1988.

Cross-Reference

Neuroradiology: THE REQUISITES, pp 156-159.

Comment

This case shows an intraventricular blood clot with thrombus casting the lateral, third, and fourth ventricles. There is secondary acute hydrocephalus. Intraventricular hemorrhage is common in the setting of closed head injury, occurring in 2% to 40% of patients, depending on the severity of injury. Traumatic intraventricular hemorrhage is most commonly associated with diffuse axonal injury, particularly of the corpus callosum, and may also be seen with injury to the septum pellucidum due to tearing of small subependymal veins along these structures.

Nontraumatic causes of intraventricular hemorrhage include rupture of large intraparenchymal hematomas related to a variety of disease processes (e.g., hypertension or amyloid angiopathy in the elderly). In patients presenting with intraventricular hemorrhage in the absence of other findings to suggest a cause, vascular abnormalities such as choroidal AVMs must be excluded, and angiography is usually indicated for further evaluation. Ruptured aneurysms of the posterior inferior cerebellar artery may also present with intraventricular hemorrhage, although the hemorrhage is usually located preferentially in the fourth ventricle. Whereas intraventricular hemorrhage in the setting of hypertension is common because of rupture of deep gray matter hematomas into the ventricular system, isolated intraventricular hemorrhage in the absence of a parenchymal bleed is unusual. In this case, angiography shows chronic occlusion of the proximal left middle cerebral artery, narrowing of the supraclinoid internal carotid artery with enlarged lenticulostriate collaterals, and filling of some distal middle cerebral artery branches through meningeal collaterals. This patient presented with hypertension (220/110 mm Hg) and it is presumed that the intraventricular hemorrhage is related to hypertension complicating moyamoya disease.

Notes

Right Cerebral Convexity Hypodense and Isodense Subdural Hematoma

1. Epidural hematoma.

2. Anemia (serum hemoglobin ≤10 g/dl), a tear in the pia-arachnoid resulting in dilution of the erythrocytes with CSF, and coagulopathies.

3. Epidural hematoma. The dura is adherent to and forms the endosteum of the inner table of the calvaria. This relationship of the dura to the intracranial suture results in the biconvex configuration of most epidural hematomas.

4. Birth injury, child abuse, and coagulopathies (e.g., vitamin K deficiency).

Reference

Gentry LR, Godersky JC, Thompson B, Dunn VD: Prospective comparative study of intermediate-field MR and CT in the evaluation of closed head trauma, *AJNR Am J Neuroradiol* 9:91-100, 1988, and *AJR Am J Roentgenol* 150:673-682, 1988.

Cross-Reference

Neuroradiology: THE REQUISITES, pp 152-156.

Comment

Acute subdural hematomas in young patients are usually the result of closed head injury (e.g., motor vehicle accident), whereas in elderly patients most are related to falls. Subdural hematomas are typically caused by tearing of the bridging veins that cross the subdural compartment, extending from the pia to the venous sinuses. Tearing of these veins is due to motion of the brain relative to the fixed dural sinuses. Most subdural hematomas are located along the supratentorial convexities; however, they may also occur in the posterior fossa and along the tentorium cerebelli. Symptoms of isolated subdural hematomas are in part related to associated injuries of the underlying brain.

Imaging features of subdural hematomas depend on their age. Acute (hours to days old) hematomas are typically hyperdense "crescentic" extracerebral collections. Subacute (days to weeks old) hematomas tend to be isodense to gray matter; therefore it is easy to miss them after a quick glance of a CT scan. In order to escape being fooled, compare the size of the sulci over the left and right cerebral convexities. Absence of sulci or asymmetric sulci should raise suspicion. Always check that the sulci extend to the inner table of the calvaria, and evaluate the gray-white matter interface for inward buckling. The latter two findings are especially useful with bilateral, isodense subdural hematomas as one may be fooled by the marked symmetry of the right and left convexities. Chronic (weeks to months old) hematomas are usually hypodense. Fluid levels within these hematomas may be caused by interval bleeding. Calcification along the dural membrane may also occur.

Notes

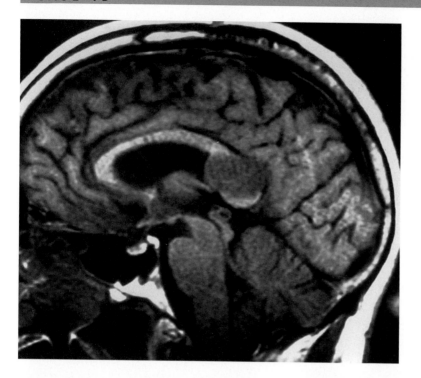

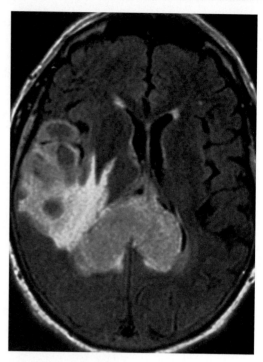

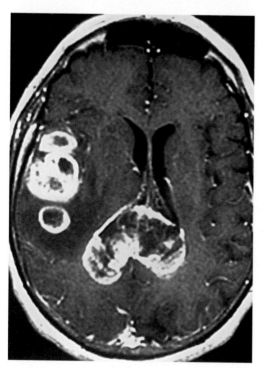

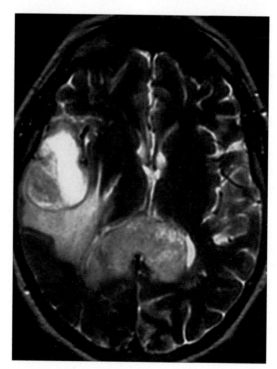

1. What mass lesions have a predilection for involving the corpus callosum?

2. Why is the corpus callosum relatively resistant to edema?

3. Besides the corpus callosum, what other white matter tracts are a common conduit of spread of glial neoplasms from one cerebral hemisphere to the contralateral side?

4. What are the MRI findings in gliomatosis cerebri?

Glioblastoma Multiforme of the Corpus Callosum—"Butterfly Glioma"

1. Neoplasms (GBM, lymphoma, and much less commonly metastatic disease), demyelinating disease, and traumatic shear injury.

2. Because of the orientation and compact nature of the white matter fibers making up the corpus callosum.

3. The anterior and posterior commissures.

4. Gliomatosis cerebri is an uncommon condition referring to an extensive infiltrating glioma. The imaging findings are often out of proportion to those on histologic evaluation. MRI shows extensive involvement of both the gray and white matter. There is frequently mild diffuse sulcal and ventricular effacement. This condition is often associated with minimal or no enhancement.

Reference

Spagnoli MV, Grossman RI, Packer RJ, et al: Magnetic resonance imaging determination of gliomatosis cerebri, *Neuroradiology* 29:15-18, 1987.

Cross-Reference

Neuroradiology: THE REQUISITES, pp 87-90.

Comment

This case demonstrates findings characteristic of a butterfly glioma. The sagittal T1W image shows expansion of the splenium. Abnormal signal intensity and a mass also are present in the right temporal lobe. Enhanced images reveal marked necrosis of the splenial and right temporal lobe lesions. The T2W images show abnormal signal intensity in the white matter surrounding the temporal lobe mass, which extends into the corpus striatum and is contiguous with the signal abnormality in the corpus callosum. Multicentric gliomas are uncommon, occurring in 1% to 5% of GBM cases. They may represent true separate lesions; however, more often they represent contiguous spread of tumor (which is likely the case in this patient). Multicentric gliomas may be synchronous (multiple lesions detected at the time of presentation) or metachronous (occurring at different times and discontinuous on pathology). It may be difficult to distinguish such gliomas from metastases on imaging. When separate lesions are identified, it is important to evaluate for the presence of continuity between the separate lesions on the basis of abnormal T2W signal intensity. However, the connection may not be apparent on imaging but only on pathologic evaluation. There is an increased association of multicentric gliomas in neurofibromatosis type I. In this case a thin rind of subependymal enhancement is present along the lateral ventricles and septum pellucidum. Of the infiltrative astrocytic tumors, GBM is most commonly associated with subependymal spread.

Notes

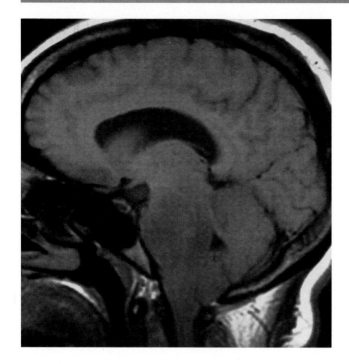

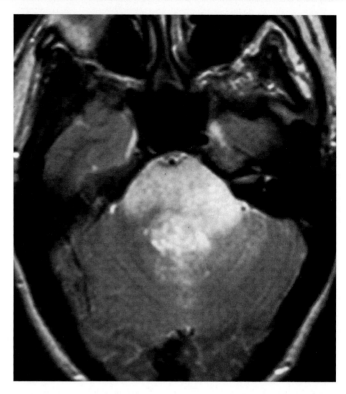

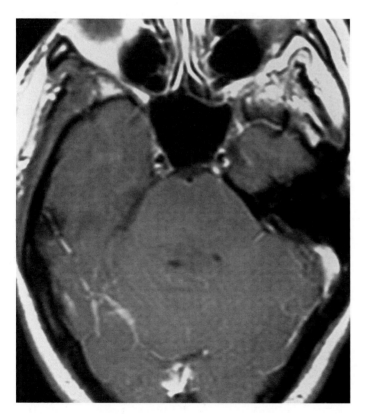

1. What is the differential diagnosis in this pediatric patient?

2. What part of the brain stem is most commonly affected with astrocytomas?

3. How do brainstem gliomas present clinically?

4. What is the typical location of a posterior fossa ependymoma?

Brainstem Astrocytoma

1. Astrocytoma, tuberculosis, rhomboencephalitis, demyelin-ating disease (e.g., acute disseminated encephalomyelitis), and lymphoma.

2. The pons.

3. Because of their infiltrative nature, as well as the anatomy of the brain stem, the initial clinical presentation of brain stem gliomas is usually related to cranial nerve deficits, ataxia, or long tract signs. Hydrocephalus is a common but relatively late manifestation.

4. The fourth ventricle.

Reference

Lee BC, Kneeland JB, Walker RW, Posner JB, Cahill PT, Deck MD: MR imaging of brainstem tumors, *AJNR Am J Neuro-radiol* 6:159-163, 1985.

Cross-Reference

Neuroradiology: THE REQUISITES, pp 83-85.

Comment

Magnetic resonance imaging has emerged as the imaging modality of choice for evaluation of brainstem abnormalities. Its multiplanar capabilities, improved resolution, and relative ab-sence of scanning artifacts, which are frequently present on CT scans, have resulted in improved detection of abnormalities in the posterior fossa. In addition, MRI is useful for planning radiation therapy in brainstem tumors. Given the infiltrative nature of these lesions and their location, radiation therapy remains the main therapeutic option. In cases in which tumor is exophytic, the exophytic portion can often be resected.

This case demonstrates the typical appearance of a brainstem astrocytoma, including high signal intensity on T2W images; marked expansion of the brain stem, most notably the pons but also extending into the pontomedullary junction and the middle cerebellar peduncles; effacement of the prepontine cistern; and invagination (encasement) of the basilar artery. The enhance-ment pattern of brainstem gliomas is quite variable, ranging from regions of avid nodular enhancement to minimal or no enhancement (as in this case).

Approximately 80% of brainstem gliomas occur during childhood, with the remaining 20% presenting in adulthood. Brainstem astrocytomas comprise approximately 15% of pos-terior fossa tumors in children. Most often these tumors are of the diffuse fibrillary subtype; however, more than half of them eventually demonstrate regions of anaplastic transformation and have a poor long-term prognosis.

Notes

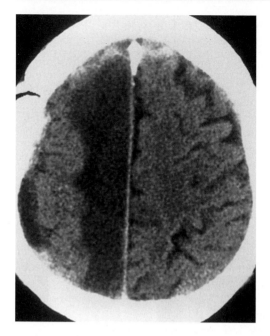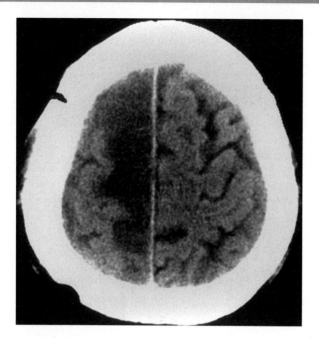

1. From which segment of the anterior cerebral artery do the medial lenticulostriate arteries arise?
2. What structures in the basal ganglia does the recurrent artery of Heubner supply?
3. What neurologic symptoms may occur secondary to anterior cerebral artery infarctions?
4. The lateral lenticulostriate arteries arise from which major vessel?

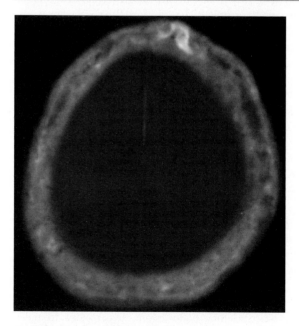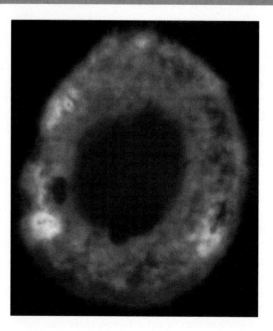

1. What is the differential diagnosis?
2. What is the name of the characteristic radiologic appearance that typifies the osteolytic phase of this disease in the calvaria?
3. How can Paget's disease be distinguished from fibrous dysplasia?
4. What neoplasm is associated with Paget's disease involving the calvaria?

Subacute Infarction in the Right Anterior Cerebral Artery Territory

1. The A-1 segment.

2. The head and anteromedial portion of the caudate nucleus and the anterior limb of the internal capsule.

3. Motor function and sensation to the contralateral leg (precentral and postcentral gyrus, respectively), olfaction, and mood swings/personality changes (cingulate gyrus).

4. The middle cerebral artery.

Reference

Kazui S, Sawada T, Naritomi H, Kuriyama Y, Yamaguchi T: Angiographic evaluation of brain infarction limited to the anterior cerebral artery territory, *Stroke* 24:549-553, 1993.

Cross-Reference

Neuroradiology, THE REQUISITES, pp 57-58, 106-110.

Comment

This case shows the characteristic appearance of a subacute stroke in the anterior cerebral artery territory. There is loss of gray-white matter differentiation and hypodensity in the medial right frontal lobe extending to the parietal lobe. There is mild mass effect. Incidentally, this patient underwent a prior craniotomy for evacuation of a right subdural hematoma.

The major cause of ischemic cerebrovascular disease is atherosclerosis. There are several reasons for performing an unenhanced head CT (and, when necessary, MRI) in the setting of an acute stroke. Among the most important are to exclude acute hemorrhage before treatment, or a nonischemic cause for the patient's symptoms. Other lesions may occasionally present with symptoms that mimic a stroke. In patients with a clinical presentation characteristic of an ischemic event, CT is performed to determine whether there is evidence of an acute infarction (early loss of gray-white matter differentiation or sulcal effacement) or associated acute hemorrhage. There has been an increasing role for the use of lytic therapy (intravenous systemic or intraarterial urokinase). The presence of acute blood and/or evidence on CT of an acute stroke are relative contraindications for this treatment. Angiography has a secondary role in the evaluation of stroke. Typically, angiography is not used in the acute setting to establish the presence of a stroke; however, it is helpful in answering specific questions. Angiography may be performed to assess for a hemodynamically significant stenosis in the cervical internal carotid artery to determine whether corrective surgery is needed. In younger patients, angiography may be performed to determine the cause of a stroke (premature atherosclerosis, dissection, or an underlying dysplasia of the vasculature).

Notes

Paget's Disease of the Calvaria

1. Paget's disease, metastatic disease, and fibrous dysplasia.

2. Osteoporosis circumscripta. Osteolysis is most commonly seen in the frontal or occipital region.

3. Paget's is a disease of middle-aged and elderly persons, whereas fibrous dysplasia is typically seen in children and young adults. In contrast to fibrous dysplasia, extensive involvement of the facial bones is uncommon in Paget's disease. Paget's disease causes cortical thickening, compared with fibrous dysplasia in which the cortex is relatively spared.

4. Giant cell tumors.

Reference

Altman RD: Musculoskeletal manifestations of Paget's disease of bone, *Arthritis Rheum* 23:1121-1127, 1980.

Cross-Reference

Neuroradiology: THE REQUISITES, pp 352, 390.

Comment

Paget's disease is more common in men than in women. It is often an incidental finding detected on radiographs obtained for other reasons. Patients may be symptomatic depending on the distribution of disease. Involvement of the calvaria may present with enlarging head size. Involvement of the skull base resulting in platybasia may result in neurologic symptoms (muscle weakness and paralysis). The cause of Paget's disease is unknown; however, a viral etiology is favored.

Radiologically, Paget's disease has multiple stages, including an initial osteolytic phase characterized by osteoclastic activity with resorption of normal bone. This phase is followed by excessive and sporadic new bone formation as a result of osteoblastic activity. Eventually, Paget's disease enters its inactive stage.

Neoplastic involvement within pagetoid bone is not uncommon and includes sarcomatous degeneration, giant cell tumor, superimposed hematologic neoplasms (myeloma, lymphoma), and metastatic disease. Giant cell tumors are typically confined to the skull and less often to the facial bones. It is speculated that the increased blood flow within pagetoid bone may make it more susceptible to deposition of metastases. Clinically the development of neoplastic disease in pagetoid bone should be suspected if there is increased pain or an associated soft tissue mass.

The differential diagnosis of Paget's disease of the skull includes other sclerotic bone lesions, hyperostosis frontalis, fibrous dysplasia, and metastatic disease. In the elderly, metastatic disease may have the cotton-wool appearance of Paget's disease (prostate cancer in men and breast cancer in women).

Notes

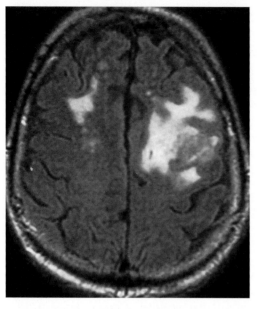 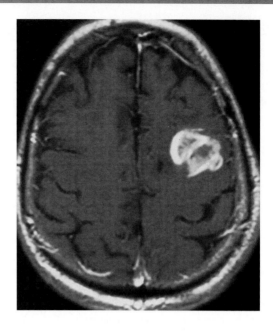

1. What is the differential diagnosis?
2. What other MRI findings might be useful in differentiating among these possibilities?
3. What glial neoplasm is most commonly associated with hemorrhage?
4. What are the likely histologic correlates of T2W signal abnormality in the white matter surrounding a glioma?

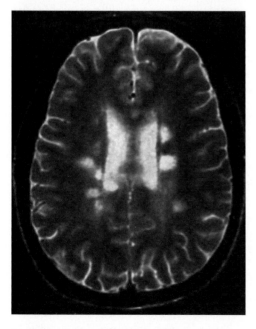

1. What is the differential diagnosis?
2. How are Virchow-Robin spaces distinguished from white matter lesions?
3. What is the pathologic hallmark of an acute, active multiple sclerosis plaque?
4. What percentage of patients with multiple sclerosis have isolated spinal cord disease?

Glioblastoma Multiforme

1. Glioma, metastasis, lymphoma, abscess.

2. Multiple lesions favor metastatic disease over a glioma, abnormal signal intensity extending into the corpus callosum favors glioma or lymphoma over metastasis, and the presence of a capsule that is high in signal intensity on unenhanced T1W images and hypointense on T2W images may suggest an abscess.

3. GBM.

4. Edema and tumor. MRI cannot delineate the exact margins of a glial neoplasm and cannot separate edema from tumor because GBMs grow by infiltrating along the white matter tracts.

Reference

Earnest F IV, Kelly PJ, Scheithauer BW, et al: Cerebral astrocytomas: histopathologic correlation of MR and CT contrast enhancement with stereotactic biopsy, *Radiology* 166:823-827, 1988.

Cross-Reference

Neuroradiology: THE REQUISITES, p 87.

Comment

Most GBMs enhance and usually demonstrate heterogeneity because of the presence of necrosis and/or hemorrhage. Enhancement may extend into the adjacent white matter. There are several reasons to administer intravenous contrast. In a newly identified brain tumor in which biopsy is anticipated, regions of enhancement correlate with regions of solid tumor on pathology. Therefore, contrast may be useful in identifying areas for stereotactic biopsy. In addition, enhanced images may identify tumor spread to regions that would otherwise not be noticed on unenhanced images. For instance, GBMs may spread to the leptomeninges, subarachnoid space, or subependymal region along the ventricular margins. In the postoperative setting contrast may help to distinguish surgical change from residual tumor. It is common practice to perform MRI within 24 to 48 hours following tumor resection. Enhancement in the surgical bed is suspicious for residual tumor. Tumors typically enhance within this time interval, whereas granulation tissue and scar do not; however, scar may occasionally enhance quite early in the postoperative setting. Granulation/scar tissue usually develops within 48 to 72 hours following surgery, and differentiating scar from tumor in MRI scans performed after this time interval becomes increasingly difficult. Because hemorrhage is usually present in the operative bed, it is also important to acquire unenhanced T1W images in the same plane and at the same levels as the contrast study in order to distinguish blood products from enhancement.

Notes

Multiple Sclerosis

1. Vasculopathies (small vessel ischemic disease, vasculitis, hypertension, migraines), demyelinating disease, and inflammatory processes (Lyme disease, sarcoid).

2. Dilated perivascular spaces follow the signal intensity of CSF on all pulse sequences. FLAIR or proton density weighted images are best at distinguishing perivascular spaces (which are isointense to CSF) from white matter lesions (which are hyperintense).

3. Perivenous inflammatory changes.

4. Approximately 8% to 12%. In patients presenting with myelopathy and an MRI study that reveals a cord lesion, multiple sclerosis should be considered.

Reference

Loevner LA, Grossman RI, McGowan JC, Ramer KN, Cohen JA: Characterization of multiple sclerosis plaques with T1-weighted MR and quantitative magnetization transfer, *AJNR Am J Neuroradiol* 16:1473-1479, 1995.

Cross-Reference

Neuroradiology: THE REQUISITES, pp 202-212, 480-481.

Comment

Most acquired diseases involving the white matter have similar MRI findings. Patient history and physical examination are of paramount importance in limiting the differential diagnosis.

Multiple sclerosis affects the oligodendrocytes. In the acute stage, plaques have an inflammatory reaction with edema, cellular infiltration, and a spectrum of demyelination. Plaques tend to be in a perivenous distribution. Chronic lesions show astrocytic hypoplasia, resolution of the cellular infiltration, and loss of myelin. The diagnosis of multiple sclerosis remains a clinical one; however, findings on MRI may be extremely helpful in supporting the diagnosis, as well as in measuring disease burden. On T1W images, plaques may be isointense to hypointense to brain. Hypointense lesions most likely are associated with gliosis and significant myelin loss. Lesions in the periventricular white matter may be obscured on T2W imaging if they are isointense to the CSF. Proton density or FLAIR imaging is particularly helpful in identifying lesions in the periventricular region. Lesions at the callosal-septal interface are highly suggestive of multiple sclerosis. Contrast administration allows separation of lesions with an abnormal blood-brain barrier (enhancing lesions) from those with an intact blood-brain barrier (nonenhancing lesions). MRI is more sensitive in detecting active disease in that enhancing lesions may be identified in clinically silent areas of the brain.

Notes

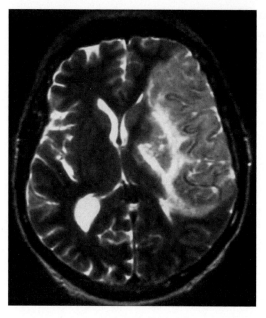 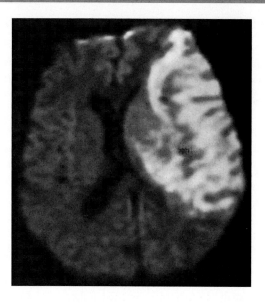

1. What type of MRI is the second figure in this case?
2. In the context of acute infarction, what is meant by the term "penumbra"?
3. What functional MRI techniques may be used to detect ischemic tissue in the setting of acute stroke?
4. Which type of MRI assesses the transit of intravenous gadolinium during the first pass of this contrast agent through the brain?

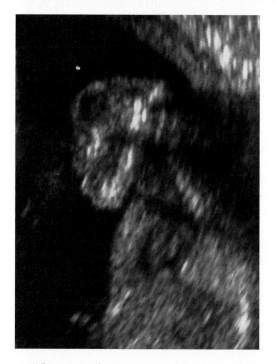

1. This anomaly represents the most common type of what developmental defect?
2. What sonographic findings are characteristic of this entity?
3. What other anomalies are associated with this condition?
4. Is this condition associated with maldevelopment of cartilage or membranous bone?

Acute Middle Cerebral Artery Territory Stroke

1. Diffusion imaging.

2. Normal brain tissue surrounding a region of infarcted brain that is at increased risk for ischemic injury.

3. Perfusion and diffusion imaging.

4. Perfusion imaging.

Reference

Beauchamp NJ Jr, Ulug AM, Passe TJ, van Zijl PCM: MR diffusion imaging in stroke: review and controversies, *Radio-Graphics* 18:1269-1283, 1998.

Cross-Reference

Neuroradiology: THE REQUISITES, pp 58-59, 105-114.

Comment

Computed tomography is usually the first study obtained in the evaluation of acute stroke. In early strokes, thrombolytic therapy may be employed either intravenously or intraarterially. Before interventions with clot busters, detection of acute hemorrhage and/or infarction is important because these conditions are relative contraindications to such therapy.

Magnetic resonance imaging is more sensitive than CT in detecting acute infarcts. MRI has also shown extension of infarctions on follow-up examinations. It is identification of this "penumbra" (brain tissue at risk for irreversible ischemia) that is at the heart of further development of MRI techniques. One wants to protect this tissue from ischemia by applying appropriate interventions. Furthermore, in order to deliver protective agents, perfusion to this tissue is necessary. Tissue perfusion may be assessed with perfusion imaging. Rapid imaging is performed both before and during the bolus injection of gadolinium. On first pass through the cerebral vasculature, there is a drop in measured signal intensity due to the T2* effects of this agent. Using mathematic models, this decrease in signal intensity may be converted to concentration of contrast over time. Tissue perfusion may also be assessed with diffusion imaging which measures movement of water molecules. In this sequence a 180° pulse is flanked by strong diffusion gradients. The greater the distance a water molecule travels, the more signal loss will occur due to dephasing. In the CNS, water molecules have a predilection to move more readily in the direction of axons. This directional preference is termed *anisotropic diffusion*. The direction in which a diffusion gradient is applied will determine the end result. Diffusion imaging is the most sensitive indicator of ischemia, with the image becoming abnormal within minutes of onset. Mismatches between abnormal diffusion and perfusion imaging may indicate brain at risk.

Notes

Anencephaly

1. Open neural tube defect.

2. Failure to identify the normal bony calvaria, as well as normal brain tissue above the osseous ridges of the orbit (acrania).

3. Among the most common are spinal abnormalities, which occur in approximately 50% of anencephalic fetuses. Spinal anomalies may range from spina bifida to severe dysraphism, which may be associated with a myelomeningocele.

4. "Acrania," or absence of the cranial vault, is caused by failure of development of membranous bone. However, bones formed from cartilage such as the skull base and the orbits develop normally.

Reference

Johnson A, Losure TA, Weiner S: Early diagnosis of fetal anencephaly, *J Clin Ultrasound* 13:503-505, 1985.

Cross-Reference

Neuroradiology: THE REQUISITES, p 250.

Comment

Anencephaly is the most common congenital anomaly of the CNS and the most common open neural tube defect. As with all neural tube defects, anencephaly is more common in girls by a ratio of approximately 4:1. Most women seeking prenatal care are screened for maternal serum alpha-fetoprotein (AFP) levels. When these serum levels are abnormal, amniocentesis is often performed to measure the AFP level in the amniotic fluid. In a woman who has previously given birth to a child with an open neural tube defect, the recurrence risk is high and these patients in particular must be carefully screened during each subsequent pregnancy. Neural tube defects are not the only cause of elevated maternal serum AFP; it can also be elevated in the setting of twin gestations, fetal demise, or when the gestational dates are wrong (interpretation of normal AFP is based on gestational age/last menstrual period). In addition, elevated maternal serum AFP may be present in other congenital anomalies, including omphalocele and gastroschisis. Therefore in the setting of elevated AFP, in addition to clinical correlation, it is also important to provide a second level of testing (prenatal sonography) that assesses the fetus for anomalies.

In anencephaly, the prosencephalon is absent; however, portions of the mesencephalon and rhombencephalon are present. The large calvarial defect (acrania) is covered by a thick angiomatous stroma, but not bone or normal skin. Virtually all cases of anencephaly are incompatible with life.

Notes

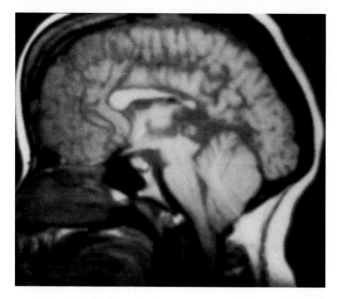

1. What findings would you expect to find on skull radiographs in this patient?
2. What cervical spine anomalies are frequently associated with these malformations?
3. Which type of Chiari malformation is associated with a myelomeningocele?
4. What are the accepted normal limits in children and adults for the inferior position of the cerebellar tonsils relative to the foramen magnum?

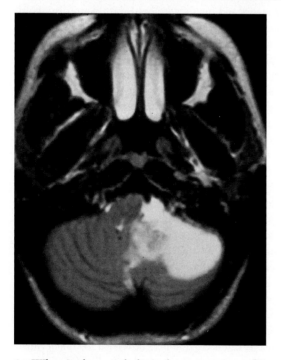 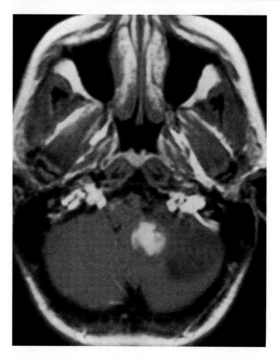

1. What is the usual clinical presentation of intraaxial posterior fossa masses?
2. In a pediatric patient, what is the most likely diagnosis?
3. What are common sites of origin of these neoplasms in the supratentorial compartment?
4. What disorder is associated with pilocytic astrocytomas involving the visual pathway?

Chiari II Malformation

1. A small posterior fossa, a large foramen magnum, and scalloping of the petrous bones and clivus. Patients may have a "Luckenschadel" or "lacunar" skull, which represents a bone dysplasia that typically resolves during the early months of infancy.

2. Klippel-Feil syndrome, partial fusion of C2 and C3, occipitalization of the atlas (partial or complete fusion of C1 with the occiput), and a hypoplastic ring of C1.

3. Chiari II malformation.

4. Cerebellar tonsil position relative to the foramen magnum varies with age. In children younger than 10 years of age, 6 mm or less is considered within normal limits. In adulthood, 3 mm or less is normal variation. Typically, low lying tonsils that are within normal variation are rounded in contour.

Reference

Naidich TP, McLone DG, Fulling KH: The Chiari II malformation: part IV. The hindbrain deformity, *Neuroradiology* 25:179-197, 1983.

Cross-Reference

Neuroradiology: THE REQUISITES, pp 261-262, 264.

Comment

Chiari malformations typically occur during the first 3 to 4 weeks of gestational life and are dorsal induction–neural tube defects. Chiari II malformations are the most common symptomatic form in which the vermis, cerebellar tonsils, and medulla are herniated into the foramen magnum and upper cervical canal. The cerebellum herniates up through the tentorial incisura ("towering cerebellum"), the cerebellar hemispheres wrap around the brain stem and the tectum is "beaked." The fourth ventricle is elongated and displaced inferiorly. Chiari II malformations are associated with a spectrum of supratentorial anomalies, including dysgenesis of the corpus callosum (most commonly splenial anomalies) and heterotopias. Myelomeningoceles are seen in virtually all Chiari II malformations and more than 50% of cases are associated with syringohydromyelia. In Chiari I malformations there is herniation of the cerebellar tonsils, which are pointed (peg-like) in configuration into the cervical spinal canal. The remainder of the cerebellum, brain stem, and fourth ventricle are normal in location. Whereas syringohydromyelia is frequently seen in Chiari I malformations, myelomeningoceles are not.

Chiari III malformations have the same findings as Chiari II malformations but also include herniation of the posterior fossa contents into a high cervical and/or occipital encephalocele. There is no associated lumbosacral myelomeningocele.

Notes

Juvenile Pilocytic Astrocytoma of the Cerebellum

1. Symptoms related to mass effect, including hydrocephalus and ataxia.

2. Pilocytic astrocytoma.

3. Optic nerve/chiasm, hypothalamus, and the inferior aspect (floor) of the third ventricle.

4. Neurofibromatosis type 1.

Reference

Yachnis AT: Neuropathology of pediatric brain tumors, *Semin Pediatr Neurol* 4:282-291, 1997.

Cross-Reference

Neuroradiology: THE REQUISITES, pp 83, 291-292, 511.

Comment

Astrocytomas are the most common intracranial tumors in children, accounting for up to 50% of such neoplasms. Approximately two thirds are located in the posterior fossa. Depending on the series cited, cerebellar astrocytomas and medulloblastomas are the most common infratentorial neoplasms in children. Approximately 80% of all cerebellar astrocytomas in children are of the pilocytic variety. Most patients with pilocytic astrocytomas have normal karyotypes; however, long arm deletions of chromosome 17 have been associated. It is important that both radiologists and neuropathologists be able to distinguish pilocytic astrocytomas from the less common but more aggressive anaplastic fibrillary types because prognosis and management are distinctly different. Pilocytic astrocytomas represent one of the more benign forms of glial neoplasms and are classified as circumscribed gliomas by the WHO. Histologically, tightly packed, piloid processes arising from tumor cells are typical, as are microscopic and macroscopic cysts. Eosinophilic granular bodies and Rosenthal fibers (astrocytic processes) are also present. The prognosis is usually excellent following surgical management. Conversely, higher grade infiltrative astrocytomas have a poor prognosis.

The pilocytic astrocytoma has a characteristic appearance. Typically these tumors are well-circumscribed masses that usually arise within the cerebellar hemisphere (but may arise in the midline), with a unilocular cyst and an enhancing solid mural nodule. Usually the cystic component follows the signal characteristics of CSF on all MR imaging pulse sequences; however, cysts with a high protein content may be hyperintense relative to CSF on T1W, proton density, or FLAIR images. The wall of the cyst does not usually enhance; however, rim enhancement of the cyst can occur and may be related to enhancement of normal adjacent cerebellar parenchyma. Calcification and hemorrhage are uncommon in juvenile pilocytic astrocytomas.

Notes

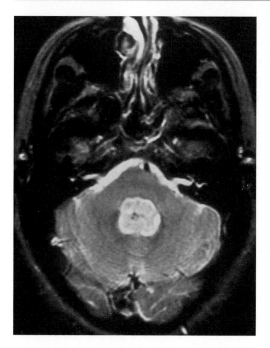
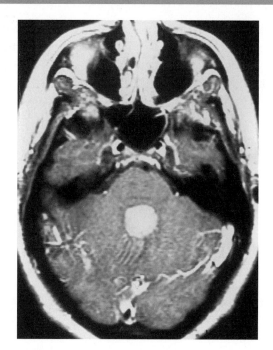

1. What is the differential diagnosis in this case?
2. In children, what is the most common fourth ventricle mass?
3. What are potential causes of hydrocephalus in patients with choroid plexus papillomas?
4. What is the cause of regions of hypointensity on MRI scans in choroid plexus papillomas?

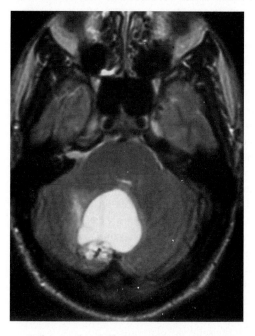
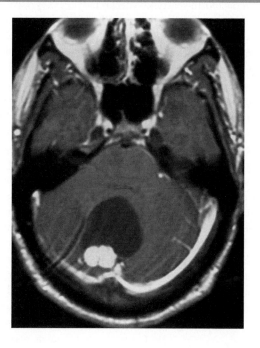

1. What is the differential diagnosis?
2. What clinical factors help to distinguish a hemangioblastoma from a pilocytic astrocytoma?
3. What characteristic imaging finding in this case helps in differentiating a hemangioblastoma from a pilocytic astrocytoma?
4. What neurocutaneous syndrome is associated with multiple hemangioblastomas?

Choroid Plexus Papilloma of the Fourth Ventricle

1. Fourth ventricular meningioma, choroid plexus papilloma, metastasis, and hemangioma. In the pediatric population ependymoma must also be considered.

2. Ependymoma.

3. Overproduction of CSF or obstruction to CSF flow related to adhesions from proteinaceous and/or hemorrhagic material blocking the subarachnoid cisterns and/or ventricular outlets.

4. Calcification, vascular flow voids, and/or tumoral hemorrhage.

Reference

Hopper KD, Foley LC, Nieves NL, Smirniotopoulos JG: The intraventricular extension of choroid plexus papillomas, *AJNR Am J Neuroradiol* 8:469-472, 1987.

Cross-Reference

Neuroradiology: THE REQUISITES, pp 78-79.

Comment

Choroid plexus papillomas are epithelial tumors arising from the surface of the choroid plexus. Overall, they occur most commonly in the lateral ventricles (45%). They may also arise within the fourth ventricle (approximately 40%) and the third ventricle (approximately 10%). In adults the majority of choroid plexus papillomas occur in the fourth ventricle, whereas in children 80% arise in the atria/trigone of the lateral ventricles. Choroid plexus papillomas may cause hydrocephalus as a result of overproduction of CSF and/or obstructive hydrocephalus related to blockage of outflow from the ventricular system. In addition, large tumors will cause focal expansion of the ventricle they fill; they may also cause trapping.

Pathologically, these tumors are comprised of vascularized connective tissue and frond-like papillae lined by a single layer of epithelial cells. Calcification, hemorrhage, and cysts are frequently present. On imaging, many of these pathologic features are evident. Calcification is readily identified on CT, as are regions of large cyst formation. On MRI, regions of hypointensity may correspond to calcium, vessels, and/or blood products. Tumors that are very cystic will be hyperintense on T2W imaging, whereas those with large areas of blood products from old hemorrhages may be hypointense on T2W imaging. Following contrast administration, choroid plexus papillomas enhance avidly. The enhancement pattern may be homogenous or heterogeneous depending on the degree of cyst formation, calcification, and the presence of hemorrhage.

Notes

Isolated Hemangioblastoma

1. Hemangioblastoma, pilocytic astrocytoma, and vascular metastasis.

2. The age of the patient. Pilocytic astrocytomas tend to occur in children, whereas isolated cerebellar hemangioblastomas usually present in young adults.

3. The presence of tumor vessels (flow voids on MRI) within the solid nidus. Vessels may also be present in vascular metastases such as renal cell and thyroid carcinomas.

4. von Hippel-Lindau disease.

Reference

Lee SR, Sanches J, Mark AS, Dillon WP, Norman D, Newton TH: Posterior fossa hemangioblastomas: MR imaging, *Radiology* 171:463-468, 1989.

Cross-Reference

Neuroradiology: THE REQUISITES, pp 81-82.

Comment

Cerebellar hemangioblastomas are benign neoplasms that represent the most common primary infratentorial neoplasm in adults. They are more common in men, and presentation is typically during adulthood (except when associated with von Hippel-Lindau disease, where presentation may occur in late adolescence). Patients may present with headache, nausea and vomiting, ataxia, and vertigo. Although these neoplasms typically have a vascular nidus, subarachnoid hemorrhage is an uncommon presentation. More than 80% of posterior fossa hemangioblastomas occur in the cerebellum. They may also occur in the spinal cord or medulla (in the region of the area postrema). Cerebral hemangioblastomas are unusual, representing less than 2% of all hemangioblastomas, and are usually indicative of von Hippel-Lindau disease (posterior fossa tumors are also usually present).

There are two characteristic imaging appearances of cerebellar hemangioblastomas. The first is that of a solid and cystic mass (occurring in more than 50% of cases). In most cases there is no enhancement around the cyst wall. The solid vascular mural nodule associated with the cyst avidly enhances, and the nodule usually abuts the pial surface. Frequently, the solid nodule will have within or around it large vessels that are recognized on MRI as serpentine regions of signal void consistent with flow. Alternatively, hemangioblastomas may present as poorly demarcated, avidly enhancing masses typically associated with numerous vascular flow voids (up to 40% of cases).

Management is typically surgical resection, which is considered curative. Recurrence may occur if there has been incomplete resection of the solid vascular nidus.

Notes

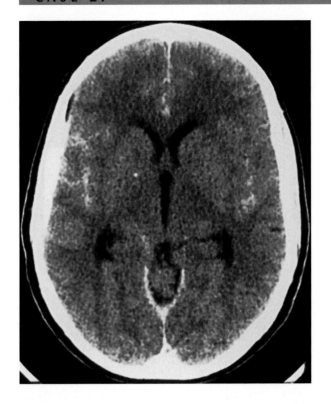
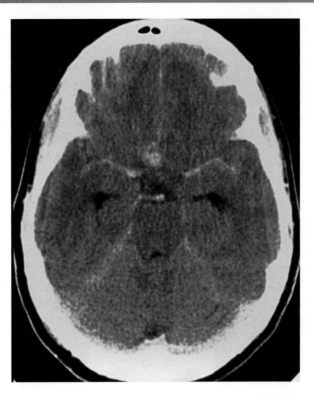

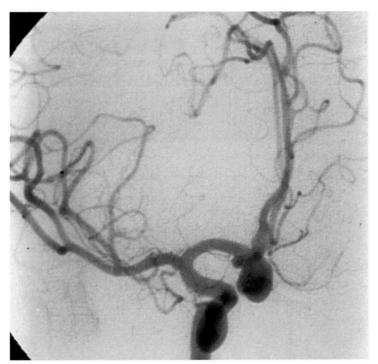

1. What is the most common anatomic variant associated with aneurysms arising from the anterior communicating artery?

2. At what time following an acute subarachnoid hemorrhage is symptomatic vasospasm most likely to occur?

3. In patients with acute onset pupil involving third nerve palsy, catheter angiography is indicated to exclude aneurysms of which arteries?

4. What CT findings are highly suggestive of rupture of an anterior communicating artery aneurysm?

Acute Subarachnoid Hemorrhage/Rupture of an Anterior Communicating Artery Aneurysm

1. A hypoplastic A-1 segment. Others include duplication or fenestrations of the anterior communicating artery and azygous variation of the anterior cerebral arteries.

2. Between the fifth and twelfth days.

3. The posterior communicating artery and, less frequently, the superior cerebellar artery. Pupillary dilation, ptosis, and strabismus because of compression of cranial nerve III may be present.

4. Bilaterally symmetric subarachnoid hemorrhage, hemorrhage within the interhemispheric fissure, frontal lobe hematoma, and/or septal/intraventricular hemorrhage.

Reference

Bagley LJ, Hurst RW: Angiographic evaluation of aneurysms affecting the central nervous system, *Neuroimaging Clin North Am* 7:721-737, 1997.

Cross-Reference

Neuroradiology: THE REQUISITES, pp 136-139.

Comment

Berry or saccular aneurysms represent focal dilations most commonly found at branching points of parent vessels. They are the result of a congenital weakness or deficiency in the elastica and media of the arterial wall. The most frequent sites for ruptured aneurysms include (in descending order of frequency) the anterior communicating artery complex, the origin of the posterior communicating artery, the middle cerebral artery, and the vertebrobasilar circulation. Multiple aneurysms may occur in up to 15% to 20% of cases. Although most aneurysms are sporadic in nature, there is an increased incidence in certain conditions such as connective tissue disorders/collagen vascular disease (fibromuscular dysplasia, moyamoya, Ehlers-Danlos syndrome, and polycystic kidney disease).

The first CT image shows bilateral acute subarachnoid hemorrhage, most notably in the Sylvian cisterns and the anterior interhemispheric fissure in a pattern consistent with rupture of an anterior communicating artery aneurysm. The second image was obtained before surgery and immediately following cerebral angiography (and is therefore effectively an enhanced examination confirmed by enhancement of the circle of Willis). An anterior communicating artery aneurysm at the anterior portion of the suprasellar cistern can be seen. Evaluation of a patient with suspected acute subarachnoid hemorrhage should always begin with an unenhanced CT head study.

Notes

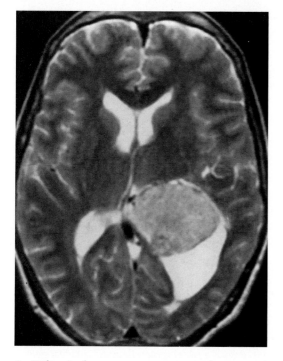 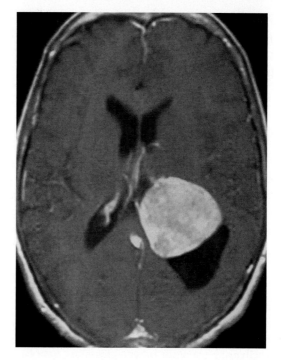

1. What is the most common neoplasm to arise in the trigone of the lateral ventricle in a pediatric patient?

2. When assessing patients with intraventricular masses, what are the two most important factors in differentiating among the possible neoplasms?

3. What is the most common location of intraventricular meningiomas in adults?

4. What is the characteristic location of a subependymal giant cell astrocytoma?

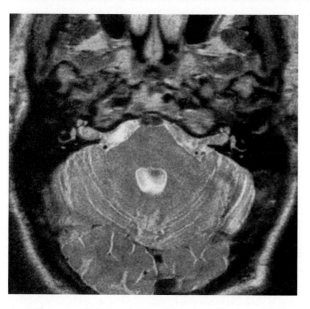 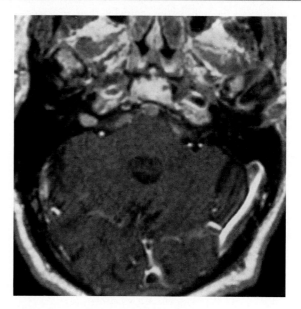

1. What are the two major divisions of cranial nerve VIII, and where do they course in the internal auditory canal?

2. What structure separates the internal auditory canal (IAC) into superior and inferior portions?

3. What cystic lesions may occur in the cerebellopontine angle?

4. The presence of bilateral vestibular schwannomas is indicative of what disorder?

Intraventricular Meningioma

1. Choroid plexus papilloma.

2. The age of the patient (child vs. adult) and the location of the mass (lateral, third, or fourth ventricle).

3. Along the choroid plexus of the atrium of the lateral ventricle.

4. Along the foramen of Monro.

Reference
Lang I, Jackson A, Strang FA: Intraventricular hemorrhage caused by intraventricular meningioma: CT appearance, *AJNR Am J Neuroradiol* 16:1378-1381, 1995.

Cross-Reference
Neuroradiology: THE REQUISITES, pp 511-512.

Comment
These images demonstrate a well-demarcated mass lesion in the atrium of the left lateral ventricle along the glomus of the choroid plexus. On T2W imaging the lesion is mildly hyperintense to the brain parenchyma; however, it is hypointense to CSF. Following contrast administration, there is homogeneous, avid enhancement. In adults, this is the typical appearance of an intraventricular meningioma and the most common location for these neoplasms, which are speculated to arise from arachnoid rests within the choroid. Like choroid plexus papillomas, intraventricular meningiomas occur slightly more often on the left. When large enough, these meningiomas may trap a particular segment of the lateral ventricle (such as the temporal horn), resulting in focal dilation. Also, when they are large enough that the tumor compresses the walls of the ventricles, there may be resultant edema in the adjacent brain parenchyma. Their appearance on CT is similar to that of other intracranial meningiomas. Differential considerations of a mass in this location in adults include glial neoplasms (astrocytomas, ependymomas) and a metastasis to the choroid plexus. Choroid plexus papillomas can usually be eliminated as a diagnostic consideration because they occur most commonly in children and because in adults they are found more frequently within the fourth ventricle.

Notes

Vestibular Schwannoma of the Internal Auditory Canal

1. The cochlear and vestibular divisions. The vestibular branches run in the superior and inferior portions of the posterior IAC, whereas the cochlear division runs in the anteroinferior portion of the IAC.

2. The crista falciformis.

3. Epidermoid and arachnoid cysts.

4. Neurofibromatosis type 2.

Reference
Mulkens TH, Parizel PM, Martin JJ, et al: Acoustic schwannoma: MR findings in 84 tumors, *AJR Am J Roentgenol* 160:395-398, 1993.

Cross-Reference
Neuroradiology: THE REQUISITES, pp 53, 73-74.

Comment
Schwannomas arise most commonly along cranial nerve VIII (the vestibular nerve is more common than the cochlear nerve). Cranial nerves V and VII are the next most common sites for schwannomas. In the IAC and cerebellopontine angle, the differential diagnosis of an enhancing mass is usually in distinguishing a schwannoma from a meningioma. Features favoring a schwannoma are extension of a cerebellopontine angle mass into the IAC, flaring of the porus acusticus (the opening of the IAC), and the absence of dural enhancement. Meningiomas occasionally extend into the IAC (which is not expanded), are typically associated with a dural tail (although a dural tail is not diagnostic of a meningioma), and are frequently centered superior or inferior and anterior or posterior to the porus acusticus. In this case, an enhancing mass contained within the IAC highly favors a schwannoma (the IAC is mildly expanded suggesting slow growth of the mass). The T2W image is high resolution with a 512×512 matrix. Although on close observation the mass may be seen by the keen eye, this case illustrates the importance of administering gadolinium to clinch the diagnosis, especially in cases of small lesions or lesions isolated to the IAC.

Schwannomas comprise more than 90% of purely intracanalicular lesions. However, only 5% to 15% are located exclusively within the IAC, whereas approximately 15% of acoustic schwannomas present only in the cerebellopontine angle cistern. About 75% of acoustic schwannomas involve both structures.

On MRI, schwannomas have variable signal intensity depending on their cellularity, water content, and the presence of necrosis. Small lesions (<2 cm) typically are mildly hypointense compared with brain parenchyma, and enhancement is present and usually homogeneous. Lesions larger than 2 cm frequently undergo necrosis, resulting in heterogeneous enhancement.

Notes

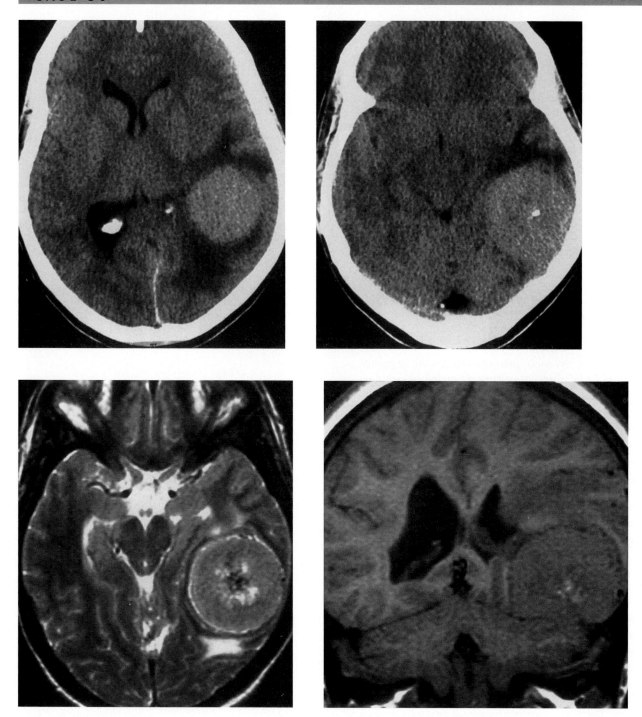

1. Is the mass intraaxial or extraaxial in location?
2. What findings on MRI are indicative of an extraaxial mass?
3. What conditions are associated with multiple meningiomas?
4. What percentage of meningiomas undergo cystic or fatty degeneration?

Meningioma

1. Extraaxial.

2. A cleft or "pseudocapsule" (CSF, dura, and/or vessels) that separates the mass from the brain (as in this case); buckling of the gray matter; a mass that is broad-based against a dural surface (in this case the mass is broad-based along the tentorium cerebelli).

3. Prior radiation therapy, neurofibromatosis type 2, basal cell nevus syndrome.

4. Approximately 5% to 10%.

Reference

Sheporaitis LA, Osborn AG, Smirniotopoulos JG, et al: Intracranial meningioma, *AJNR Am J Neuroradiol* 13: 29-37, 1992.

Cross-Reference

Neuroradiology: THE REQUISITES, pp 68-73.

Comment

Meningiomas are the most common intracranial, extraaxial neoplasm. Although there are a variety of histologies, including fibroblastic, angioblastic, syncytial, and transitional types, prognosis is not primarily dependent on the histology but rather on the location of the meningioma. Large meningiomas occurring over the cerebral convexities may be treated with embolization followed by surgery with minimal neurologic deficit; however, meningiomas as small as 1 cm involving the cavernous sinus may be very symptomatic and present a more challenging treatment dilemma. Meningiomas occur most commonly in middle-aged women; however, they are also found frequently in men. Most meningiomas are sporadic, isolated lesions. Multiple meningiomas may be familial or may be seen in patients with prior radiation therapy to the brain, neurofibromatosis type 2, and basal cell nevus (Gorlin-Goltz) syndrome.

On unenhanced CT, more than 50% of meningiomas are hyperdense (as in this case). Approximately 20% to 25% are associated with calcification and/or a reaction in the adjacent bone (hyperostosis is more common than osteolysis). On MRI, meningiomas are often isointense to gray matter on T1W and T2W sequences; however, they may be hyperintense on T2W imaging. Meningiomas typically have avid, homogeneous enhancement. The most important clue to making the diagnosis of a meningioma is in establishing that the mass is extraaxial in location. One finding consistent with an extraaxial location is the presence of a "pseudocapsule," which may represent CSF, dura, and/or vessels along the piaarachnoid. Although the presence of an enhancing dural tail is highly suggestive of meningioma, this is a nonspecific finding and may be seen in other disease processes.

Notes

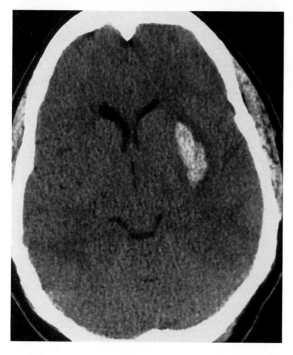

1. What is the most common cause of nontraumatic intracranial hemorrhage in adults?
2. What is responsible for the high signal intensity on T1W images in subacute hemorrhage?
3. What are the three most common locations for hypertensive bleeds?
4. What is responsible for the low signal intensity on both T1W and T2W images in chronic hemorrhages?

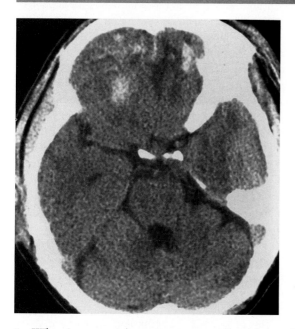

1. What intracranial structures normally enhance following the intravenous administration of contrast material?
2. What is the cause of the parenchymal hemorrhages in this case?
3. What are characteristic locations for cortical contusions in the setting of acceleration/deceleration injuries (e.g., MVAs)?
4. What are potential causes for blood-fluid levels in a traumatized brain?

Hypertensive Intracerebral Hemorrhage

1. Hypertension.

2. Methemoglobin and high protein content.

3. The basal ganglia (especially the putamen), the thalamus, and the pons, in descending order of frequency.

4. Susceptibility effects from hemosiderin and ferritin.

Reference

Chan S, Kartha K, Yoon SS, Desmond DW, Hilal SK: Multifocal hypointense cerebral lesions on gradient-echo MR are associated with chronic hypertension, *AJNR Am J Neuroradiol* 17:1821-1827, 1996.

Cross-Reference

Neuroradiology: THE REQUISITES, pp 130-131.

Comment

This case is a characteristic illustration of a basal ganglionic hypertensive hemorrhage. In adults the most common cause of nontraumatic intracerebral hemorrhage is hypertension. Hemorrhages related to high blood pressure have a predilection to involve the deep gray matter (basal ganglia and thalamus) and brain stem, which are supplied by perforating vessels arising from the cerebral and basilar arteries. Rupture of microaneurysms (Charcot-Bouchard) arising from the deep perforating vessels may be the basis of hypertensive hemorrhages in a subset of patients. Approximately two thirds of hypertensive hemorrhages occur in the basal ganglia. Rupture into the ventricular system may be present in up to one half of these patients and is associated with a poor prognosis.

The MRI evaluation of intracerebral hemorrhage is complex, and the imaging appearance is related to a multitude of factors. In the acute setting (hours to a few days), hemorrhage may be isointense to hypointense on both T1W and T2W images because of deoxyhemoglobin. In the early subacute phase (2 days to 1 week), hemorrhage is hyperintense on T1W imaging and hypointense on T2W imaging as a result of high protein concentrations and intracellular methemoglobin. In the late subacute phase (1 week to months), hemorrhage is hyperintense on both T1W and T2W imaging. Finally, in the chronic setting (months to years) hemorrhage is hypointense due to susceptibility effects of hemosiderin and ferritin.

Notes

Traumatic Hemorrhagic Contusion

1. Those without a blood brain barrier (choroid plexus, pituitary stalk, mucous membranes, extraocular muscles, cavernous sinus, vessels). It is important to be able to determine whether images are enhanced because acute hemorrhage has a similar density to iodinated contrast material.

2. Trauma.

3. The anterior and inferior portions of the temporal and frontal lobes, as well as the occipital poles.

4. Hemorrhage into injured necrotic brain or blood dyscrasias (abnormal coagulation).

References

Wysoki MG, Nassar CJ, Koenigsberg RA, Novelline RA, Faro SH, Faerber EN: Head trauma: CT scan interpretation by radiology residents versus staff radiologists, *Radiology* 208: 125-128, 1998.

Gentry LR, Gordersky JC, Thompson B: MR imaging of head trauma: review of the distribution and radiopathologic features of traumatic lesions, *AJNR Am J Neuroradiol* 9:101-110, 1988.

Cross-Reference

Neuroradiology: THE REQUISITES, pp 156-157.

Comment

Hemorrhagic contusions are among the most common traumatic brain injuries. They tend to occur along the superficial surfaces of the brain and are the result of acceleration/deceleration forces that cause the brain to rub along surfaces where there are prominent osseous ridges or dural reflections. Therefore the anterior and inferior portions of the temporal and frontal lobes typically are contused as the surface of the brain rubs against the floor and anterior wall of the anterior cranial fossa and the sphenoid wings and temporal bones, respectively. Hemorrhagic contusions may also occur in the setting of penetrating trauma (gun and knife club types of injuries, depressed skull fractures, or iatrogenic causes). Contusions may also occur along the convexities of the cerebral hemispheres adjacent to the midline as a result of the brain rubbing against the rigid falx or the surface of the inner table of the calvaria.

Imaging findings will depend on when the patient is imaged relative to the time of injury. In the acute setting, hemorrhages are hyperdense and are frequently associated with surrounding hypodensity representing edema. Acute hemorrhage is hypointense on T2W and gradient echo MRI. Long-term follow-up shows resolution of the hemorrhage, encephalomalacia in the area of traumatized brain, and hemosiderin in the trauma bed.

Notes

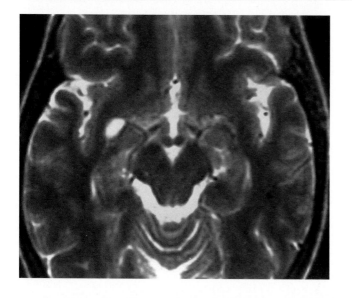
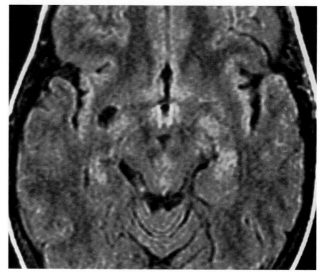
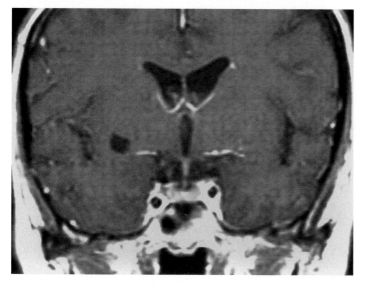

1. What is the differential diagnosis?
2. What CNS infection is associated with dilated Virchow-Robin spaces and pseudocysts within the basal ganglia?
3. Do lacunar infarcts typically occur in the upper half or the bottom half of the putamen?
4. Virchow-Robin spaces are extensions of what CSF space?

Virchow-Robin Perivascular Space

1. Lacunar infarct, perivascular space, developmental cyst, and cystic neoplasm.

2. *Cryptococcus* (especially in immunocompromised patients).

3. The upper half.

4. The subarachnoid space.

Reference
Jungreis CA, Kanal E, Hirsch WL, Martinez AJ, Moossy J: Normal perivascular spaces mimicking lacunar infarction: MR imaging, *Radiology* 169:101-104, 1988.

Cross-Reference
Neuroradiology: THE REQUISITES, p 211.

Comment
This case illustrates the typical appearance of a Virchow-Robin perivascular space. Diagnostic considerations primarily include lacunar infarct; however, developmental cysts and cystic neoplasms could potentially share many of the same imaging features. Dilated perivascular spaces can usually be distinguished from a lacunar infarct on the basis of typical imaging findings. Lacunar infarcts tend to occur in the upper half of the putamen, whereas perivascular spaces occur along the inferior half. In addition, whereas perivascular spaces are usually isointense to CSF on all pulse sequences, this is not the case with lacunar infarcts unless they have undergone cystic degeneration. Even when cystic, lacunar infarcts may have a thin surrounding hyperintense rim on proton density and FLAIR images representing gliosis. Dilated perivascular spaces are not associated with edema or enhancement, have a characteristic location along the anterior commissures, and are frequently bilateral and symmetric. In addition to the basal ganglia, they also occur in the cerebral peduncles and in the white matter at the cerebral convexities.

   Perivascular spaces are extensions of the subarachnoid space that follow the perforating vessels at the base of the brain into the basal ganglia. Virchow-Robin spaces may range from 1 to 15 mm in size. They tend to enlarge with age and in the presence of hypertension. This makes sense because most vessels (including those along the perivascular spaces) become more ectatic under both of these circumstances. In addition, just as the subarachnoid spaces become more prominent as one ages in that the perivascular spaces are extensions of the subarachnoid space, it makes sense that they enlarge in a similar manner. Given the extension of the perivascular spaces from the subarachnoid space into the brain, they are a conduit for the spread of a variety of inflammatory and neoplastic processes (e.g., *Cryptococcus*, sarcoid, and carcinomatosis).

Notes

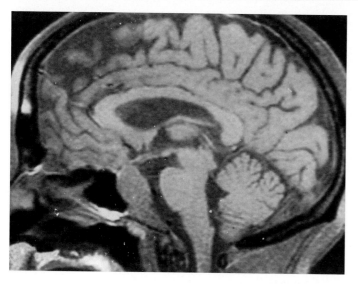
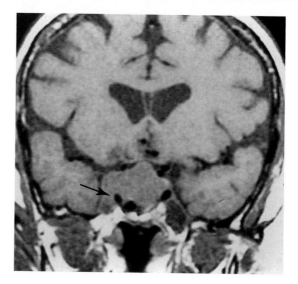

1. From what anatomic location is the lesion in this case arising?
2. What is the name of the structure *(arrow)* that the mass secondarily invades?
3. What is the classic visual symptom associated with these lesions?
4. What was the clinical presentation of this patient?

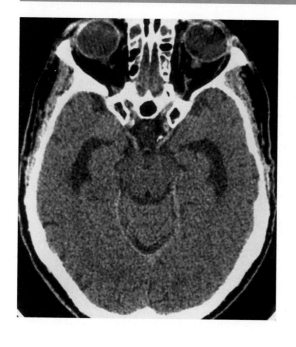
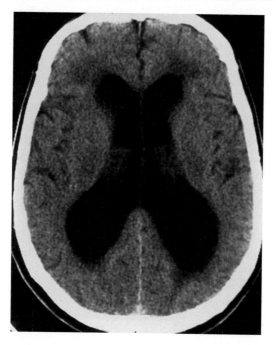

1. What is the imaging finding?
2. In noncommunicating hydrocephalus, where is the level of obstruction?
3. Colloid cysts typically cause obstruction at what level of the ventricular system?
4. In children, what midline neoplasms typically present with hydrocephalus because of obstruction of the fourth ventricle?

Macroadenoma Presenting With Multiple Cranial Neuropathies

1. The pituitary gland.

2. The cavernous sinus.

3. Bitemporal hemianopsia (tunnel vision).

4. Multiple cranial neuropathies caused by invasion of the right cavernous sinus.

Reference
Scotti G, Yu CY, Dillon WP, et al: MR imaging of cavernous sinus involvement by pituitary adenomas, *AJR Am J Roentgenol* 151:799-806, 1988.

Cross-Reference
Neuroradiology: THE REQUISITES, pp 313-314.

Comment
There is a macroadenoma (>10 mm) arising in the pituitary gland with secondary extension into the suprasellar cistern and right cavernous sinus *(arrows)*. In addition, on the sagittal T1W image, inferior extension is noted into the sphenoid sinus and the clivus. The clival extension is nicely demonstrated by the replacement of the normal high signal intensity fatty marrow on the unenhanced T1W image by abnormal hypointense tissue (likely tumor and edema). Although approximately 75% of pituitary adenomas present as a result of endocrine dysfunction, macroadenomas often present with signs and symptoms related to mass effect. These include headache, visual symptoms (characteristically bitemporal hemianopsia), and cranial nerve palsies, as in this case.

In the vast majority of cases, enhanced imaging is not necessary to evaluate macroadenomas. MRI, particularly unenhanced T1W images in the sagittal and coronal planes, is excellent for showing extension outside of the pituitary sella, including superior extension into the suprasellar cistern, inferior extension into the sphenoid sinus or skull base (clivus), and lateral extension into the cavernous sinus. Adenomas may encase the cavernous internal carotid artery, but unlike meningiomas they do not usually result in significant narrowing. In a study examining cavernous sinus involvement by pituitary adenomas, Scotti and colleagues found that invasion was unilateral in all cases and most commonly occurred with prolactin or adrenocorticotropic hormone secreting adenomas located laterally in the gland. The most specific sign of cavernous sinus invasion was encasement of the carotid artery.

Notes

Communicating Hydrocephalus Secondary to Prior Meningitis

1. Enlargement of the ventricles.

2. The ventricular system.

3. The foramen of Monro.

4. Primitive neuroectodermal tumors (medulloblastoma) and ependymomas.

Reference
Gammal TE, Allen MB Jr, Brooks BS, Mark EK: MR evaluation of hydrocephalus, *AJR Am J Roentgenol* 149:807-813, 1987.

Cross-Reference
Neuroradiology: THE REQUISITES, pp 240-242.

Comment
Obstructive hydrocephalus can be categorized as communicating or noncommunicating. Noncommunicating hydrocephalus is normally related to obstruction at some level of the ventricular system and is commonly related to neoplasms; however, obstruction of CSF flow within the ventricular system may be a complication of infection, hemorrhage, or congenital lesions (synechiae, webs, arachnoid cysts). Communicating hydrocephalus, as in this case, typically results from obstruction at the level of the arachnoid villi, foramen magnum, or tentorial incisura. Common causes of communicating hydrocephalus include inflammation of the meninges such as in meningitis (the patient in this case had prior bacterial meningitis), ventriculitis, subarachnoid hemorrhage, and carcinomatous meningitis. Obstruction of the arachnoid villi in these situations is usually related to high protein concentrations, hemorrhage, and/or hypercellularity of the CSF.

On imaging, dilation of the anterior third ventricle in particular is most indicative of hydrocephalus and should not be present in normal subjects or patients with atrophy. Elevation and thinning of the corpus callosum, best appreciated on sagittal MRI, are present in over 75% of cases of hydrocephalus. Acute hydrocephalus may manifest with hypodensity around the ventricles on CT scans or T2W in the periventricular white matter on MRI as a result of transependymal spread of CSF. Compensated long-standing hydrocephalus usually does not present with this finding unless there is acute hydrocephalus superimposed on chronic disease. Treatment of noncommunicating and communicating hydrocephalus is different. Noncommunicating hydrocephalus often requires surgery (e.g., resection of a neoplasm), whereas communicating hydrocephalus is usually treated with shunting.

Notes

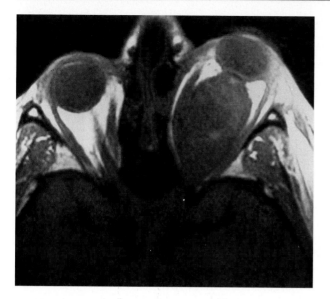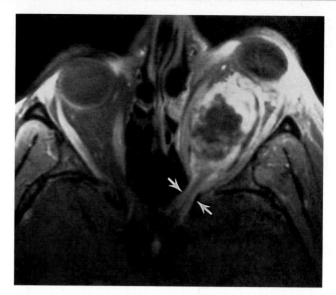

1. From what structure is the mass arising?
2. What imaging plane would best confirm this?
3. What is the name of the osseous channel *(arrows)* through which this nerve passes?
4. What is the characteristic early presentation of optic meningiomas?

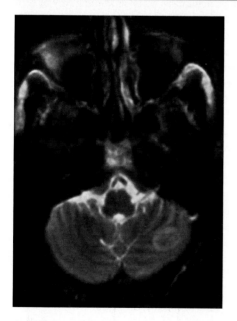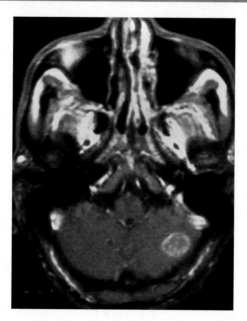

1. What is the pertinent radiologic finding on the T2W image?
2. What is the characteristic appearance on T2W images of a cavernoma?
3. What are the signal characteristics of melanoma on T1W and T2W imaging?
4. What are the most common systemic neoplasms to metastasize to the brain?

Optic Nerve Glioma

1. The optic nerve.

2. Coronal.

3. The optic canal.

4. Decreased visual acuity (this symptoms occurs relatively late in optic nerve gliomas).

Reference

Weber AL, Klufas R, Pless M: Imaging evaluation of the optic nerve and visual pathway including cranial nerves affecting the visual pathway, *Neuroimaging Clin North Am* 6:143-177, 1996.

Cross-Reference

Neuroradiology: THE REQUISITES, pp 290-294.

Comment

The images show a large necrotic mass arising from the optic nerve. There is mild expansion of the orbit, suggesting that this is a long-standing process. There is also proptosis. Importantly, there is extension of enhancing tumor around the nerve in the optic canal *(arrows)* and extending to the prechiasmatic portion of the optic nerve in the intracranial compartment. It is important that all patients with optic nerve gliomas have a head MRI to assess for intracranial extension along the optic pathways (tumors may extend back to the lateral geniculate body and optic radiations). The differential diagnosis of an enlarged optic nerve sheath complex includes neoplasm (glioma, meningioma, metastases, hematologic malignancies, and nerve sheath tumors). Inflammatory conditions may also present with an enlarged optic nerve sheath complex; these conditions include optic neuritis (multiple sclerosis), infection (tuberculosis, syphilis), sarcoid, and pseudotumor.

Most optic nerve gliomas present in childhood (either associated with neurofibromatosis type 1 or as isolated sporadic lesions). In addition, the vast majority of these neoplasms in children are low grade juvenile pilocytic astrocytomas. Many of these tumors are asymptomatic early in their development, frequently delaying diagnosis until later in disease. Loss of visual acuity is a late finding; by contrast, visual acuity loss is a relatively early presentation in meningioma.

Notes

Hemorrhagic Metastasis (Renal Cell Carcinoma)

1. A rounded, hypointense mass in the left cerebellar hemisphere.

2. A demarcated lesion with central high signal intensity and a complete peripheral rim of hypointensity related to hemosiderin.

3. Melanotic melanomas are frequently hyperintense on T1W images, and there is often T2W shortening resulting in an isointense to hypointense appearance as well.

4. Lung and breast followed by melanoma.

Reference

Atlas SW, Grossman RI, Gomori JM, et al: Hemorrhagic intracranial malignant neoplasms: spin-echo MR imaging, *Radiology* 164:71-77, 1987.

Cross-Reference

Neuroradiology: THE REQUISITES, pp 79-82.

Comment

This case demonstrates a demarcated hypointense mass in the left cerebellar hemisphere that shows heterogeneous but prominent enhancement following contrast. This is a typical appearance of a hemorrhagic metastasis. T2W shortening may be seen not only with blood products but also as a result of the paramagnetic effect of melanin, as well as in the presence of calcification, hypercellularity, or proteinaceous material. In this patient, the lesion is hemorrhagic metastatic renal cell carcinoma. Even though vascular metastases, such as renal and thyroid carcinoma, and melanoma and choriocarcinoma have a propensity to bleed, because breast and lung carcinoma are so much more common, a hemorrhagic metastasis is still more likely to be related to one of these latter cancers. In the case of a single cerebral hemorrhagic mass, primary brain tumors such as GBM should be considered; however, primary brain tumors in the posterior fossa are unusual in adults (representing less than 1% to 2% of posterior fossa neoplasms). The most common infratentorial neoplasm in adults is metastatic disease.

Notes

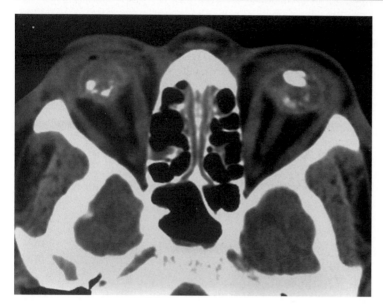

1. What ocular neoplasms/masses are associated with calcification?
2. Calcification related to drusen characteristically occurs at what location in the globe?
3. What is the cause of the entity presented in this case?
4. What metabolic abnormality is associated with ocular calcifications?

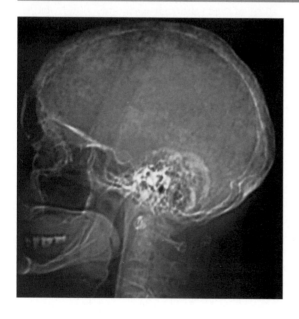 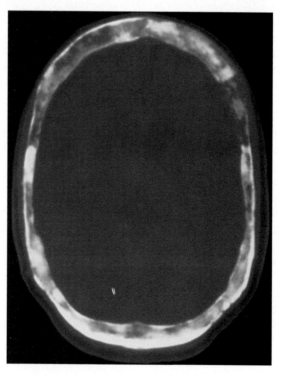

1. Which imaging modality is most sensitive in detecting abnormalities of cortical bone?
2. Which imaging modality is most sensitive in detecting marrow abnormalities?
3. What is the differential diagnosis in this case?
4. What finding on the current examination is suggestive of an aggressive process as opposed to Paget's disease?

Phthisis Bulbi

1. Retinoblastomas, astrocytic hamartomas, and choroidal osteomas.

2. At the insertion of the optic nerve head/optic disk.

3. Previous trauma or infection.

4. Hypercalcemic states.

Reference

Brant-Zawadzki M, Enzmann DR: Orbital computed tomography: calcific densities of the posterior globe, *J Comput Assist Tomogr* 3:503-508, 1979.

Cross-Reference

Neuroradiology: THE REQUISITES, pp 283-285, 289.

Comment

This case demonstrates the characteristic appearance of phthisis bulbi, which refers to calcification and/or ossification of a thickened sclera within a shrunken, atrophic globe. Phthisis bulbi represents extensive degenerative changes of the globe related to a spectrum of insults; however, it is most commonly seen in the setting of prior trauma or inflammation/infection. Phthisis bulbi may also be easily recognized on MRI because of the configuration of the globe in combination with the peripheral posterior hyperintensity on T1W images and corresponding hypointensity on T2W images (resulting from deposition of paramagnetic ions and calcification).

Intraocular calcification may be present in a variety of conditions. Metabolic disorders associated with hypercalcemia (hyperparathyroidism) not uncommonly may have calcification along the posterior sclera. A variety of degenerative conditions may be associated with ocular calcification, the most common being optic nerve drusen in which there is calcification of the optic disk at the level of the insertion of the optic nerve. Other degenerative conditions associated with such calcification include phthisis bulbi, prior retinal detachment, and retinopathy of prematurity (retrolental fibroplasia). Masses associated with calcification include retinoblastoma, choroidal osteoma (seen most often in young women) and astrocytic hamartoma (seen in tuberous sclerosis and neurofibromatosis). Ocular calcification may also be seen in association with congenital vascular lesions, as in Sturge-Weber and von Hippel-Lindau syndromes. Finally, ocular calcification may be seen in the setting of infection, often associated with *Toxocara* species and cytomegalovirus. Establishing the correct diagnosis in patients with ocular calcification is frequently possible and depends on other associated radiologic findings, unilateral versus bilateral disease, and correlation with clinical history.

Notes

Calvarial Metastases—Breast Carcinoma

1. CT.

2. MRI.

3. Blastic metastases, Paget's disease.

4. Destruction of the cortex. In Paget's disease of the calvaria, there is typically cortical thickening without destruction.

Reference

Daffner RH, Lupetin AR, Dash N, Deeb ZL, Sefczek RJ, Schapiro RL: MRI in the detection of malignant infiltration of bone marrow, *AJR Am J Roentgenol* 146:353-358, 1986.

Cross-Reference

Neuroradiology: THE REQUISITES, p 332.

Comment

This case illustrates mixed blastic and lytic metastases in a woman with breast carcinoma. Other carcinomas that may present with blastic metastases include prostate carcinoma (the most common cause of blastic metastases in men) and less commonly carcinoid; Hodgkin's lymphoma; and mucinous carcinomas of the lung, colon, and bladder. In older patients, blastic and/or mixed metastases (blastic and lytic) can be mistaken for the "cotton-wool" appearance of diffuse calvarial Paget's disease. On close examination of a CT scan these can often be distinguished, although sometimes other imaging modalities may be necessary. In addition to having regions of sclerosis and/or lysis, Paget's disease is usually associated with thickening of the diploic space, as well as cortical thickening. In contrast, metastatic disease (as in this case) is typically not associated with bony expansion and there is usually no cortical thickening. In this case, particularly in the left hemicalvaria in the frontotemporal region, erosion and destruction of the cortical margin of the outer table suggest an aggressive process. When there is a question, particularly in a patient without a known systemic malignancy, a bone scan may be performed. In most instances, both Paget's disease and metastatic disease will be "hot" on nuclear scintigraphy; however, the reason to perform the bone scan is not to assess the calvaria but rather to assess the remainder of the skeleton for evidence of additional foci of metastatic disease. Paget's disease is not infrequently polyostotic (involves multiple sites). However, plain radiographs of additional pagetoid lesions detected on bone scans usually have a characteristic appearance.

Notes

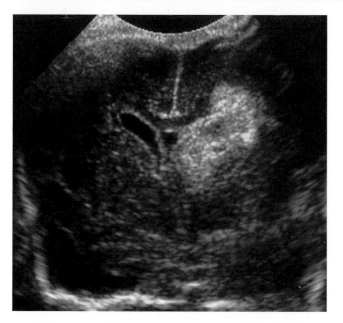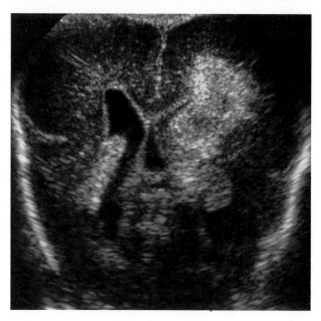

1. What are the most significant risk factors in developing this lesion in the perinatal period?
2. What are common causes of intracranial hemorrhage in full-term infants in the perinatal period?
3. What are the anatomic boundaries of traumatic extracranial cephalohematomas?
4. What is meant by a grade II germinal matrix hemorrhage?

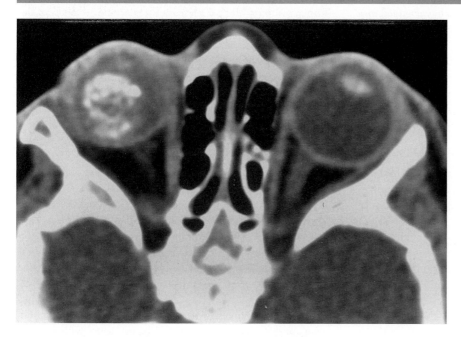

1. What are causes of intraocular calcification in children?
2. What is meant by the "third eye" in trilateral retinoblastoma?
3. How are retinoblastomas differentiated from other causes of intraocular calcifications in children?
4. What is the most common clinical presentation of retinoblastoma?

Germinal Matrix Hemorrhage*

1. Prematurity and low birth weight.

2. Traumatic delivery and ischemic/hypoxic insult.

3. Cephalohematomas are subperiosteal hemorrhages contained by the cranial sutures.

4. The hemorrhage extends into the ventricular system; however, the ventricles are normal in size (no hydrocephalus).

Reference

Rorke LB, Zimmerman RA: Prematurity, post-maturity, and destructive lesions in utero, *AJNR Am J Neuroradiol* 13:517-536, 1992.

Cross-Reference

Neuroradiology: THE REQUISITES, p 266.

Comment

The germinal matrix represents the site of neuronal precursors in the subependymal region of the ventricular system from where neuronal migration occurs to form the cerebral cortex. Premature low-birth-weight infants are at highest risk for developing perinatal germinal matrix hemorrhages. These hemorrhages are often present in the immediate postpartum period; however, they may occur for up to 3 to 4 weeks following delivery. Germinal matrix hemorrhages may be graded on a scale of I to IV. Grade I is hemorrhage confined to the germinal matrix, grade II is a germinal matrix hemorrhage that has extended into the ventricles (the ventricles are normal in size initially), grade III refers to intraventricular extension with ventriculomegaly, and grade IV to extension of hemorrhage into the cerebrum. Usually germinal matrix hemorrhages are readily identified on sonographic evaluation through the anterior fontanelle in infants at risk. Similarly, premature infants at risk for such bleeds are followed up with ultrasound on a regular basis in the perinatal period.

Most cranial hemorrhages in full-term infants are related to birth trauma or ischemic injury. Traumatic vaginal deliveries may result in subgaleal hematomas and/or cephalohematomas. Less commonly, traumatic delivery may result in intracranial hemorrhage, which may include subdural hematomas (most common along the tentorium cerebelli and posterior interhemispheric fissure) and subarachnoid and parenchymal bleeds. Hemorrhagic infarction related to ischemia is among the most common causes of nontraumatic hemorrhage in the perinatal period.

Notes

Retinoblastoma*

1. Retinoblastoma, persistent hyperplastic primary vitreous, toxocaral endophthalmitis, Coats' disease (congenital retinal telangiectasia), and retrolental fibroplasia.

2. Pineoblastoma of the pineal gland.

3. Most retinoblastomas present before the age of 3 years; before 3 years of age, however, calcification is usually absent in other conditions associated with ocular calcification.

4. Leukokoria.

References

Barkhof F, Smeets M, vander Valk P, Tan KE, Hoogenraad F, Peeters J, Valk J: MR imaging in retinoblastoma, *Eur Radiol* 7:726-731. 1997.

Potter PD, Shields CL, Shields JA, Flanders AE: The role of magnetic resonance imaging in children with intraocular tumors and simulating lesions, *Ophthalmology* 103:1774-1783, 1996.

Cross-Reference

Neuroradiology: THE REQUISITES, pp 284-286.

Comment

Retinoblastoma represents the most common intraocular tumor in childhood. The typical clinical presentation is leukokoria, an abnormal pupillary reflex characterized by a "white" pupil. Other common clinical presentations include strabismus, decreased visual acuity, or eye pain (which may be related to glaucoma). The majority of retinoblastomas (98%) present before 3 years of age. Retinoblastomas most commonly represent isolated sporadic tumors; however, they may be heritable in an autosomal dominant pattern. Up to 30% to 40% of patients with retinoblastoma have bilateral tumors; familial disease should be considered in these cases.

Because the radiologic hallmark of retinoblastoma is the presence of intraocular calcification before the age of 3 years, CT remains the best imaging modality for the detection of retinoblastoma. MRI is not as sensitive in detecting calcification. CT is also important in assessing the other eye for small calcifications. Not all retinoblastomas (particularly small ones) have calcification, so the absence of calcification does not entirely exclude the possibility of retinoblastoma. MRI plays an important role in assessing these patients as retinoblastoma may spread along the nerves and vessels to the retrobulbar orbit, and there may be subarachnoid seeding. Both modes of transmission may result in intracranial dissemination of disease. Therefore patients with retinoblastoma should be evaluated with MRI to determine the extent of disease. A small percentage (<5%) of patients with bilateral retinoblastomas may present with pineoblastoma of the pineal gland ("third eye").

Notes

---

*Figures for Case 40 courtesy Jill Langer, MD.

*Figure for Case 41 courtesy Robert A. Zimmerman, MD.

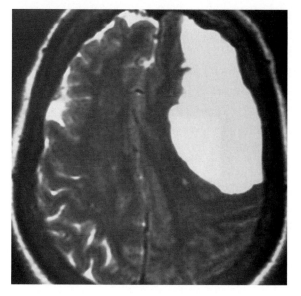
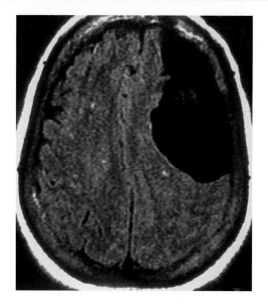

1. Is the mass intraaxial or extraaxial?
2. What imaging findings differentiate an extraaxial from an intraaxial mass?
3. What is the differential diagnosis of a cystic mass in this location?
4. Are most arachnoid cysts congenital or acquired?

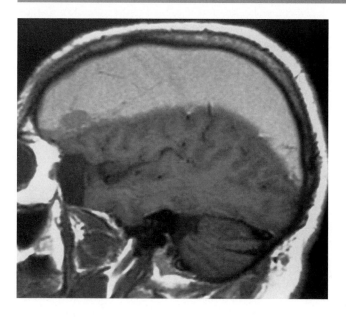
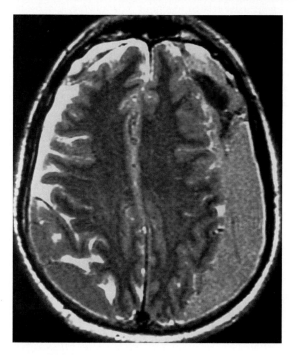

1. What structure or type of hemoglobin is diamagnetic?
2. What are the signal characteristics on T1W and T2W imaging of acute subdural hematomas?
3. What patients are at increased risk for bilateral, complex subdural hematomas?
4. What are the MRI signal characteristics of subacute (weeks to months old) hematomas?

Arachnoid Cyst

1. Extraaxial.

2. There is buckling of the gray and white matter of the left frontal lobe, and the lateral aspect of the mass is broad based against the dural surface/inner table of the calvaria.

3. Arachnoid or epidermoid cysts.

4. Congenital.

Reference

Gandy SE, Heier LA: Clinical and magnetic resonance features of primary intracranial arachnoid cysts, *Ann Neurol* 21:342-348, 1987.

Cross-Reference

Neuroradiology: THE REQUISITES, pp 77, 247-249, 261.

Comment

Most intracranial arachnoid cysts are congenital and are derived from the meninx primitiva, which envelops the developing CNS. As CSF fills the subarachnoid spaces, the meninx is resorbed. At the same time a cleft may develop between layers of the arachnoid membrane and may behave like a one-way ball-valve mechanism in which there is preferential flow of CSF into this cleft, resulting in formation of a cyst. Less commonly, arachnoid cysts may be acquired as a result of adhesions in the subarachnoid space related to a prior inflammatory process or hemorrhage.

The most common location for an arachnoid cyst is the middle cranial fossa. Other common locations include the cerebral convexities (most commonly the frontal convexity as in this case), the basal cisterns (suprasellar, cerebellopontine angle, and quadrigeminal), and the retrocerebellar region. On CT and MRI, arachnoid cysts usually follow the density or intensity of CSF, respectively. When large enough, cysts may cause smooth remodeling of the inner table of the bony calvaria and osseous expansion. There may also be hypogenesis of the underlying brain parenchyma (most commonly described in the temporal lobe with middle cranial fossa cysts). Calcification is unusual, and enhancement should not be present. The major differential consideration is an epidermoid cyst. On unenhanced T1W images an internal matrix, although subtle, is typically evident in epidermoid cysts. On intermediate (long TR/short TE) or FLAIR images arachnoid cysts follow the signal intensity characteristics of CSF, whereas epidermoid cysts tend to be hyperintense relative to CSF. In addition, on diffusion weighted images arachnoid cysts are hypointense (like the ventricles) resulting from an increased apparent diffusion constant (ADC), whereas epidermoid cysts do not have an increased ADC.

Notes

Complex Subdural Hematoma

1. Oxyhemoglobin. Diamagnetic materials have no unpaired electrons.

2. Hypointense (isointense to gray matter).

3. Elderly patients with atrophy and recurrent falls, as well as patients following shunting for hydrocephalus.

4. Hyperintense on T1W (methemoglobin) and hyperintense on T2W imaging.

Reference

Gomori JM, Grossman RI: Mechanisms responsible for the MR appearance and evolution of intracranial hemorrhage, *RadioGraphics* 8:427-440, 1988.

Cross-Reference

Neuroradiology: THE REQUISITES, pp 121-126, 152-155.

Comment

The appearance of blood products on MRI is dependent on several factors, most importantly the structure of hemoglobin at the time of imaging. Oxyhemoglobin (oxygen bound to the iron of hemoglobin) is diamagnetic because it effectively has no unpaired electrons. On giving up its oxygen, deoxyhemoglobin is formed and hemoglobin undergoes a small but significant structural change such that water molecules in the vicinity of the deoxyhemoglobin are unable to bind to the iron. Deoxyhemoglobin has four unpaired electrons and may be oxidized to methemoglobin. Methemoglobin has five unpaired electrons, and water molecules are able to bind to the iron atom.

Susceptibility effects, proton-electron dipole-dipole interactions, and other factors contribute to the variable signal characteristics of blood products on MRI. When placed in a magnetic field, certain substances may induce an additional smaller magnetic field that may add to the externally applied field. This phenomenon may be seen with paramagnetic substances (deoxyhemoglobin and methemoglobin). Alternatively, other substances when placed in a magnetic field may induce magnetic fields that subtract from the externally applied field (seen with diamagnetic materials such as oxyhemoglobin). Susceptibility effects of blood products depends on the proportionality constant between the strength of the applied magnetic field and the induced magnetic field.

Methemoglobin induces a local magnetic field significantly greater than that of a proton. Therefore if a proton gets close enough to this field a spin transition may occur. In order to have a proton-electron dipole-dipole interaction, water must bind to heme. Even though the number of heme molecules is small relative to that of water, the exchange rate of water molecules is quite rapid compared with the repetition time; hence many water molecules are bound to heme during MRI. Proton-electron dipole-dipole interactions result in shortening of T1 and T2.

Notes

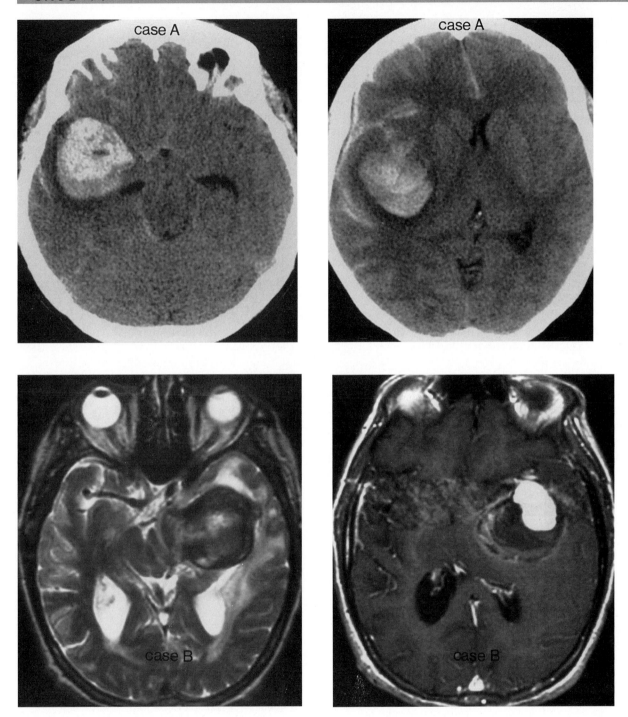

case A

case A

case B

case B

1. What is the clinical presentation of these lesions?

2. What is the definition of a "giant aneurysm"?

3. What are common vessels of origin of these lesions?

4. What is the shortcoming or pitfall of catheter angiography in the evaluation of giant aneurysms?

Giant Middle Cerebral Artery Aneurysm

1. Symptoms related to subarachnoid hemorrhage or mass effect (headache, nausea, vomiting).

2. An aneurysm with a maximal diameter larger than 2.5 cm.

3. Middle cerebral artery, cavernous internal carotid artery, and tip of the basilar artery.

4. Although angiography will adequately assess the patent lumen, it cannot evaluate the true size of these aneurysms because the thrombosed portions are not visualized.

References

Velthuis BK, Rinkel GJE, Ramos LMP, et al: Subarachnoid hemorrhage: aneurysm detection and preoperative evaluation with CT angiography, *Radiology* 208:423-430, 1998.

Atlas SW, Grossman RI, Goldberg HI, et al: Partially thrombosed giant intracranial aneurysms: correlation of MR and pathologic findings, *Radiology* 162:111-114, 1987.

Cross-Reference

Neuroradiology: THE REQUISITES, pp 136-139.

Comment

The middle cerebral artery bifurcation or trifurcation has a propensity for the development of giant aneurysms. Giant aneurysms may present with subarachnoid hemorrhage or symptoms caused by mass effect related to aneurysm size or intraparenchymal rupture/hematoma. The patient in case A presented both with the "worst headache of life" related to subarachnoid hemorrhage and left hemiparesis. The patient in case B presented with seizures.

Thrombus may form within large aneurysms and may be a source of distal emboli. Unenhanced CT in case A shows a hyperdense giant aneurysm. At its periphery there is heterogeneous density related to thrombus. On MRI giant aneurysms have a characteristic appearance as in case B. Findings include signal void consistent with flow in the patent lumen, phase artifact related to flow, and heterogeneous signal intensity representing thrombus of varying ages.

Recent investigations with CT angiography (CTA) in the setting of subarachnoid hemorrhage have shown detection rates for aneurysms as high as 93% to 96%. False negative examinations may be related to CTA technique, aneurysm size (especially those less than 5 mm), and aneurysm location. Aneurysms originating from the posterior communicating artery, the infraclinoid internal carotid artery, and the ophthalmic artery that are in close proximity to bone especially may go undetected. Advantages of CTA include its rapidity, noninvasiveness, and that it may provide preoperative information regarding the relationship of an aneurysm to adjacent bony landmarks. However, presently catheter angiography remains the standard for evaluating subarachnoid hemorrhage.

Notes

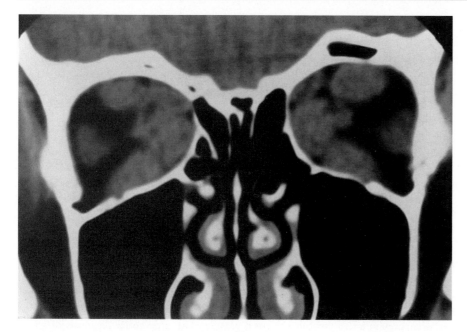

1. What are vascular causes of enlargement of the extraocular muscles?
2. How often does the entity in this case involve the orbits bilaterally?
3. Isolated involvement of what extraocular muscle is extremely rare in thyroid ophthalmopathy?
4. In thyroid eye disease, what portion of the extraocular muscles is characteristically spared?

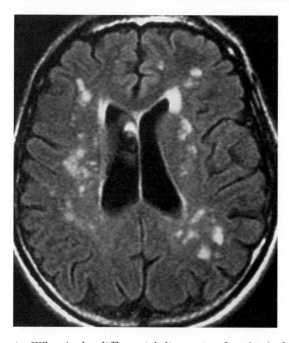

1. What is the differential diagnosis of multiple foci of T2W hyperintensity in the white matter?
2. What inflammatory conditions have a predilection to involve the corpus callosum?
3. What are the two most common risk factors for the development of small vessel ischemic disease?
4. Involvement of what structures in addition to the white matter is frequently present in small vessel ischemic disease?

Thyroid Ophthalmopathy

1. Carotid-cavernous fistula, thrombosis of the superior ophthalmic vein, cavernous sinus thrombosis, and AVMs.

2. In approximately 90% of cases.

3. The lateral rectus muscle.

4. The tendinous insertions.

Reference

Ulmer JL, Logani SC, Mark LP, Hamilton CA, Prost RW, Garman JN: Near-resonance saturation pulse imaging of the extraocular muscles in thyroid-related ophthalmopathy, *AJNR Am J Neuroradiol* 19:943-950, 1998.

Cross-Reference

Neuroradiology: THE REQUISITES, p 296.

Comment

Thyroid ophthalmopathy is more common in women by a ratio of 4:1 and is frequently asymptomatic; however, when present it may be seen in euthyroid or hyperthyroid states. Clinical signs and symptoms may include proptosis, lid retraction, decreased ocular range of motion, visual loss resulting from compression of the optic nerve in the orbital apex, and/or corneal exposure caused by eyelid retraction. Pain is uncommon. The most common cause of unilateral or bilateral exophthalmos in adults is thyroid ophthalmopathy. The incidence of bilateral disease may be as high as 90% of cases. Most patients evaluated with CT or MRI carry a known diagnosis of thyroid ophthalmopathy, and the role of imaging is to assess for the presence of optic nerve compression in the orbital apex by enlarged muscles. When there is compromise of vision in cases failing to respond to medical therapy, orbital decompression by removal of the osseous walls around the orbital apex may be necessary.

Magnetic resonance imaging may also be useful in evaluating patients with ophthalmopathy without laboratory or clinical evidence of thyroid disease. The most common patterns of extraocular muscle involvement are enlargement of all of the extraocular muscles or of the inferior and medial rectus muscles only. Isolated involvement of the lateral rectus muscle is unusual and when present should raise suspicion for a different disease process such as myositis or pseudotumor. Characteristically, in thyroid ophthalmopathy there is enlargement of the muscle bellies with sparing of the tendinous insertions. In late stages of disease fibrosis resulting in contraction of the muscle bellies may be evident, and there may be fatty replacement of the muscles.

Notes

Small Vessel Ischemic Disease

1. Demyelinating disease, small vessel ischemic disease, migraine headaches, vasculitis, and other inflammatory conditions.

2. Demyelinating disease (multiple sclerosis).

3. Aging and hypertension.

4. The basal ganglia, thalami, and pons.

Reference

Brown JJ, Hesselink JR, Rothrock JF: MR and CT of lacunar infarcts, *AJR Am J Roentgenol* 151:367-372, 1988.

Cross-Reference

Neuroradiology: THE REQUISITES, pp 210-211.

Comment

This case illustrates numerous foci of increased T2W signal intensity within the periventricular white matter, as well as within the basal ganglia. The differential diagnosis of white matter lesions on MRI is broad and includes inflammatory processes such as demyelinating disease (e.g., multiple sclerosis, acute disseminated encephalomyelitis), infectious disease (e.g., Lyme disease), vasculitis, and small vessel ischemic disease (the most common of all of the entities). Imaging findings that may favor small vessel ischemic disease include proportionate involvement of the deep gray matter (the globus pallidus, caudate, putamen, and thalami) and pons, as well as the absence of mass effect and enhancement. Enhancement is more likely to be present in inflammatory conditions, including demyelinating disease. When assessing patients with white matter lesions, the patient's age and clinical history are of paramount importance. Like everything else, small vessel ischemic disease increases in frequency with age. In addition, hypertension, smoking, hyperlipidemia, and insulin-dependent diabetes mellitus may accelerate the development of small vessel disease.

The white matter lesions associated with small vessel ischemic disease have been referred to as *leukoaraiosis,* and the histologic correlate is that of myelin pallor and gliosis. In addition, dilated perivascular spaces are frequently noted. Patients symptomatic from small vessel ischemic disease will frequently present with neurologic symptoms related to lacunar infarctions in the deep gray matter. These infarctions often have a characteristic symptom complex depending on lesion location in these structures. However, the majority of lesions related to small vessel ischemic disease are probably asymptomatic because they may be in clinically silent areas. Patients with long-standing sequelae of small vessel ischemic disease may present with progressive dementia (multiinfarct dementia) on a chronic basis. In this situation, patients typically present with unexplained progressive dementia rather than focal neurologic symptoms.

Notes

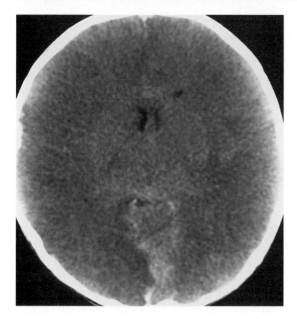

1. In the absence of known significant head trauma, the radiologist must be highly suspect of what diagnosis?
2. What other cranial manifestation is frequently present in child abuse?
3. What finding in the eyes is characteristic of this diagnosis?
4. What is the cause of a leptomeningeal cyst?

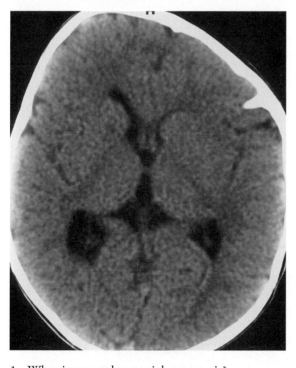
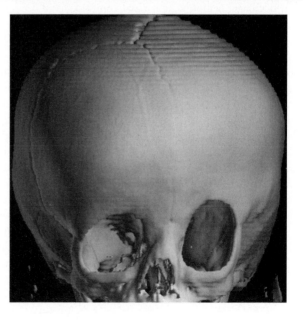

1. What is meant by cranial synostosis?
2. What is the most common suture to close prematurely?
3. Trigonocephaly and hypotelorism are characteristic of premature closure of which suture?
4. Plagiocephaly refers to what pattern of craniosynostosis?

Nonaccidental Trauma—Child Abuse*

1. Child abuse (nonaccidental trauma).

2. Skull fractures (particularly depressed or multiple fractures).

3. Retinal hemorrhages.

4. Skull fracture complicated by a dural tear.

Reference

Sato Y, Yuh WTC, Smith WL, et al: Head injury in child abuse: evaluation with MR imaging, *Radiology* 173:653-657, 1989.

Cross-Reference

Neuroradiology: THE REQUISITES, pp 164-165.

Comment

The presence of skull fractures and/or intracranial hemorrhage, particularly in infants in the absence of known trauma to explain such injuries, should raise the suspicion of child abuse (nonaccidental trauma). There are more than 1 million reported cases of child abuse each year, and head trauma is among the leading causes of morbidity and death in these children. Brain injury may be the result of direct trauma, aggressive shaking, or strangulation/suffocation. There is often little or no evidence of external trauma. The most common type of intracranial hemorrhage in the setting of child abuse is a subdural hematoma, although subarachnoid hemorrhage, epidural hematoma, intraventricular hemorrhage, hemorrhagic cortical contusion, and diffuse axonal injury are all manifestations of nonaccidental trauma. Bilateral retinal hemorrhages are highly suggestive of child abuse (shaken baby syndrome). In the absence of significant head trauma, the presence of skull fractures (especially bilateral, depressed, and/or occipital fractures), which are found in as many as 45% of nonaccidental trauma cases, should raise the suspicion for child abuse. Because it is not fully developed, the infant skull is extremely pliable, hence it is relatively resistant to fracture. In the worse case, diffuse cerebral edema resulting in mass effect and herniation is not uncommon in abused children. Cerebral infarction may occur as a result of strangulation, or vascular compromise may be caused by intracranial mass effect. Infarctions in multiple vascular territories should be viewed with suspicion.

Notes

Craniosynostosis—Left Coronal Suture*

1. Premature closure of cranial suture(s).

2. Sagittal synostosis.

3. The metopic.

4. Premature closure of one of the paired sutures (coronal, lambdoid, or, much less frequently, temporosquamousal).

Reference

Mafee MF, Valvassori GE: Radiology of the craniofacial anomalies, *Otolaryngol Clin North Am* 14:939-988, 1981.

Cross-Reference

Neuroradiology: THE REQUISITES, pp 262-263, 264.

Comment

Craniostenosis, or craniosynostosis, refers to premature closure of one or more of the cranial sutures. Isolated premature closure of the sagittal suture is most common, occurring in more than 50% of cases of craniosynostosis. Unilateral or bilateral premature closure of the coronal suture(s) is the next most common, followed by premature closure of the metopic suture. The lambdoid suture undergoes premature closure in less than 1% of craniostenosis cases. Depending on the suture(s) involved, there are characteristic deformities of the skull and orbit. Premature closure of the sagittal suture results in a head that has limited growth in the transverse dimension. This results in dolichocephaly (scaphocephaly), in which there is an increase in head size in the anteroposterior dimension.

Plagiocephaly refers to premature closure of a single coronal or lambdoid suture (or occasionally the temporosquamousal suture). In the majority of cases, plagiocephaly is seen with closure of a single coronal suture, resulting in elevation of the lesser wing of the sphenoid bone and leading to the "harlequin" appearance of the orbit. Premature closure of both coronal sutures results in brachycephaly. Early fusion of the metopic suture in the frontal region results in trigonocephaly, or simply a "triangular" configuration of the head. Craniosynostosis is usually an isolated abnormality, although it may be associated with a variety of congenital syndromes. Such conditions include Apert's syndrome, which is associated with a "clover-leaf" deformity of the skull resulting from closure of the coronal, lambdoid, and sagittal sutures. Other syndromes associated with craniostenosis are hypophosphatasia, Crouzon's disease (craniofacial dysostosis), and Treacher Collins syndrome (mandibulofacial dysostosis).

Notes

---

*Figure for Case 47 courtesy Jill Hunter, MD.

*Figures for Case 48 courtesy Jill Hunter, MD.

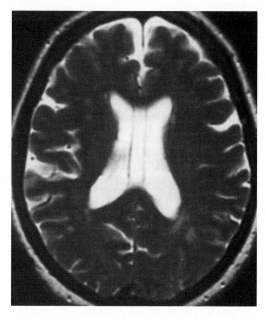

1. What is the anatomic landmark that demarcates the cavum septum pellucidum from a cavum vergae?
2. Development of the corpus callosum is intimately associated with development of what other structure?
3. What structures traverse the cistern of the velum interpositum?
4. What is the normal volume of CSF surrounding the CNS?

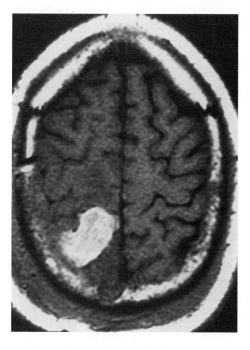 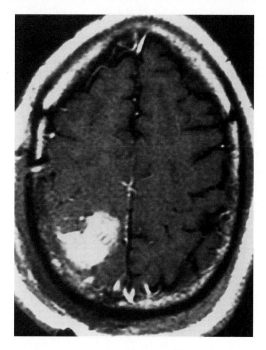

1. Over what time period does granulation tissue develop in an operative bed?
2. When is the best time to image a patient following resection of a brain tumor in order to assess for residual neoplasm?
3. Why does granulation tissue typically enhance?
4. Regarding radiation injury, is hemorrhage most commonly present in early, early delayed, or late delayed radiation injury?

Cavum Septum Pellucidum

1. The columns of the fornix.

2. The septum pellucidum.

3. The internal cerebral veins and vein of Galen.

4. Approximately 150 ml.

References

Silbert PL, Gubbay SS, Vaughan RJ: Cavum septum pellucidum and obstructive hydrocephalus, *J Neurol Neurosurg Psychiatry* 56:820-822, 1993.

Degreef G, Lantos G, Bogerts B, Ashtari M, Lieberman J: Abnormalities of the septum pellucidum on MR scans in first-episode schizophrenic patients, *AJNR Am J Neuroradiol* 13:835-840, 1992.

Cross-Reference

Neuroradiology: THE REQUISITES, pp 36-37.

Comment

The cavum pellucidum is bordered superiorly by the corpus callosum and posteriorly by the body of the fornix. The portion of the cavum extending posterior to the columns of the fornix is called the *cavum vergae*. The cavum septum pellucidum and cavum vergae are potential cavities that lie between the membranes of the septum pellucidum. They most commonly represent a normal anatomic variant. On obstetric ultrasound, the cavum septum pellucidum is present in essentially all fetuses. During the latter half of gestation, the cavum septum pellucidum decreases in size. However, at birth approximately 80% of term infants have a small residual cavum septum pellucidum that continues to decrease in size as the child ages. Review of the literature shows considerable variation in the reported prevalence of a cavum septum pellucidum/cavum vergae in normal adults. Autopsy studies have also shown significant variability (range, 3% to 30%). When a cavum septum pellucidum and cavum vergae are present concomitantly, they usually communicate with one another. However, they do not typically communicate with the ventricular system. A persistent cavum septum pellucidum is usually asymptomatic. Cysts may arise in this location and exert mass effect. In addition, enlargement of the cavum septum pellucidum with intermittent obstruction of the foramen of Monro resulting in hydrocephalus has rarely been reported. Cysts may be treated with surgical resection, shunting of the cyst, or fenestration. The cistern of the velum interpositum is located above the third ventricle, and the internal cerebral veins and Galen's vein traverse it.

Notes

Postoperative—Brain Tumor Resection

1. Usually within 3 to 4 days.

2. Within 48 hours following surgery (before scar tissue develops).

3. Because it tends to be highly vascularized.

4. Late delayed.

Reference

Dolinskas CA, Simeone FA: Surgical site after resection of a meningioma, *AJNR Am J Neuroradiol* 19:419-426, 1998.

Cross-Reference

Neuroradiology: THE REQUISITES, pp 99-100.

Comment

A common indication for MRI is assessment for residual neoplasm in patients following resection of a brain tumor. Detection of residual neoplasm will affect patient prognosis and decisions regarding therapy (repeat surgery and/or the addition of radiation or chemotherapy). In addition to containing fibrous tissue, granulation tissue is often highly vascularized; therefore it enhances on imaging. Because granulation tissue is dynamic in nature, it may enhance for months to years following surgery. Typically granulation tissue develops within the first 3 days following surgery. MRI is more sensitive than CT in detecting enhancing scar. In patients with enhancing tumors before surgical resection, postoperative imaging is often performed within 48 to 72 hours following surgery. This is because typically within the first 2 to 3 days following surgery granulation tissue is just developing and frequently does not enhance. Therefore enhancing tissue on these initial postoperative scans should cause suspicions for residual neoplasm. Imaging performed after this time may result in confusion in distinguishing granulation tissue from residual tumor. Because patients frequently have hemorrhage in the operative bed following tumor resection, it is important that enhanced images be compared with unenhanced T1W images obtained in the same plane and location as the postcontrast images. Ultimately, the best way to distinguish residual tumor from granulation tissue and/or blood is to perform sequential imaging. Postoperative hematoma resolves, and granulation tissue typically decreases in size over time. In contrast, residual tumor grows. Other factors that may help point toward residual tumor is increasing T2W signal abnormality (edema) in the brain parenchyma adjacent to regions of enhancement.

Notes

Fair Game

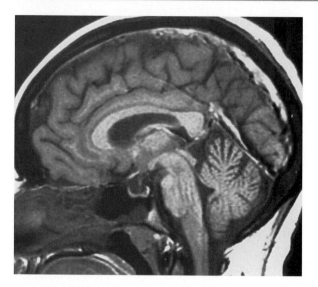
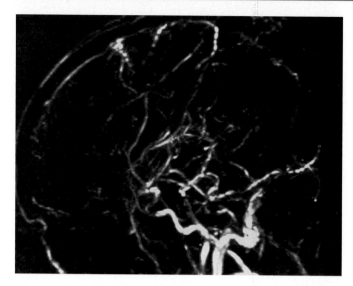

1. What is your diagnosis?

2. What systemic disorders are associated with this condition?

3. What is the most serious complication associated with venous thrombosis?

4. How can you distinguish methemoglobin within thrombus from flow-related enhancement on T1W imaging?

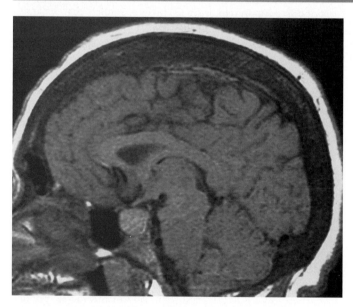

1. What was the clinical presentation in this patient?

2. What is the physical appearance of a patient with hyperpituitary gigantism?

3. What is pituitary apoplexy?

4. What treatment is associated with an increased incidence of hemorrhage within an adenoma?

Superior Sagittal and Straight Sinus Thrombosis With Partial Recanalization

1. Superior sagittal and straight sinus thrombosis.

2. Dehydration, hypercoagulable states (deficiency of antithrombin-III, protein S or C, nephrotic syndrome, use of oral contraceptives, antiphospholipid antibodies, homocystinuria, L-asparaginase), underlying malignancy, pregnancy, and infection (meningitis).

3. Hemorrhagic venous infarction.

4. Methemoglobin is high in signal intensity on T1W imaging in any plane, whereas flow-related enhancement produces high signal intensity in the first few sections of the sequence in vessels that run perpendicular to the imaging plane. When in doubt, do a phase contrast study.

Reference

Dormont D, Sag K, Biondi A, Wechsler B, Marsault C: Gadolinium-enhanced MR of chronic dural sinus thrombosis, *AJNR Am J Neuroradiol* 16:1347-1352, 1995.

Cross-Reference

Neuroradiology: THE REQUISITES, pp 131-132.

Comment

Dural sinus thrombosis and venous infarction are commonly underdiagnosed because of lack of consideration of these entities. Sinus thrombosis has a spectrum of clinical presentations, including headache and papilledema related to increased intracranial pressure, as well as focal neurologic deficits and seizures in cases complicated by intraparenchymal hemorrhage or venous infarction. Venous thrombosis is associated with a variety of underlying systemic disorders as discussed above. In the differential diagnosis of intracerebral hemorrhage in the absence of known risk factors (e.g., trauma or hypertension), the presence of bilateral and/or subcortical hemorrhages that are not in arterial vascular distributions should raise suspicion for sinus thrombosis complicated by venous infarction.

With the advent of MRI, diagnosing venous thrombosis has become easier. In the setting of acute thrombosis, deoxyhemoglobin is hypointense on T2W imaging and may be mistaken for normal blood flow. In the acute setting, flow-sensitive gradient echo imaging may distinguish normal blood flow, which is of high signal intensity, from acute thrombosis, which is hypointense because of lack of flow. In cases of subacute thrombosis, methemoglobin within the clot appears hyperintense on both T1W and T2W images. Flow-sensitive time-of-flight gradient echo images often are not helpful because both the methemoglobin in the thrombus and blood flow are hyperintense. In this situation, phase-contrast MRA is helpful because it provides suppression of high signal from the hemorrhage such that only flow is demonstrated on these images.

Notes

Pituitary Adenoma With Acromegaly

1. Acromegaly.

2. In children the growth plates are still open, and there is stimulation of endochondral bone formation at the physeal growth plate that results in excessive, proportional bone growth. Such patients are tall.

3. A clinical syndrome manifested by the acute onset of headache, nausea and vomiting, visual disturbance, cranial neuropathies, and/or a change in mental status. It is most commonly associated with hemorrhage within an adenoma, although it has been described with infarction. However, most pituitary hemorrhages are asymptomatic.

4. Bromocriptine.

Reference

Marro B, Zouaoui A, Sahel M, et al: MRI of pituitary adenomas in acromegaly, *Neuroradiology* 39:394-399, 1997.

Cross-Reference

Neuroradiology: THE REQUISITES, pp 313-315.

Comment

Pituitary adenomas are slow-growing, benign epithelial neoplasms arising from the anterior lobe of the gland. They are typically demarcated with a "pseudocapsule" that separates them from the normal gland. Pituitary adenomas larger than 10 mm in size are referred to as *macroadenomas,* and those less than 10 mm in diameter are referred to as *microadenomas.* Many adenomas are incidental findings (asymptomatic).

The clinical presentation of pituitary adenomas depends on their size, the presence of hormone secretion resulting in endocrine hyperfunction, and the presence of extension beyond the sella. In vivo, approximately 75% of pituitary adenomas are hormonally active (however, in autopsy series nonsecreting adenomas are much more common). The most common clinically significant secreting adenoma is the prolactinoma (which arises from the prolactin-secreting cells [lactotrophs]). Hormonally active pituitary adenomas arising from somatotrophs, the growth hormone-secreting cells, cause acromegaly in adults and gigantism in children. In acromegaly, endochondral and periosteal bone formation are stimulated, as is proliferation of connective tissue. These changes result in bone overgrowth and increased soft tissue thickness, especially in the "acral" regions (feet, hands, mandible). There is enlargement of the mandible, thickening of the cranial vault, and frontal bossing (the result of enlargement of the frontal sinuses and prominence of the supraorbital ridges). Adenomas that are not hormonally active may become symptomatic because of their size and extrasellar extension. Suprasellar extension may result in headache and visual disturbance (bitemporal hemianopsia), and extension into the cavernous sinus may result in cranial neuropathies.

Notes

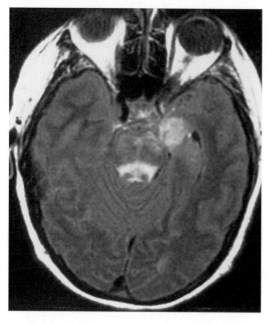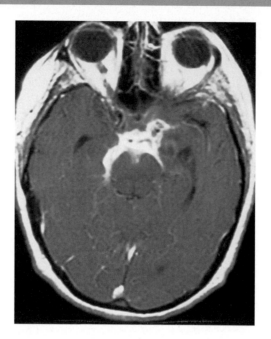

1. What are the major MRI findings?

2. What disease processes affect the basilar meninges?

3. In cases of meningitis with associated hydrocephalus, is hydrocephalus normally communicating or noncommunicating?

4. What primary CNS neoplasms have a predilection for subarachnoid seeding?

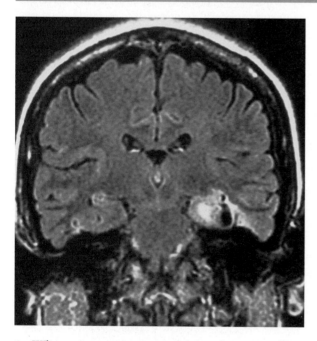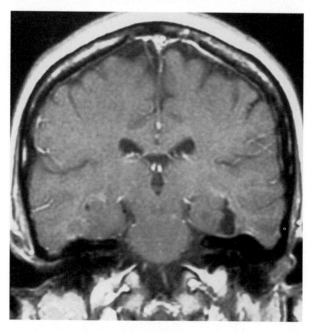

1. What primary supratentorial neoplasms usually presenting in children and young adults frequently have both solid and cystic components?

2. In mesial temporal sclerosis, what structures are usually affected?

3. What MRI findings help differentiate mesial temporal sclerosis from a neoplasm?

4. What is the most common location of a ganglioglioma?

Tuberculosis—Basilar Meningitis and Arteritis

1. Diffuse enhancement of the basal cisterns, T2W high signal intensity in the midbrain, and a ring enhancing lesion in the medial left temporal lobe.

2. Infection (e.g., tuberculosis, neurosyphilis, pyogenic infections, *Cryptococcus*), sarcoid, leptomeningeal seeding of tumor (e.g., carcinomatous from systemic malignancies or primary brain tumors), lymphoma, and chemical meningitis (e.g., drugs, pantopaque, fat from ruptured dermoids).

3. Communicating because of blockage of the basal cisterns from an inflammatory exudate. Occasionally, hydrocephalus may be secondary to mass effect from a parenchymal lesion or from entrapment of a ventricle related to ependymitis.

4. Primitive neuroectodermal tumors (medulloblastoma, pineoblastoma), germinoma, glial neoplasms (GBM, oligodendroglioma), and choroid plexus papilloma.

References

Singer MB, Atlas SW, Drayer BP: Subarachnoid space disease: diagnosis with fluid-attenuated inversion-recovery MR imaging and comparison with gadolinium-enhanced spin-echo MR imaging—blinded reader study, *Radiology* 208:417-422, 1998.

Jinkins JR, Gupta R, Chang KH, Rodriguez-Carbajal J: MR imaging of central nervous system tuberculosis, *Radiol Clin North Am* 33:771-786, 1995.

Cross-Reference

Neuroradiology: THE REQUISITES, pp 187-189.

Comment

Over the last decade there has been an increased incidence of tuberculosis in the United States. This may in part be related to the acquired immunodeficiency syndrome (AIDS) epidemic. Up to 5% of patients with tuberculosis develop CNS disease (up to 10% of patients with AIDS have CNS manifestations). Tuberculous infection in children is usually related to primary infection, whereas in adults it is usually caused by postprimary infection.

Central nervous system tuberculosis may have a variety of clinical and radiologic presentations, including tuberculous meningitis, cerebritis, abscess formation, and tuberculoma. FLAIR imaging has shown a high sensitivity in the detection of subarachnoid and leptomeningeal disease, which is hyperintense in involved areas. CNS tuberculosis is normally related to hematogenous dissemination from a systemic source such as the lung, genitourinary system, and gastrointestinal tract. Arteritis may be seen in up to one third of patients with basilar meningitis. This is because the vessels coursing through this inflammatory exudate may become directly involved. Consequences of arteritis include spasm and infarction.

Notes

Ganglioglioma

1. Astrocytoma, ganglioglioma, and pleomorphic xanthoastrocytoma.

2. The parahippocampus and the limbic system.

3. Although both have signal abnormalities, mesial temporal sclerosis is usually associated with volume loss, including ex vacuo dilation of the temporal horn, whereas most neoplasms (unless very small) are associated with mass effect.

4. The temporal lobe, followed by the frontal lobe.

Reference

Castillo M, Davis PC, Takei Y, Hoffman JC Jr: Intracranial ganglioglioma: MR, CT, and clinical findings in 18 patients, *AJNR Am J Neuroradiol* 11:109-114, 1990.

Cross-Reference

Neuroradiology: THE REQUISITES, p 95.

Comment

Gangliogliomas and ganglioneuromas are slow-growing, benign tumors that most commonly affect children and young adults. Gangliogliomas have a predominance of glial tissue and typically occur in the cerebrum, most commonly arising in the temporal lobe, followed by the frontal lobe, parietal lobe, occipital lobe, and region of the hypothalamus/third ventricle. They may also be infratentorial, arising within the cerebellum or brain stem. Gangliogliomas are typically circumscribed tumors that occur peripherally or superficially in the brain parenchyma. They are usually cystic (purely cystic or cystic with solid components), although solid tumors without cyst formation may occur. Calcification is frequently present, and these neoplasms may demonstrate variable contrast enhancement ranging from mild to marked. However, contrast enhancement need not be present. Because gangliogliomas are composed of both glial (usually astrocytes) and neural elements, they may undergo malignant degeneration. When neuronal elements make up the majority of the mass, the neoplasm is referred to as a *ganglioneuroma*. In contrast, gangliocytomas comprise mature ganglion cells, although they rarely have glial elements and therefore have no potential for malignant change.

In children and young adults, the main differential considerations for ganglioglioma on imaging studies include low grade astrocytoma, juvenile pilocytic astrocytoma, dysembryoplastic neuroepithelial tumor (DNET), and pleomorphic xanthoastrocytoma. Unlike gangliogliomas, pilocytic astrocytomas and pleomorphic xanthoastrocytomas rarely have calcification.

Notes

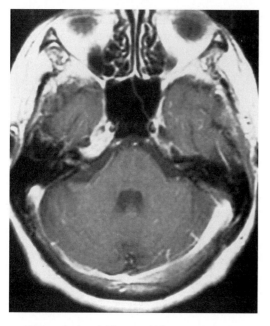
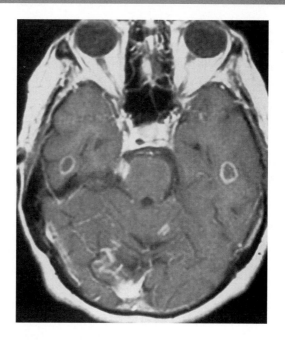

1. What is the differential diagnosis?
2. What is the most sensitive radiologic examination to detect meningeal disease?
3. What are the most common extracranial malignancies to involve the leptomeninges?
4. Blockage of the basal cisterns and arachnoid villi may result in what condition?

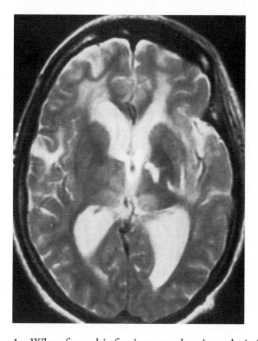
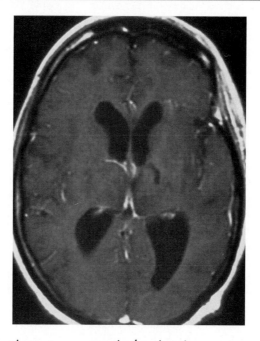

1. What fungal infections predominantly infect immunocompromised patients?
2. What fungal infections may occur in both immunocompetent and immunocompromised patients?
3. Why is there a lower incidence of both hydrocephalus and enhancement of parenchymal lesions in immunocompromised patients infected with *Cryptococcus* compared with the immunocompetent patients with the same infection?
4. What imaging finding in the basal ganglia, brain stem, and cerebral hemispheres is highly suggestive (but not diagnostic) of cryptococcosis?

Subarachnoid Seeding—Leptomeningeal Carcinomatosis

1. Carcinomatous meningitis, CSF seeding from a primary CNS malignancy, inflammatory/granulomatous disease (sarcoidosis, tuberculosis), and infectious meningitis.

2. Contrast-enhanced MRI.

3. Leukemia, lymphoma, adenocarcinomas (particularly of the breast and lung), and melanoma.

4. Communicating hydrocephalus.

Reference

Sze G, Soletsky S, Bronen R, Krol G: MR imaging of the cranial meninges with emphasis on contrast enhancement and meningeal carcinomatosis, *AJNR Am J Neuroradiol* 10:965-975, 1989.

Cross-Reference

Neuroradiology: THE REQUISITES, pp 487-489.

Comment

Leptomeningeal carcinomatosis is a relatively uncommon presentation of metastatic disease to the CNS in patients with extracranial malignancies. Carcinomatous meningitis is reported in approximately 2% to 3% of patients with such malignancies; as treatment for cancer improves and patients live longer, however, it is likely that the incidence of subarachnoid seeding from systemic malignancies will increase. Patients may present with nonspecific symptoms, including headache and meningeal signs; however, they may also present with cranial neuropathies and symptoms related to communicating hydrocephalus. Histologic examination of leptomeningeal spread typically demonstrates metastatic cellular infiltrates within the subarachnoid space.

Contrast-enhanced CT is insensitive for the detection of leptomeningeal spread. Contrast-enhanced MRI is currently the imaging modality of choice for detecting subarachnoid seeding; however, it is not always sensitive either. Lumbar puncture to obtain CSF for cytologic evaluation for malignant cells remains the gold standard for diagnosing carcinomatous meningitis (serial punctures may be necessary).

In this case, enhancement can be seen within the IACs bilaterally, particularly on the right. In addition, there is enhancing soft tissue filling Meckel's cave on the right, more superiorly there is enhancement of the cisternal portion of cranial nerve V. Linear enhancement along the folia of the cerebellar vermis can also be seen, as can two ring enhancing intraparenchymal brain metastases within the temporal lobes (it is possible that one of these lesions was the source of the pia-arachnoid metastases). Although not present in this case, in patients with carcinomatous meningitis one may also see enhancement along the perivascular spaces within the brain parenchyma and along the ependymal surface of the ventricles.

Notes

Central Nervous System Cryptococcosis

1. *Candida, Aspergillus,* and *Mucor.*

2. *Cryptococcus, Coccidioides,* and *Histoplasma.*

3. This likely reflects the inability of these patients to mount significant inflammatory and cell-mediated immune responses.

4. Dilated perivascular (Virchow-Robin) spaces.

Reference

Mathews VP, Alo PL, Glass JD, Kumar AJ, McArthur JC: AIDS-related CNS cryptococcosis: radiologic-pathologic correlation, *AJNR Am J Neuroradiol* 13:1477-1486, 1992.

Cross-Reference

Neuroradiology: THE REQUISITES, pp 190-191.

Comment

This examination demonstrates mild communicating hydrocephalus with dilation of the lateral ventricles. There are focal regions of high signal intensity in the basal ganglia without associated enhancement representing dilated perivascular spaces. In addition, there are more focal, poorly defined regions of increased T2W signal intensity within the basal ganglia and thalami bilaterally (regions of parenchymal abnormality at the gray-white matter interface in the cerebrum were also present [images not shown]). In this patient with human immunodeficiency virus (HIV) infection, the paucity of enhancement may be related to the inability to mount an inflammatory reaction given the immunodeficient state of the patient. The CT and MRI findings are often nonspecific and are unable to distinguish among the various fungal infections, as well as toxoplasmosis and tuberculosis. Lymphoma in the setting of AIDS must also be considered.

Fungal infection in the CNS results in granulomatous changes that may affect the intracranial vasculature, meninges, and/or brain parenchyma. In patients with cryptococcosis, CT and MRI are often unremarkable. Alternatively, a spectrum of imaging findings may occur, including dilated perivascular spaces; parenchymal cryptococcomas (more common in the deep gray matter of the basal ganglia and thalami than in the cerebral cortex); and, less commonly, miliary disease with parenchymal, leptomeningeal, and intraventricular nodules. The diagnosis of CNS cryptococcosis may be established by analysis of the CSF with Indian ink, detection of cryptococcal antigen, and/or positive fungal cultures.

Notes

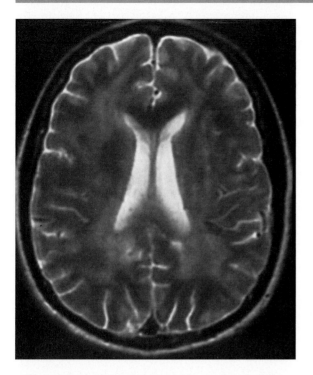
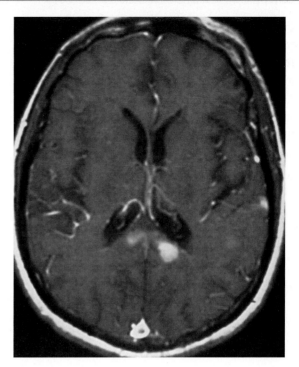

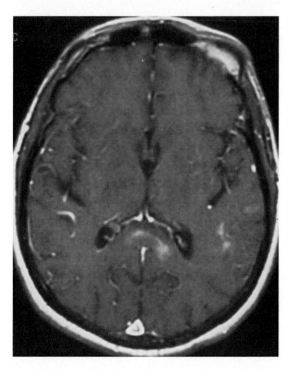

1. In this patient with HIV infection, what are the diagnostic considerations for the enhancing lesions within the splenium and subcortical white matter of the left temporal lobe?

2. What areas of the brain are typically involved in this entity?

3. In patients with systemic lymphoma, what is the most common pattern of CNS involvement?

4. What is the typical pattern of enhancement of primary CNS lymphoma?

Primary Central Nervous System Lymphoma in a Patient With Acquired Immunodeficiency Syndrome

1. Neoplasm (lymphoma), demyelinating disease (progressive multifocal leukoencephalopathy [PML]), and infection.

2. Deep gray matter, corpus callosum, periventricular white matter, and the subependymal region.

3. Subarachnoid (leptomeningeal) involvement.

4. Usually solid; however, in the AIDS population ring enhancement of lesions is also frequently seen.

Reference

Johnson BA, Fram EK, Johnson PC, Jacobowitz R: The variable MR appearance of primary lymphoma of the central nervous system: comparison with histopathologic features, *AJNR Am J Neuroradiol* 18:563-572, 1997.

Cross-Reference

Neuroradiology: THE REQUISITES, p 186.

Comment

Primary CNS lymphoma is a relatively uncommon neoplasm; however, with the AIDS epidemic the incidence has doubled to tripled over the last 10 to 15 years. Primary CNS lymphoma is most commonly seen in patients with AIDS, although it may also be seen in other immunocompromised patients, including those who have undergone organ transplantation or those on chronic systemic immunosuppressive therapy. Lesions are typically seen in the supratentorial compartment; although far less common, lesions in the posterior fossa may also occur.

On imaging, primary CNS lymphoma may have a spectrum of appearances. On unenhanced CT, masses may be hyperdense (this is slightly less common in the AIDS population). Typical lesion distribution includes the periventricular white matter, the corpus callosum, and the deep gray matter structures. MRI signal characteristics are variable; however, like other small cell, hypercellular tumors, they may be relatively isointense to brain parenchyma (gray matter) on T1W and T2W sequences. Following contrast, lesion enhancement is typically more solid in nature; in the setting of HIV infection, however, peripheral or ring enhancement of lesions is common. In that the majority of parenchymal lymphomatous masses are believed to contact the meninges or ependyma, enhancement along the subependymal surface of the ventricles or along the perivascular spaces should make lymphoma highly suspect in immunocompromised patients (sarcoid can have a similar appearance). It is important to know whether a patient has been on steroids before imaging because steroid therapy may have a marked impact on imaging findings (enhancement may be absent and imaging studies relatively unremarkable).

Notes

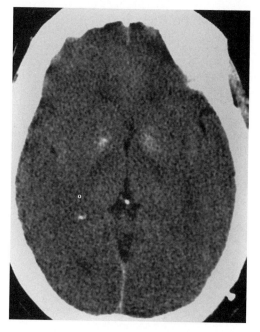 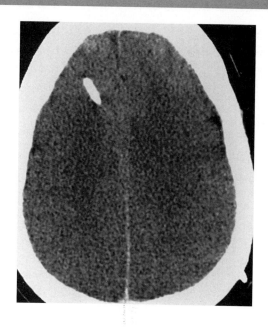

1. What are the major imaging findings?

2. What is the watershed territory in fetuses and newborns?

3. What are common causes of anoxic-ischemic encephalopathy?

4. What are the pathologic findings in adults with global hypoxic-ischemic encephalopathy?

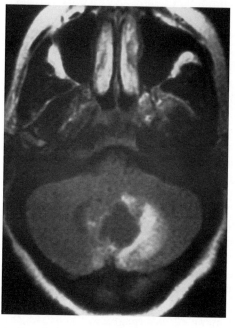 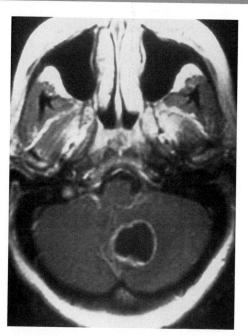

1. In adults, what is the most common neoplastic mass in the cerebellum?

2. In children, what is the most common neoplasm arising within the cerebellar hemisphere?

3. What is the most common primary cerebellar neoplasm in adults?

4. What are the most common primary carcinomas to metastasize to the cerebellum?

CASE 58

Global Anoxic Brain Injury

1. Diffuse loss of gray-white matter differentiation and sulcal/cisternal effacement.

2. The deep periventricular white matter. Therefore radiologic and pathologic manifestations of global hypoxic-ischemic injury are present within the deep white matter and result in periventricular leukomalacia.

3. Global perfusional abnormalities, although disturbances in oxygenation may result in the same picture (including prolonged severe hypotension, respiratory arrest, asphyxia, and carbon monoxide inhalation).

4. In severe cases, generalized cortical laminar necrosis. Involvement of the globus pallidus, putamen, and caudate nuclei is common. The other common pattern of abnormality is arterial infarcts in the watershed territories at the confluence between the anterior, middle, and posterior cerebral artery territories.

Reference

Castillo M, Scatliff JH, Kwock L, et al: Postmortem MR imaging of lobar cerebral infarction with pathologic and in vivo correlation, *RadioGraphics* 16:241-250, 1996.

Cross-Reference

Neuroradiology: THE REQUISITES, p 214.

Comment

Global hypoxic-ischemic injury is typically related to decreased perfusion; less commonly it may be related to a disturbance in blood oxygenation. Postanoxic encephalopathy typically occurs after a period in which a diffuse episode of cerebral hypoperfusion has occurred. The patient may have a lucid interval but over a 1- to 2-week period undergo a precipitous decline that may result in even death. In this scenario, the pathologic changes are most pronounced in the white matter where there is demyelination and necrosis. Carbon monoxide poisoning may produce a similar clinical course and radiologic appearance.

In the acute setting of global hypoxic-ischemic injury, unenhanced CT may demonstrate global loss of gray-white matter differentiation, diffuse parenchymal hypodensity, and sulcal effacement as in this case. The high density in the globus pallidus bilaterally represents incidental senescent calcification. On MRI, T2W hyperintensity may be seen in the watershed territories (acute watershed ischemia may demonstrate contrast enhancement in the early stages). In laminar necrosis, T2W hyperintensity may be seen globally throughout the cortex. Imaging in the subacute phase may demonstrate cortical hemorrhage in the setting of laminar necrosis, which is commonly of high signal intensity on unenhanced T1W images. In the subacute to chronic stages, hypointensity in the cortex and on gradient echo images may be noted.

Notes

CASE 59

Isolated Metastases to the Cerebellum—Breast Carcinoma

1. Metastatic disease.

2. Astrocytoma (pilocytic variety).

3. Hemangioblastoma.

4. Lung and breast. However, melanoma, thyroid, and renal cancer not uncommonly result in cerebellar metastases. More often than not, patients with metastases in the posterior fossa will also have lesions in the supratentorial compartment.

Reference

Smalley SR, Laws ER Jr, O'Fallon JR, Shaw EG, Schray MF: Resection for solitary brain metastasis: role of adjuvant radiation and prognostic variables in 229 patients, *J Neurosurg* 77:531-540, 1992.

Cross-Reference

Neuroradiology: THE REQUISITES, pp 79-82.

Comment

Infratentorial masses typically arise within the cerebellum and less frequently the fourth ventricle. Importantly, lesions occurring in this location are distinctly different in the pediatric and adult populations. In children the most common neoplasms arising in the posterior fossa in descending order of frequency are pilocytic astrocytoma, medulloblastoma (primitive neuroectodermal tumors), ependymoma, and brainstem glioma. In adults the most common space-occupying mass arising within the cerebellum is a stroke. Of the neoplastic processes, metastases are most common. Astrocytomas and medulloblastomas rarely occur in the adult population (comprising less than 1% to 2% of posterior fossa tumors in adults).

There is nothing characteristic about the imaging appearance of metastases within the posterior fossa. Like in the cerebral hemispheres, they are typically demarcated, rounded masses. Following contrast, they demonstrate a spectrum of patterns of enhancement (from solid to rim enhancement). When metastases are large enough to be detected on CT, they are typically hypodense unless they are hemorrhagic (in which case they are hyperdense). MRI is much more accurate in detecting posterior fossa lesions. On MRI many metastases are hypointense on T1W imaging and hyperintense on T2W imaging; however, when there is hemorrhage, calcification, dense cellularity, and/or proteinaceous material, lesions may be hypointense on T2W imaging. When masses are hyperintense on unenhanced T1W imaging, hemorrhagic metastases (which are also frequently hyperintense on T2W imaging) or melanoma (which is typically hypointense on T2W imaging) should be considered.

Notes

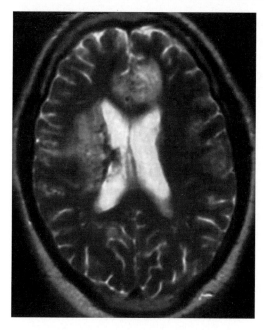 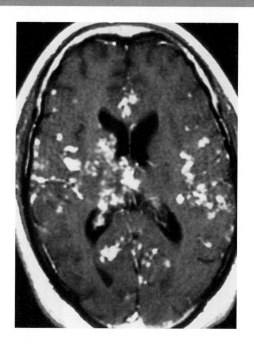

1. What are the major MRI findings?

2. What are the main diagnostic considerations in this 48-year-old patient with parenchymal and leptomeningeal disease?

3. Approximately what percentage of patients with systemic sarcoidosis develop CNS involvement?

4. What findings may be present in the CSF in CNS sarcoidosis?

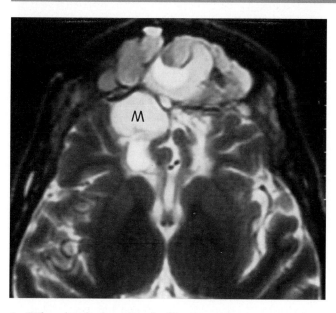 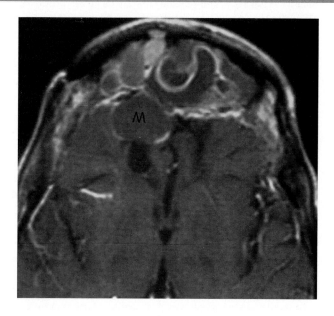

1. What are the imaging findings?

2. What determines the signal characteristics of these lesions on MRI?

3. What is the cause of formation of these lesions, and what underlying risk factors contribute to this?

4. What complications may occur with frontal sinus mucoceles?

Central Nervous System Sarcoidosis

1. Multifocal regions of increased T2W signal intensity within the basal ganglia, cortex, and subcortical white matter (some of these enhance); diffuse nodular enhancement of the leptomeninges; and enhancement along the ependyma of the lateral ventricles.

2. Infectious and noninfectious inflammatory conditions (such as tuberculosis and sarcoidosis, respectively), non-Hodgkin's lymphoma, and carcinomatous meningitis.

3. Approximately 5% to 15%.

4. Cerebral spinal fluid findings are nonspecific for sarcoidosis but include elevated protein, increased cells (predominantly lymphocytes), and decreased glucose.

Reference

Lexa FJ, Grossman RI: MR of sarcoidosis in the head and spine: spectrum of manifestations and radiographic response to steroid therapy, *AJNR Am J Neuroradiol* 15:973-982, 1994.

Cross-Reference

Neuroradiology: THE REQUISITES, pp 116, 196-197.

Comment

Sarcoidosis is a systemic disorder characterized pathologically by noncaseating granulomas. Typical presentation is in the third and fourth decades of life. Sarcoidosis is slightly more common in women than in men. CNS involvement has been reported in 5% to 15% of cases, and isolated CNS involvement is rare (occurring in less than 2% to 4% of patients). Multiple patterns of CNS involvement have been described. The most common of these is a chronic meningitis with a predilection for the leptomeninges of the basal cisterns. These patients may present with chronic meningeal symptoms, cranial neuropathies (especially involving the facial and optic nerves), or symptoms related to involvement of the hypothalamus and pituitary stalk. Imaging findings are best demonstrated with MRI and include nodular enhancement of the leptomeninges that tends to be most pronounced in the basal cisterns (but may be seen in any of the subarachnoid spaces). There may be enhancing tissue around the hypothalamus/pituitary stalk. Another common pattern of CNS sarcoid is parenchymal brain involvement with multifocal regions of abnormality that may occur as a result of direct extension from leptomeningeal disease or disease along the Virchow-Robin spaces, or there may be granulomas in the brain. White matter lesions mimicking multiple sclerosis may be present because of disease extension along the perivascular spaces or related to sarcoid-induced small vessel vasculitis. Less commonly, dural-based disease may be the predominant imaging finding and may be mistaken for a meningioma. This case illustrates a somewhat typical imaging appearance of neurosarcoid.

Notes

Multiple Frontal Sinus Mucoceles With Extension Into the Anterior Cranial Fossa in a Patient With Prior Trauma (Motor Vehicle Accident)

1. Multiple frontal sinus expansile masses with variable T1W and T2W signal intensities that rim enhance, and encephalomalacia in the inferior frontal lobes bilaterally.

2. Their protein concentration and viscosity. They are commonly observed to be hyperintense on both T1W and T2W images.

3. Obstruction of a sinus ostium or a compartment of a septated sinus. Underlying risk factors for the development of mucoceles include a history of sinusitis, trauma, allergies, and/or instrumentation.

4. Secondary infection (mucopyocele) or direct extension into the anterior cranial fossa *(M),* as in this case. In the setting of trauma, risk factors for extension into the anterior cranial fossa include fracture of the posterior wall of the frontal sinus. Alternatively, as a mucocele continues to expand, it may directly erode the posterior frontal sinus table, allowing for intracranial extension.

Reference

Van Tassel P, Lee YY, Jing BS, De Pena CA: Mucoceles of the paranasal sinuses: MR imaging with CT correlation, *AJR Am J Roentgenol* 153:407-412, 1989.

Cross-Reference

Neuroradiology: THE REQUISITES, pp 299-300, 368.

Comment

Mucoceles develop from obstruction of sinus ostia and represent mucoid secretions encased by mucus-secreting epithelium (the sinus mucosa). Mucoceles occur most commonly in the frontal sinuses, although they are also seen in the ethmoid air cells (anterior more common than posterior). They are least common in the sphenoid sinus. Patients frequently have a history of chronic sinusitis, trauma, and/or sinus surgical intervention. Mucoceles are usually not infected; when symptomatic, they present with signs and symptoms related to the mass effect of the lesion. Mucoceles in the frontal sinus may present with frontal bossing, headache, or orbital pain. Frontal and frontoethmoidal mucoceles may cause symptoms related to orbital extension, including proptosis and diplopia.

In the radiologic evaluation of mucoceles, CT best demonstrates the osseous changes of the sinus walls, which may be remodeled and expanded, thinned, and with large mucoceles partially eroded or dehiscent. However, MRI best detects its interface with the intraorbital and intracranial structures. When necessary, enhanced MRI is useful in distinguishing a mucocele (which demonstrates peripheral enhancement) from a neoplasm (which typically demonstrates solid enhancement).

Notes

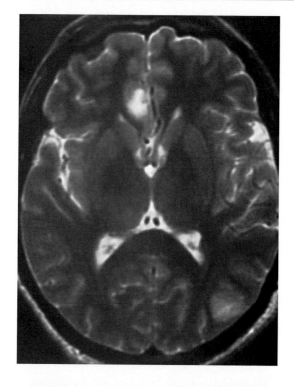

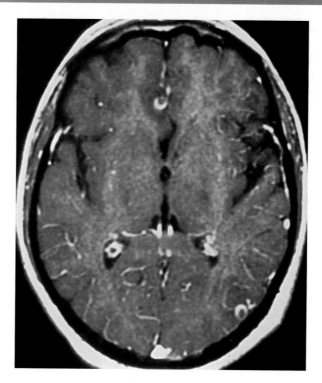

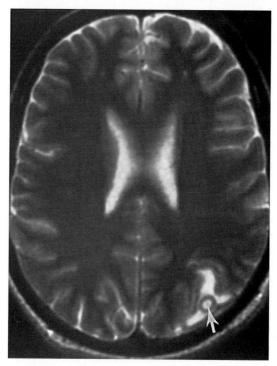

1. What is the differential diagnosis?

2. What is the most likely diagnosis?

3. What factors determine the clinical presentation of patients with this entity?

4. What is the most common location of intraventricular neurocysticercosis?

Cysticercosis of the Central Nervous System

1. The differential diagnosis of multiple superficial (cortical and gray-white matter junction) lesions includes an infectious or inflammatory process (e.g., septic emboli, abscesses, and cysticercosis) and metastatic disease.

2. Cysticercosis.

3. They are dependent on the stage of infestation, as well as the site(s) of parasitic involvement. Initial cerebral infection and the mature cystic phase of the infection when the larvae are alive are frequently asymptomatic. Patients may be most symptomatic as the larvae die because the larvae incite a significant inflammatory reaction.

4. The fourth ventricle.

References

Sheth TN, Pilon L, Keystone J, Kucharczyk W: Persistent MR contrast enhancement of calcified neurocysticercosis lesions, *AJNR Am J Neuroradiol* 19:79-82, 1998.

Suss RA, Maravilla KR, Thompson J: MR imaging of intracranial cysticercosis: comparison with CT and anatomopathologic features, *AJNR Am J Neuroradiol* 7:235-242, 1986.

Cross-Reference

Neuroradiology: THE REQUISITES, pp 193-196.

Comment

Cysticercosis is the most common parasitic infection of the CNS. It usually involves the intracranial compartment, although it may involve the spinal contents. Cysticercosis is endemic in Central and South America, parts of Asia, Mexico, and India. The pork tapeworm *(Taenia solium)* is the causative agent. Humans may become the definitive host by eating inadequately cooked pork that harbors the larvae of the pork tapeworm (cysticerci). These larvae develop into tapeworms in the small intestine that release eggs that pass into the stool. If humans ingest food or water contaminated by these ova, they may serve as an intermediate host. In the stomach the ova release oncospheres (primary larvae), which enter the bloodstream through the gastrointestinal mucosa. These primary larvae may deposit within muscle and subcutaneous tissue, although they have a propensity to infect the CNS. There are multiple patterns of neurocysticercosis, including the parenchymal pattern (larvae penetrate directly into the brain), the intraventricular pattern (involves the ependyma and/or choroid plexus), and the subarachnoid pattern (involves the meninges). In mixed neurocysticercosis there is involvement of the parenchyma, ventricles, and/or subarachnoid spaces. Patients with parenchymal involvement may present with seizures and focal neurologic signs. Intraventricular involvement may be symptomatic if there is obstructive hydrocephalus, and meningeal involvement may result in communicating hydrocephalus.

There is a spectrum of radiologic appearances depending on the stage of disease; however, imaging findings are frequently characteristic. In the initial stage of cerebral infection, the larvae result in small edematous lesions that are hypodense on CT and hyperintense on T2W images. The cysticerci then develop into cysts that range in size from millimeters to centimeters and contain a scolex. There may be mild surrounding edema in the brain, as in this case. On the more cephalad T2W image in this case, the left parietal lobe lesion has a characteristic appearance, with a defined capsule with a hypointense rim and a small 1-mm hypointense focus *(arrow)* representing the scolex. As the cysts die, there is an intense inflammatory reaction in the adjacent brain parenchyma that may result in prominent edema and mass effect. It is at this time that patients may be most symptomatic, presenting with seizures or focal neurologic signs. After years of infestation the cysts finally collapse and often calcify. Recently, rim enhancement has been described in as many as 38% of calcified lesions (this is in contrast to prior reports in which calcified lesions were reported not to enhance).

Notes

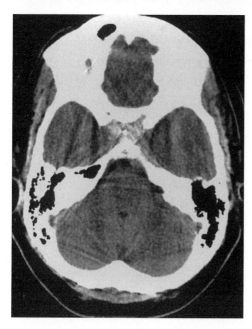
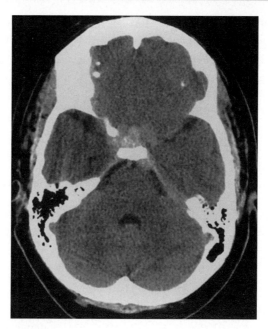

1. What are causes of a hyperdense mass on unenhanced CT?

2. What masses in the sellar and suprasellar regions may appear hyperdense on unenhanced CT?

3. What sellar and/or suprasellar masses are associated with calcification?

4. What imaging study could be performed to exclude an aneurysm?

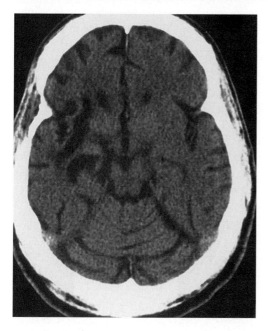
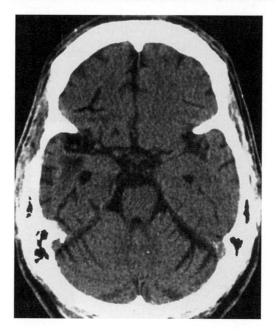

1. What is the pertinent finding in the brain stem?

2. What is the cause of this finding?

3. What should be expected on corresponding MRI?

4. What are causes of this degenerative process?

Parasellar Meningioma

1. The presence of acute hemorrhage, hypercellularity, calcium/cartilage, and/or a high protein concentration.

2. Hemorrhagic pituitary adenoma, meningioma, aneurysm, craniopharyngioma, germ cell tumor, hemorrhagic metastasis, teratoma, tuberculous granulomata.

3. Meningioma, craniopharyngioma, germ cell tumor, and aneurysm.

4. MRI or MRA.

Reference

Yeakley JW, Kulkarni MV, McArdle CB, Haar FL, Tang RA: High-resolution MR imaging of juxtasellar meningiomas with CT and angiographic correlation, *AJNR Am J Neuroradiol* 9:279-285, 1988.

Cross-Reference

Neuroradiology: THE REQUISITES, pp 316-317, 323-324.

Comment

The unenhanced CT images show a multilobular mass involving the suprasellar cistern, which is hyperdense. The mass extends over the dorsum sella and extends into the prepontine cistern on the left (above the level of the petrous apex). Differential considerations include a neoplasm such as a craniopharyngioma, meningioma, or germ cell tumor. Less likely, extension of a hemorrhagic pituitary adenoma into the suprasellar cistern or a multilobular aneurysm could appear like this. On close observation, there are small calcifications on the second image just anterior to the dorsum sella. The imaging findings are not specific for a particular diagnosis; however, in a middle-aged patient meningioma or craniopharyngioma should be placed at the top of the list of considerations. Transphenoid biopsy revealed a meningioma. Another finding that may be useful in distinguishing among the possible causes of a mass in the suprasellar cistern with this appearance is the age of the patient (germ cell tumors typically occur in younger patients, whereas craniopharyngiomas have a bimodal age distribution with lesions seen in children and a second peak in adulthood). Meningiomas tend to be seen in adults (except in the case of neurofibromatosis type 2 and even rarer syndromes that may be seen in children). Additionally, one can examine the bony structures around the sella (the tuberculum sella, anterior clinoid processes, and dorsum sella), where the presence of bone reaction (particularly osteosclerosis) favors a meningioma.

Notes

Wallerian Degeneration

1. Atrophy on the right (wallerian degeneration).

2. An old right middle cerebral artery infarct.

3. High signal intensity in the pyramidal tract on T2W images in addition to the atrophy.

4. Infarction, trauma, demyelinating disease, radiation injury, neurodegenerative disorders, and primary brain tumors.

Reference

Lexa FJ, Grossman RI, Rosenquist AC: MR of Wallerian degeneration in the feline visual system: characterization by magnetization transfer rate with histopathologic correlation, *AJNR Am J Neuroradiol* 15:201-212, 1994.

Cross-Reference

Neuroradiology: THE REQUISITES, p 217.

Comment

Wallerian degeneration is a manifestation of brain injury from a variety of causes. Degenerative changes of axons and their myelin sheaths occur along the distal axonal segment as a result of injury to the proximal axon or neuronal cell body. Among the causes of degeneration of the corticospinal tract pathways, the most common is cortical infarction (as in this case). Other injuries and neurodegenerative processes (e.g., amyotrophic lateral sclerosis) may result in wallerian degeneration. Histologically, wallerian degeneration represents several stages of progressive axonal degradation, ultimately resulting in gliosis and volume loss.

Magnetic resonance imaging is superior to CT in detecting wallerian degeneration. CT may demonstrate the later changes of atrophy of the involved corticospinal pathways within the brain stem, but it does not show the earlier changes. On MRI signal alterations on T2W and/or T1W images may be seen as early as 4 weeks following injury (some studies suggest even earlier), and in the late stages (weeks to months) signal alteration and atrophy are invariably present. In the late stages, T2W hyperintensity is accompanied by hypointensity on corresponding T1W images.

Notes

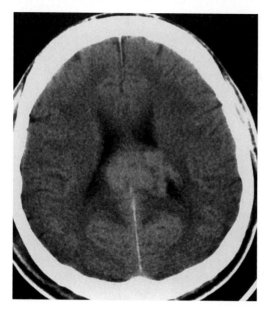 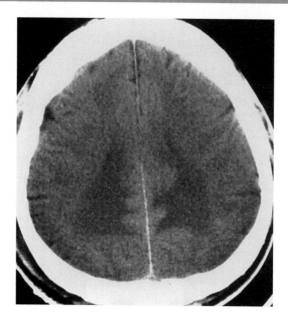

1. From what structure is the mass arising?
2. What neoplasms typically involve the corpus callosum?
3. Why is the corpus callosum relatively resistant to edema?
4. What conditions predispose a patient to the development of primary CNS lymphoma?

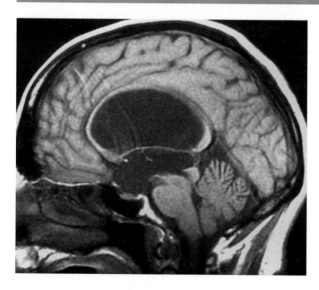 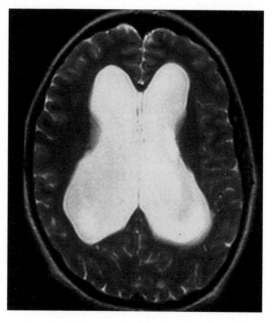

1. What is the level of ventricular obstruction in this case?
2. What can cause obstruction of the aqueduct of Sylvius?
3. What imaging study is most useful in distinguishing an intrinsic lesion of the aqueduct from extrinsic compression related to a mass lesion?
4. In communicating hydrocephalus, what is the typical level of obstruction of CSF circulation?

CASE 65

Primary Central Nervous System Lymphoma—Immunocompetent Patient

1. The corpus callosum.

2. GBM and lymphoma. Occasionally, metastases may occur here (although isolated metastases to the corpus callosum in the absence of other lesions are extremely unusual).

3. Because of the compact nature and the orientation of the white matter fibers.

4. Immunosuppression (particularly in patients with HIV), and immunosuppressive therapy for treatment of cancer or organ transplantation.

References

Yang PJ, Knake JE, Gabrielsen TO, et al: Primary and secondary histiocytic lymphoma of the brain: CT features, *Radiology* 154:683-686, 1985.

Jack CR Jr, O'Neill BP, Banks PM, Reese DF: Central nervous system lymphoma: histologic types and CT appearance, *Radiology* 167:211-215, 1988.

Cross-Reference
Neuroradiology: THE REQUISITES, pp 90-92.

Comment

Primary CNS lymphoma is uncommon, but its incidence has increased dramatically over the last decade as a result of its relatively common occurrence in patients with AIDS (affecting approximately 6%). The origin of lymphoma is unknown because the CNS does not have lymphoid tissue. It has been postulated that CNS lymphoma arises from microglial cells. Primary lymphoma is non-Hodgkin's in nature and most commonly seen in immunocompromised patients. It usually presents in the sixth and seventh decades of life.

The supratentorial compartment is most commonly involved, although involvement of the brain stem and cerebellum is not rare. The most common imaging presentation of primary CNS lymphoma is multiple masses. Focal masses in the basal ganglia, thalami, and periventricular white matter are common. Alternatively, patients may present with a single mass, as in this case. Although the standard teaching is that CNS lymphoma enhances solidly and avidly, in the setting of AIDS there is a spectrum of patterns of pathologic enhancement ranging from solid to ring-like. The patient in this case is not immunocompromised. The mass bridging the body of the corpus callosum is hyperdense on unenhanced imaging because of its cellularity. Vasogenic edema is present in the adjacent parietal white matter. The MRI signal intensity characteristics may be quite variable, ranging from marked hyperintensity to marked hypointensity (isointense to brain tissue) in cases of very cellular neoplasms. Hemorrhage is uncommon in lymphomatous masses. The differential diagnosis in this case is a GBM.

Notes

CASE 66

Aqueductal Stenosis

1. The aqueduct of Sylvius.

2. Obstruction may be congenital (webs or diaphragms within the aqueduct or gliosis). Acquired aqueductal stenosis may be intrinsic, related to clot or adhesions from prior subarachnoid hemorrhage or infection (meningitis or ventriculitis), or extrinsic on the basis of compression of the aqueduct related to tumors in this region (tectal gliomas, pineal tumors, cerebellar neoplasms, or occult cerebral vascular malformations of the brain stem).

3. MRI in the sagittal plane.

4. The arachnoid villi.

Reference

Yoshimoto Y, Ochiai C, Kawamata K, Endo M, Nagai M: Aqueductal blood clot as a cause of acute hydrocephalus in subarachnoid hemorrhage, *AJNR Am J Neuroradiol* 17:1183-1186, 1996.

Cross-Reference
Neuroradiology: THE REQUISITES, pp 238-239, 259.

Comment

This case demonstrates the characteristic findings in congenital aqueductal stenosis. There is prominent dilation of the lateral and third ventricles with a relatively normal-sized fourth ventricle. There is upward convexity or bowing of the corpus callosum related to the lateral ventricular dilation, and there is inferior bowing of the anterior recesses of the third ventricle with depression of the optic chiasm. Congenital aqueductal stenosis may be seen as an inherited X-linked recessive disorder in boys. Children may present with an enlarging head circumference. Blockage of the aqueduct may be caused by webs, septae, or gliosis.

Aqueductal stenosis is often acquired in relation to prior subarachnoid hemorrhage, meningitis or ventriculitis, or extrinsic compression from a mass or tumor. MRI is the imaging modality of choice in evaluating affected patients; sagittal MRI is particularly useful in distinguishing intrinsic aqueductal abnormalities from extrinsic mass compression. The presence or absence of aqueductal CSF flow may be evaluated using spin echo and gradient echo flow scans with gradient moment nulling. On spin echo images, hypointensity within the aqueduct (signal void) is consistent with flow, whereas on gradient echo imaging the presence of high signal intensity within the aqueduct is consistent with flow.

Notes

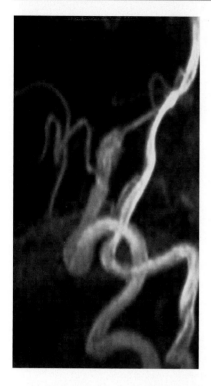
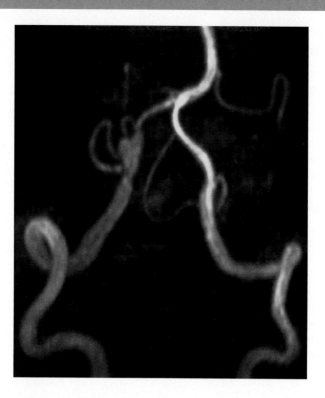

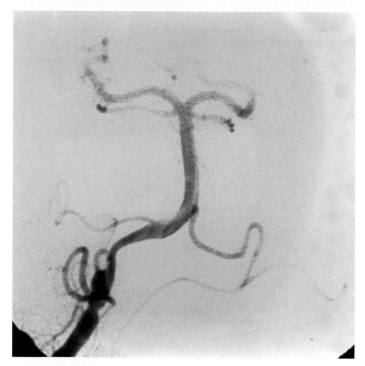

1. Do traumatic dissections more commonly affect the extracranial or intracranial vasculature?

2. What are common injuries of the vertebral arteries?

3. What are risk factors for intracranial dissections?

4. What are common complications of vascular dissections?

Right Vertebral Artery Dissection With Pseudoaneurysm

1. Extracranial.

2. Vascular dissection, laceration/rupture, and arteriovenous fistulas.

3. Trauma associated with skull base fractures (particularly the sphenoid bone, carotid canal, and petrous apex) increases the risk of injury to the internal carotid arteries. Dissections also occur in patients with vascular dysplasia (e.g., fibromuscular dysplasia, Marfan syndrome), and in patients with hypertension.

4. Transient ischemic attack and stroke related to embolic or thromboocclusive changes. Pseudoaneurysms may also occur.

Reference

Levy C, Laissy JP, Raveau V, et al: Carotid and vertebral artery dissections: three-dimensional time-of-flight MR angiography and MR imaging versus conventional angiography, *Radiology* 190:97-103, 1994.

Cross-Reference

Neuroradiology: THE REQUISITES, pp 133-135, 162-164.

Comment

The images show narrowing of the lumen of the distal right vertebral artery. Just proximal to the origin of the posteroinferior cerebellar artery there is a pseudoaneurysm complicating the dissection. Vascular dissections may be asymptomatic. When symptomatic, the symptoms may occur days to weeks after the actual injury. As a result, dissections often escape clinical detection. In addition, symptomatic lesions can be overlooked or masked by other injuries in patients with acute injuries. Therefore the key to making the diagnosis is considering it in the appropriate clinical scenario. Although CT is not a sensitive study for detecting vascular injuries, it may identify patients at increased risk (those with skull base fractures or fractures of the vertebral bodies extending through the foramen transversarium, which houses the cervical vertebral artery).

The combination of MRI and MRA is sensitive for detecting vascular injuries because these modalities assess the vascular lumen, the vessel wall, and tissues around the vessel. MRI findings include intramural hematoma, which is typically hyperintense on unenhanced T1W images, and narrowing and compromised flow in the arterial lumen (a narrowed but patent vessel can usually be distinguished from one that is occluded). Pseudoaneurysms may also be detected. The angiographic appearance of a dissection may vary and includes spasm, segmental tapering related to intramural hematoma (the hematoma is not visualized on angiography), aneurysmal dilation of the vessel, vascular occlusion, intimal flap, and/or retention of contrast material in the vessel wall.

Notes

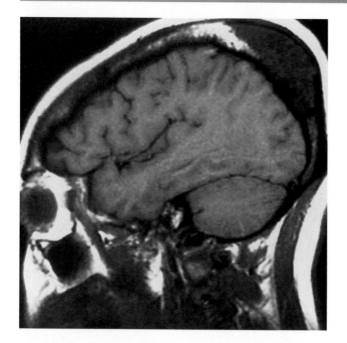

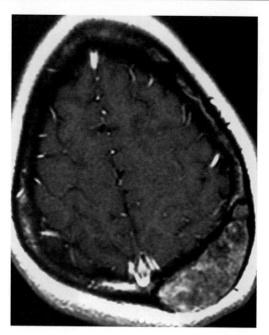

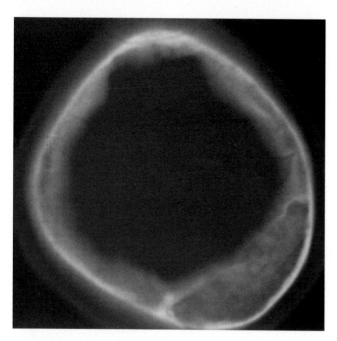

1. What is the differential diagnosis?

2. What laboratory abnormality is often seen in fibrous dysplasia and Paget's disease?

3. What are the clinical manifestations of McCune-Albright syndrome?

4. Which bones are most commonly affected in polyostotic fibrous dysplasia?

CASE 68

Fibrous Dysplasia of the Calvaria

1. Fibrous dysplasia and Paget's disease. Metastatic disease is unlikely given the imaging appearance of the lesion (an expansile mass with preservation of the inner and outer cortical tables).

2. Elevated alkaline phosphatase levels.

3. This is a form of polyostotic fibrous dysplasia that occurs in girls and is typically associated with precocious puberty and cutaneous hyperpigmentation.

4. The skull and facial bones.

Reference

Jee WH, Choi KH, Choe BY, Park JM, Shinn KS: Fibrous dysplasia: MR imaging characteristics with radiopathologic correlation, *AJR Am J Roentgenol* 167:1523-1527, 1996.

Cross-Reference

Neuroradiology: THE REQUISITES, pp 390, 425.

Comment

Fibrous dysplasia is a developmental bone disorder in which osteoblasts do not undergo normal differentiation and maturation. The cause is unknown. Fibrous dysplasia may be monostotic (a solitary lesion) or polyostotic (lesions in multiple bones or multiple lesions in one bone). Approximately 75% of cases of fibrous dysplasia are monostotic (25% polyostotic). Polyostotic fibrous dysplasia involves the skull and facial bones more frequently than does monostotic disease. Common areas of calvarial involvement include the ethmoid, maxillary, frontal, and sphenoid bones. Involvement of these bones may result in orbital abnormalities such as exophthalmos, visual disturbances, and displacement of the globe. Involvement of the temporal bone may result in hearing loss and/or vestibular dysfunction.

Fibrous dysplasia of the skull or facial bones on plain radiography may present as radiolucent or sclerotic lesions. Sclerotic lesions are more common in the calvaria, skull base, and sphenoid bones. Although Paget's disease may occur in these same locations of the calvaria, unlike fibrous dysplasia, concomitant involvement of the facial bones is less common.

In this patient there is a mass in the left parietal bone that is heterogeneous and sclerotic, giving a "ground glass" appearance. There is associated focal expansion of the diploic space. The outer cortical table of the calvaria is bowed, although there is preservation of the inner and outer cortical tables without destruction or significant thickening of the cortex. These features are typical of fibrous dysplasia. In contrast, although there may be expansion of the diploic space in patients with Paget's disease, there is normally thickening of the cortex (which may be extensively involved).

Notes

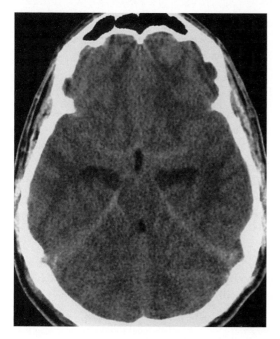
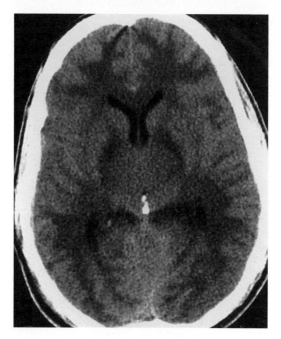

1. What basal ganglionic structure is involved in this case?

2. What toxic exposures may result in injuries or infarction to the globus pallidus?

3. Selective bilateral necrosis of the globus pallidus is specific for what pathophysiologic insult?

4. What movement disorders may be associated with pallidal lesions?

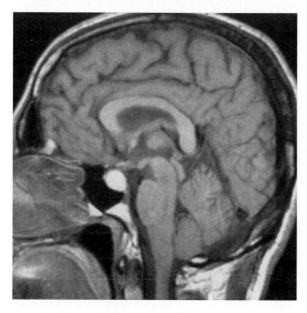
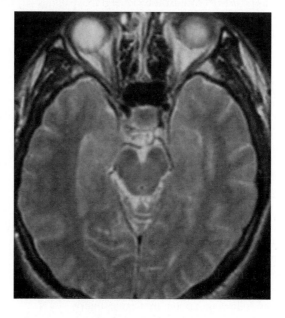

1. What is the differential diagnosis?

2. In addition to the MRI findings, the presence of what other radiologic findings would favor the diagnosis of craniopharyngioma?

3. Most Rathke's cleft cysts are localized in what part of the pituitary gland?

4. When large enough, this lesion may cause visual symptoms or hormonal dysfunction as a result of compression of what structures?

CASE 69

Carbon Monoxide Poisoning

1. The globus pallidus.

2. The most common is carbon monoxide poisoning. Other exposures that affect the globus pallidus include cyanide and manganese (hyperalimentation).

3. Anoxic/hypoxic injury.

4. Slow initiation and execution of voluntary movements (akinesia), dystonia, and increased rigidity.

Reference

Inagaki T, Ishino H, Seno H, Umegae N, Aoyama T: A long-term follow-up study of serial magnetic resonance images in patients with delayed encephalopathy after acute carbon monoxide poisoning, *Psychiatry Clin Neurosci* 51:421-423, 1997.

Cross-Reference

Neuroradiology: THE REQUISITES, pp 119, 236-237.

Comment

Injury to the brain with a particular predilection for the basal ganglia may be seen in a variety of toxic exposures, neurodegenerative processes, and metabolic disorders. Of the toxic insults, carbon monoxide, cyanide, and trichloroethane (inhalation of typewriter correction fluid) poisoning have a particular predilection to involve the globus pallidus bilaterally. The pathologic/microscopic correlate of the abnormal hypodensity on CT or T2W hyperintensity on MRI within the bilateral globus pallidus is that of necrosis caused by anoxic injury. Although carbon monoxide toxicity has a somewhat characteristic imaging appearance, the diagnosis is usually established by the clinical circumstances in which the patient is found. The diagnosis of carbon monoxide toxicity is confirmed by identification of carboxyhemoglobin in the blood.

In addition to density and intensity alterations in the globus pallidus bilaterally, other imaging manifestations of diffuse anoxic brain injury may be identified, including injury to the hippocampus (Ammon's horn) bilaterally and global cerebral swelling manifested as sulcal effacement and accentuation of the gray-white matter differentiation (as in this case). Abnormalities in the cerebellum may also be noted. Patients with carbon monoxide poisoning may experience sudden neurologic deterioration and coma approximately 2 to 3 weeks following the initial injury. Imaging often reveals accompanying white matter disease, which may be extensive and pathologically represents acute demyelination. On delayed imaging performed months to years following carbon monoxide injury, T2W hypointensity in the deep gray matter, especially the putamen, may be present and is likely due to iron deposition.

Notes

CASE 70

Rathke's Cleft Cyst

1. Rathke's cleft cyst, hemorrhagic pituitary adenoma, and craniopharyngioma.

2. Calcification, an associated soft tissue mass, and/or areas of solid enhancement.

3. Unlike pituitary adenomas, which are more frequently localized in the lateral portion of the gland, large autopsy series have shown that the vast majority of Rathke's cleft cysts are localized in the center of the gland (pars intermedia).

4. The optic chiasm and the anterior lobe of the pituitary gland, respectively.

Reference

Teramoto A, Hirakawa K, Sanno N, Osamura Y: Incidental pituitary lesions in 1000 unselected autopsy specimens, *Radiology* 193:161-164, 1994.

Cross-Reference

Neuroradiology: THE REQUISITES, pp 249, 319, 512.

Comment

In the vast majority of cases, Rathke's cleft cysts are incidental findings noted at autopsy or identified on imaging studies performed for other reasons. In a recent series of 1000 autopsy specimens, 11% of the pituitary glands had an incidental Rathke's cleft cyst. These lesions are typically localized within the pituitary sella, although they may also extend into the suprasellar region. In addition, Rathke's cleft cysts may be centered in the suprasellar cistern anterior to the hypothalamic stalk. The cysts are typically lined by a single layer of epithelium, which may contain goblet cells. The contents within the cysts are mucoid, resulting in their typical MRI appearance. Specifically, most Rathke's cleft cysts are circumscribed masses with high signal intensity on both unenhanced T1W and T2W images. Although this is the most common pattern, however, cysts may also be hypointense or isointense on either T1W or T2W images, depending on their protein concentration and viscosity. In this case, the cyst is hyperintense on unenhanced T1W imaging and hypointense on T2W imaging. Following the administration of intravenous contrast material these cysts do not enhance (although there may be mild peripheral enhancement).

Although most Rathke's cleft cysts are incidental findings, symptoms may occur with larger lesions that compress the optic chiasm (resulting in headache and visual disturbances) or pituitary gland (patients may present with diabetes insipidus or hypopituitarism).

Notes

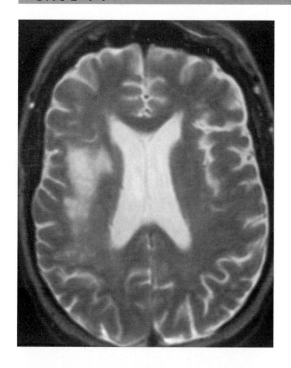

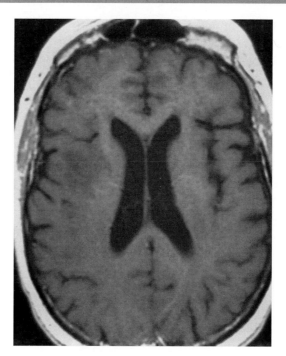

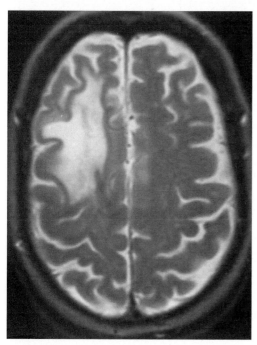

1. What is the differential diagnosis in this patient with HIV infection?

2. What imaging findings favor progressive multifocal leukoencephalopathy?

3. What are common MRI findings in HIV demyelination and infection with CMV?

4. What CNS cells are classically infected in patients with PML?

Progressive Multifocal Leukoencephalopathy

1. Demyelination related to cytomegalovirus (CMV) or direct HIV infection, encephalitides (particularly CMV), progressive multifocal leukoencephalopathy (PML), and lymphoma.

2. Asymmetric white matter involvement, subcortical and deep white matter involvement, and the absence of mass effect and enhancement.

3. These two direct viral infections of the white matter most commonly have periventricular T2W hyperintensity, which is bilateral with a more symmetric appearance.

4. The oligodendrocytes.

Reference

Whiteman ML, Post MJ, Berger JR, Tate LG, Bell MD, Limonte LP: Progressive multifocal leukoencephalopathy in 47 HIV-seropositive patients: neuroimaging with clinical and pathologic correlation, *Radiology* 187:233-240, 1993.

Cross-Reference

Neuroradiology: THE REQUISITES, pp 213-214.

Comment

Before the AIDS epidemic, PML was largely seen in a spectrum of immunocompromised patients, including those with hematologic malignancies (leukemia and lymphoma), following organ transplantation, patients taking immunosuppressive drugs, and those with autoimmune disorders. However, over the last decade the majority of cases of PML have been noted in patients with HIV infection. PML is caused by infection of the oligodendrocytes with a papovavirus (JC virus).

The clinical presentation of PML includes focal neurologic deficits (hemiparesis), visual symptoms, and a change in mental status. The infection is rapidly progressive with continued neurologic decline, CNS demyelination, and death usually occurring within 6 months to a year from the onset of symptoms.

Magnetic resonance imaging is far more sensitive in defining the number and extent of lesions in PML. On CT PML usually appears as focal region(s) of hypodensity within the white matter, usually without mass effect or enhancement. On MRI increased T2W signal intensity is noted in the involved white matter. PML has a predilection in particular to involve the subcortical white matter, although the deep white matter is also commonly involved. There is a slight preference for involvement of the parietal and occipital white matter, but any area of the brain may be affected. Although single focal lesions may be seen, multifocal lesions typically occur with a bilateral but asymmetric distribution. A unilateral multifocal distribution may also occur. Mass effect and/or enhancement are uncommon in PML, occurring in less than 5% to 10% of cases. On T1W images lesions tend to be hypointense.

Notes

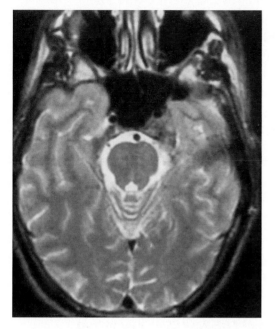
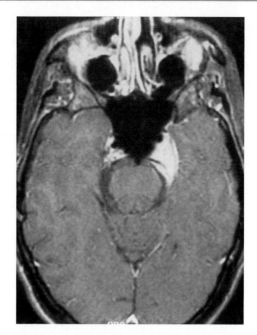

1. What is the anatomic location of the mass in these images?
2. What cranial nerves course through the cavernous sinus?
3. Which cranial nerve is most medially located within the cavernous sinus?
4. What idiopathic inflammatory condition can affect the cavernous sinus?

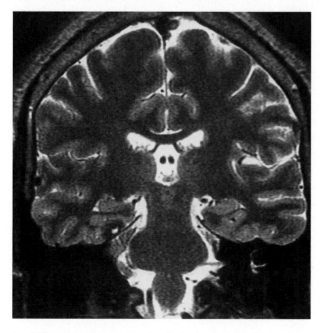
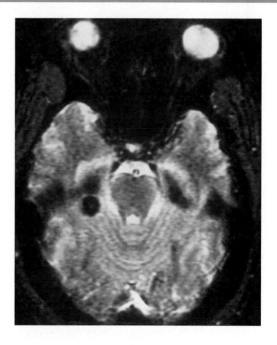

1. What was this patient's clinical presentation?
2. What does the central region of high signal intensity, which was also hyperintense on unenhanced T1W images (not shown), represent?
3. What is the differential diagnosis of this lesion, particularly when they are multiple?
4. What finding on T2W and gradient echo susceptibility images help to distinguish a cavernoma from other lesions?

CASE 72

Cavernous Sinus Mass—Lymphoma

1. The left cavernous sinus.

2. III, IV, V (first and second divisions), and VI.

3. VI; however, it remains lateral to the cavernous internal carotid artery.

4. Tolosa-Hunt syndrome.

Reference

Hirsch WL Jr, Hryshko FG, Sekhar LN, Brunberg J, Kanal E, Latchaw RE, Curtin H: Comparison of MR imaging, CT, and angiography in the evaluation of the enlarged cavernous sinus, *AJNR Am J Neuroradiol* 9:907-915, 1988.

Cross-Reference

Neuroradiology: THE REQUISITES, pp 297, 308-309, 326-330.

Comment

A variety of lesions can affect the cavernous sinus, including neoplasms primarily arising from bone (chondrosarcoma, chondroma, and chordoma) and bone metastases. Metastases and lymphoma primarily affecting the cavernous sinus and perineural spread of tumor are also common. Benign neoplasms include meningioma, schwannoma, and extension of a pituitary adenoma. A variety of vascular and inflammatory lesions may also involve the cavernous sinus.

Infectious processes include bacterial and fungal (actinomycosis, aspergillus, and mucormycosis) agents. In addition, the cavernous sinus may be affected indirectly by complications of infectious processes (e.g., cavernous sinus thrombosis). Tolosa-Hunt syndrome represents an idiopathic granulomatous inflammatory disorder that may affect the orbital apex and cavernous sinus. Histologically, Tolosa-Hunt syndrome is identical to orbital pseudotumor (differing only in location). It may present with painful ophthalmoplegia, deficits of the cranial nerves coursing through the cavernous sinus, and retroorbital pain. Like orbital pseudotumor, it responds rapidly to steroid treatment. MRI may show abnormal signal intensity or an enhancing mass within the cavernous sinus. There may be extension into the orbital apex.

These images demonstrate a mass within the left cavernous sinus that is hypointense to CSF (isointense to brain parenchyma). Enhancement extends along the lateral dural margin, as well as posteriorly along the tentorial margin (an appearance that may be seen with cavernous sinus meningiomas; however, the absence of narrowing of the cavernous-carotid artery makes meningioma an unlikely diagnosis). Neoplastic processes that may be hypointense on T2W imaging include lymphoma, meningioma, and, less commonly, plasmacytoma and schwannoma. Sarcoid may also be hypointense on T2W imaging. In this case, biopsy revealed non-Hodgkin's lymphoma.

Notes

CASE 73

Cavernous Malformation (Cavernous Hemangioma, Occult Cerebrovascular Malformation)

1. Seizures.

2. Methemoglobin.

3. Metastases (hemorrhagic or melanotic), amyloid angiopathy, previously treated infection, and regions of old hemorrhage (such as is seen with hypertension, diffuse axonal injury, or radiation therapy).

4. The presence of a complete circumferential hemosiderin ring and the absence of edema are seen with cavernomas.

Reference

Rigamonti D, Hadley MN, Drayer BP, et al: Cerebral cavernous malformations : incidence and familial occurrence, *N Engl J Med* 319:343-347, 1988.

Cross-Reference

Neuroradiology: THE REQUISITES, pp 141-142.

Comment

Cavernous malformations (CMs), also referred to as cavernomas, cavernous hemangiomas, and angiographically occult cerebrovascular malformations (OCVMs), represent a sinusoidal network of blood vessels without intervening normal brain parenchyma. Frequently gliosis is also present. On unenhanced CT CMs may be mildly hyperdense as a result of pooling of blood in the sinusoids. They may also be associated with focal calcification. On MRI CMs are recognized by their characteristic appearance representing blood products of different ages. Typically, cavernomas have a central region of high signal intensity on unenhanced T1W and T2W images representing methemoglobin, surrounded by a complete rim of hemosiderin that is hypointense on T2W and gradient echo susceptibility images (as in this case). In the absence of recent hemorrhage there should be no associated T2W signal abnormality (edema) within the surrounding brain parenchyma.

Angiographically, CMs are usually occult. Unlike other occult vascular malformations such as capillary telangiectasias and venous angiomas, these patients may present clinically with seizures or symptoms related to mass effect in cases in which there has been recent hemorrhage.

Notes

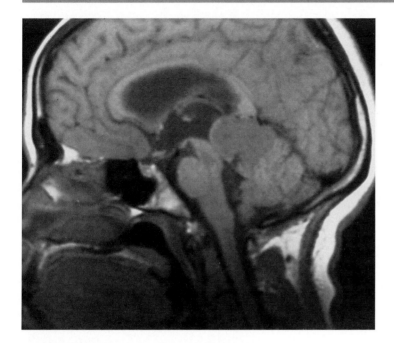

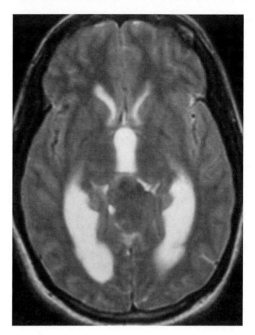

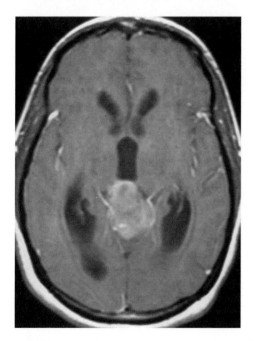

1. What vascular structures course above the pineal gland?

2. How did this young patient present clinically?

3. Pineal neoplasms in general may be divided into two categories based on their cell of origin. What are the two classes of neoplasms?

4. Which pineal neoplasm is most frequently associated with tumor seeding of the subarachnoid spaces?

Tumor of the Pineal Gland—Pineoblastoma

1. The internal cerebral veins/vein of Galen.

2. With hydrocephalus and paresis of upward gaze (Parinaud's syndrome).

3. Tumors of germ cell origin and tumors arising from pineal cells.

4. Pineoblastoma.

Reference

Smirniotopoulos JG, Rushing EJ, Mena H: Pineal region masses: differential diagnosis, *RadioGraphics* 12:577-596, 1992.

Cross-Reference

Neuroradiology: THE REQUISITES, pp 95-97.

Comment

This case shows a lobular, demarcated enhancing mass in the pineal region. There is elevation of the internal cerebral veins and compression of the tectal plate and aqueduct of Sylvius resulting in hydrocephalus. On T2W imaging the mass is isointense to white matter because of its dense cellularity. In addition to metastases to the subarachnoid spaces, when pineoblastomas are large enough they may directly invade the brain parenchyma.

Tumors of pineal cell origin (pineoblastoma and pineocytoma) comprise only 15% of pineal region masses. Unlike germ cell tumors, which show a marked predilection in males, tumors of pineal cell origin occur equally among men and women. Tumors of pineal origin frequently calcify. Calcification of the pineal gland in a child under 7 years of age should cause suspicion of tumor until proven otherwise. After 7 years of age the pineal gland begins to show calcification, which increases with age. Up to 10% of people have calcification in the pineal gland by adolescence, and up to 50% have pineal gland calcification by the age of 30 years. In cases in which the amount of calcification is small and more central, it may be difficult to determine whether it is the natural calcification of the pineal gland or calcification within tumor matrix.

Magnetic resonance imaging is most useful in characterizing masses in the pineal region. Tumors arising in the parapineal region in a child are usually gliomas arising from the tectal plate, whereas tumors arising in the parapineal region in adults may represent gliomas or meningiomas arising from the tentorium. Imaging findings and the patient's age and sex together may be useful in suggesting the correct tumor histology. Tumors of germ cell origin occur in children as do pineoblastomas, whereas pineocytomas generally seen in adults.

Notes

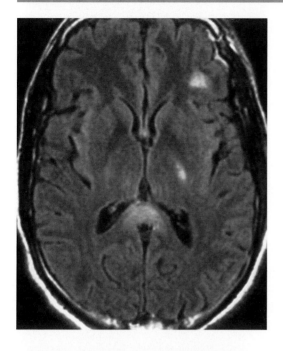
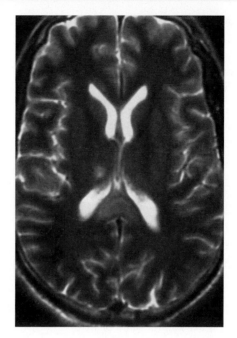

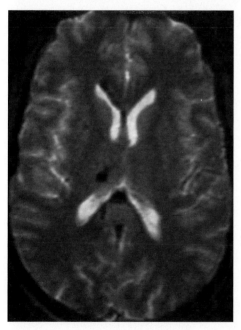

1. What are the most common locations for traumatic contusions?

2. What three anatomic locations are classically involved in diffuse axonal injury?

3. Why is the posterior and splenial region of the corpus callosum more commonly affected by shear injury than is the anterior portion?

4. In the absence of the gradient echo image, what other entities could result in a similar appearance on long TR images?

Head Trauma—Diffuse Axonal Injury

1. The frontal and temporal lobes. The anterior temporal lobes impact on the greater wing of the sphenoid bone, whereas the frontal lobes impact on the surfaces of the cribriform plate orbits, and frontal bone.

2. The lobar white matter, the corpus callosum (particularly the posterior body and splenium), and the dorsolateral aspect of the upper brain stem (midbrain and pons).

3. With rotational acceleration of the head, shear forces develop across the corpus callosum. Anteriorly there is less strain because the falx is shorter and allows transient displacement of the frontal lobes across the midline. Posteriorly, the falx is broader and more rigid, preventing motion of the cerebral hemispheres across the midline.

4. Demyelinating disease (multiple sclerosis, acute disseminated encephalomyelitis).

Reference

Mittl RL, Grossman RI, Hiehle JF, et al. Prevalence of MR evidence of diffuse axonal injury in patients with mild head injury and normal head CT findings, *AJNR Am J Neuroradiol* 15:1583-1589, 1994.

Cross-Reference

Neuroradiology: THE REQUISITES, pp 157-160.

Comment

Diffuse axonal injury is the result of shear-strain forces induced by angular rotation/acceleration of the head. Patients have loss of consciousness and cognitive impairment beginning at the moment of trauma. Diffuse axonal injury is most commonly seen in patients involved in high velocity acceleration-deceleration MVAs and is characterized by multiple focal lesions scattered throughout the lobar white matter at the gray-white matter interface. Lesions may also be seen in the corpus callosum and, in cases of severe head trauma, in the dorsolateral brain stem. Shear injuries are typically elliptic in shape, with the long axis parallel to the direction of the involved axons.

Although MRI is the most sensitive imaging modality for the evaluation of diffuse axonal injury, in the acute setting the first radiologic study should be CT because the most critical issue is to detect potentially treatable intracranial hemorrhage (subdural and epidural hematomas, large parenchymal hematomas). If there is concern for shear injury, MRI should be performed when the patient is stable. Shear injuries, unless hemorrhagic or of substantial size, frequently go undetected on CT. The presence of intraventricular hemorrhage should raise suspicion of injury to the septum pellucidum or corpus callosum. On MRI shear injuries are hyperintense on T2W images. Not infrequently these regions are associated with hemorrhage (as in this case), where on the gradient echo susceptibility image the right thalamic and corpus callosum lesions are hemorrhagic.

Notes

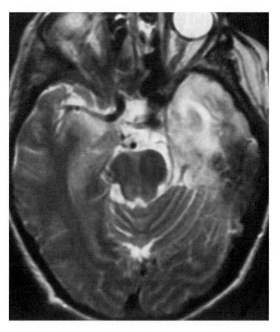
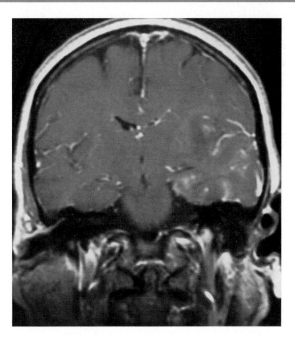

1. Which herpes simplex virus is responsible for neonatal infection?
2. What is the differential diagnosis?
3. What imaging findings are typical for herpes simplex encephalitis?
4. What group of patients is at increased risk for herpes zoster infection?

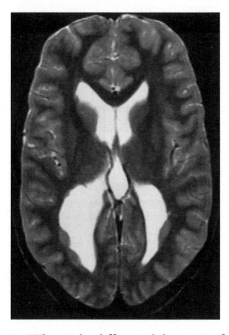
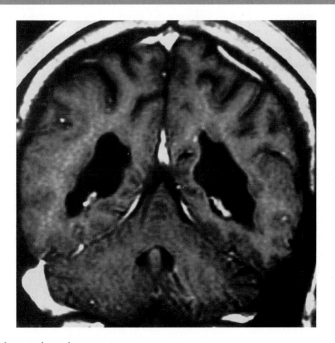

1. What is the differential diagnosis of subependymal masses?
2. What percentage of subependymal nodules in tuberous sclerosis are calcified?
3. What is the diagnosis in this case?
4. What other anomaly is present in this patient?

CASE 76

Type I Herpes Simplex Encephalitis

1. Type II, acquired either transplacentally or through the birth canal of a mother with genital herpes.

2. Encephalitis, primary neoplasm, and ischemia.

3. Medial bitemporal involvement and cortical "gyriform" enhancement.

4. Immunosuppressed patients.

Reference

Neils EW, Lukin R, Tomsick TA, Tew JM: Magnetic resonance imaging and computerized tomography scanning of herpes simplex encephalitis: report of two cases, *J Neurosurg* 67:592-594, 1987.

Cross-Reference

Neuroradiology: THE REQUISITES, pp 181-184.

Comment

Type I herpes simplex virus produces necrotizing encephalitis in adults. The clinical presentation is varied, ranging from headache, fever, and seizures to coma. Radiologic evaluation frequently reveals hypodensity with loss of gray-white matter differentiation in the temporal lobes and insular cortex on CT. Hemorrhage may also be present. The CT appearance may simulate an infarct or a primary glial neoplasm. MRI findings in the acute stages of encephalitis show hyperintensity on long TR images within the temporal and inframedial frontal lobes. There frequently is local mass effect, which is manifest by gyral expansion and sulcal effacement. Although bilateral disease is typical, herpes encephalitis usually involves the temporal lobes, insula, inferior frontal lobes, and cingulate gyrus in an asymmetric pattern. A proposed explanation for this pattern of involvement is the presence of the latent virus within the gasserian ganglion in Meckel's cave. Reactivated virus may spread along the trigeminal nerve fibers with subsequent spread along the meninges around the temporal lobes and the undersurface of the frontal lobes. Meningoencephalitis commonly results. Diagnosis may depend upon brain biopsy with a positive viral culture or identification of viral inclusion bodies. A positive herpes simplex virus polymerase chain reaction test is diagnostic, and results of this test are available before those from cultures. Cortical gyriform enhancement is often present and may be associated with meningeal enhancement.

A good outcome from herpes simplex encephalitis relies on early diagnosis, which is of course dependent on considering herpes as a diagnosis! Delay in therapy or untreated herpes has a high mortality rate (50% to 75%), with little chance of a full neurologic recovery.

Notes

CASE 77

Subependymal Heterotopia

1. Subependymal heterotopia, tuberous sclerosis, and occasionally metastases.

2. Approximately 98%.

3. Subependymal heterotopia.

4. Partial agenesis of the corpus callosum.

Reference

Barkovich AJ, Chuang SH, Norman D: MR of neuronal migration anomalies, *AJR Am J Roentgenol* 150:179-187, 1988.

Cross-Reference

Neuroradiology: THE REQUISITES, pp 256-259.

Comment

This case illustrates multiple subependymal heterotopias that are most pronounced in the occipital horns of the lateral ventricles. In subependymal heterotopia there may be nodules that are often bilaterally symmetric along the length of the lateral ventricles, or there may be just a few lesions. Heterotopias appear as masses that are isointense to gray matter on all pulse sequences and do not enhance. High signal intensity in the parenchyma surrounding the heterotopia should not occur. The differential diagnosis for subependymal heterotopia is limited, and the diagnosis is usually easily established by the stereotypic radiologic appearance. Subependymal nodules in tuberous sclerosis are readily differentiated because they do not follow the signal characteristics of gray matter, and the vast majority are calcified (hypointense on T2W and gradient echo susceptibility images). In addition, other sequelae of tuberous sclerosis are commonly present. Metastatic masses typically enhance following contrast administration. Similarly, other signs of metastatic disease are frequently present in the intracranial compartment.

Heterotopia may be associated with a spectrum of other congenital anomalies including Chiari malformations, ventral induction defects (holoprosencephaly, dysgenesis of the corpus callosum), other migrational abnormalities, and encephaloceles. In this patient there is ex vacuo enlargement of the occipital horns of the lateral ventricles (colpocephaly) as a result of underdevelopment of the surrounding deep white matter and dysgenesis of the splenium of the corpus callosum.

Notes

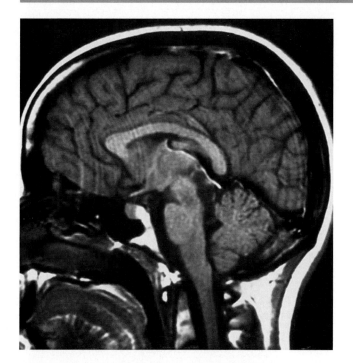
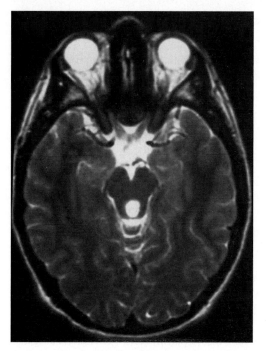
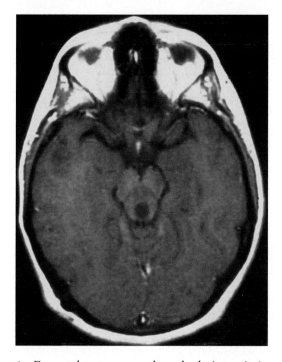

1. From what structure does the lesion arise?
2. What are the secondary imaging findings due to this lesion?
3. The tectum, or roof of the midbrain, contains what paired structures?
4. What congenital anomaly is usually associated with "beaking" of the tectum?

Glioma of the Tectum (Quadrigeminal Plate)

1. Tectum (quadrigeminal plate).

2. Obstructive hydrocephalus related to compression of the aqueduct of Sylvius.

3. The superior and inferior colliculi.

4. Chiari II malformation.

References

Sherman JL, Citrin CM, Barkovich AJ, Bower BJ: MR imaging of the mesencephalic tectum: normal and pathologic variations, *AJNR Am J Neuroradiol* 8:59-64, 1987.

Friedman DP: Extrapineal abnormalities of the tectal region: MR imaging findings, *AJR Am J Roentgenol* 159:859-866, 1992.

Cross-Reference

Neuroradiology: THE REQUISITES, pp 30, 240.

Comment

These images demonstrate an expansile mass lesion of the tectal plate that is predominantly cystic in nature. There is no significant pathologic enhancement following contrast administration. There is resultant compression of the aqueduct, as is typically seen eventually in patients with tectal gliomas. In many patients the clinical presentation is that of obstructive hydrocephalus. Gliomas arising from the tectum are usually low grade astrocytomas. They may be solid or cystic masses and have a wide spectrum of enhancement characteristics ranging from none to prominent. In that most of these are low grade neoplasms, the absence of enhancement is not surprising.

The tectum is affected more frequently by extrinsic rather than intrinsic lesions. It is often compressed (particularly the superior colliculi) along with the aqueduct of Sylvius by pineal region masses such as germ cell tumors (germinoma, embryonal carcinoma, choriocarcinoma, and teratoma), tumors of pineal origin (pineoblastoma and pineocytoma), and vein of Galen aneurysm, which may result in Parinaud's syndrome. Occasionally the tectum may be affected by demyelinating disease, vascular abnormalities, and trauma. In addition, the tectum may be abnormal in congenital malformations, most notably the Chiari II malformation in which there may be a spectrum of abnormalities ranging from collicular fusion to tectal beaking.

Notes

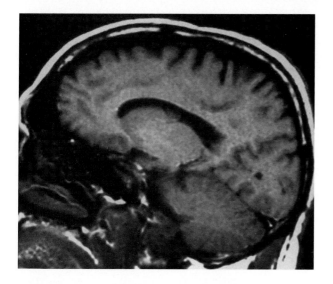
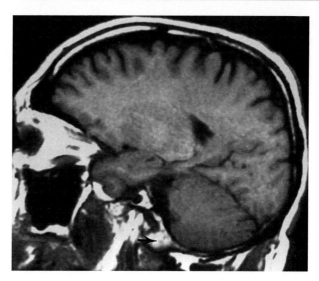

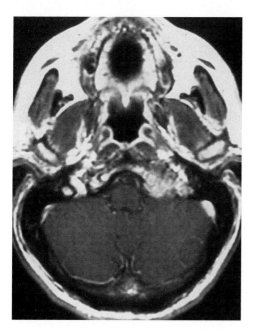

1. What structure in the first image is abnormal?

2. What are the most commonly reported lesions to affect this structure?

3. These structures are intimately related to other osseous structures at the craniovertebral junction by what important ligamentous attachments?

4. What nerves course through the hypoglossal canal and jugular foramen?

Metastatic Disease to the Occipital Condyle—Renal Cell Carcinoma

1. The occipital condyle.

2. Traumatic fractures.

3. The tectorial membrane, the superior extension of the posterior longitudinal ligament, arises from the C2 vertebral body and extends cephalad to attach to the anterior aspect of the occipital bone. The right and left alar ligaments arise from the odontoid process of C2 and attach to their respective occipital condyles.

4. Cranial nerve XII and IX, X, and XI, respectively.

Reference
Loevner LA, Yousem DM: Overlooked metastatic lesions of the occipital condyle: a missed case treasure trove, *RadioGraphics* 17:1111-1121, 1997.

Cross-Reference
Neuroradiology: THE REQUISITES, pp 436-437.

Comment
The occipital condyles and pathology affecting them are often overlooked because it is unusual for a clinician to specifically request evaluation of these structures, and because they are frequently seen only at the edge of films (the inferior sections of an axial brain MRI or CT and the lateral sections of a sagittal MRI).

In children abnormalities of the craniovertebral junction may be congenital (Chiari malformations) or acquired (traumatic, inflammatory, neoplastic). In adults acquired condyle lesions may result from trauma (fractures due to axial loading with ipsilateral flexion). Inflammatory disorders such as rheumatoid arthritis and metabolic disorders such as Paget's disease and hyperparathyroidism may result in basilar invagination.

In my experience, metastatic disease to the occipital condyle is not uncommon and probably underreported. Spread is most likely hematogenous. Most patients present with progressive occipital head and neck pain, which may be associated with cranial neuropathies related to extension of tumor into the hypoglossal canal (resulting in tongue weakness or fasciculations) or jugular foramen (resulting in neuropathies of cranial nerves IX through XI). Sagittal and axial unenhanced T1W images are most useful in identifying abnormalities of the condyles because the hyperintense fat within the marrow is an excellent intrinsic "contrast agent" and replacement of this fat with abnormal hypointense soft tissue is readily seen. In this case the left condyle is replaced by a metastasis (compare with the normal right condyle *[arrow]*). Axial T1W images are useful for identifying spread into the skull base foramina. Lesions are less conspicuous on T2W and enhanced T1W images without fat saturation (masses are isointense to the fatty marrow in the surrounding normal bone and are therefore frequently obscured).

Notes

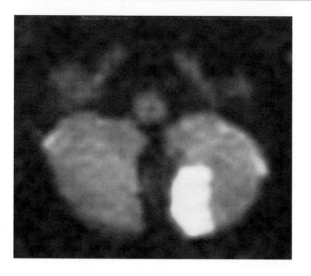
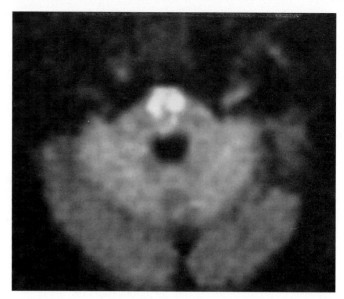

1. What type of MRI is presented in this case?

2. What vascular territories are affected?

3. The posterior inferior cerebellar artery typically arises from what vessel?

4. Which vessel arising from the posterior circulation typically courses in the cerebellopontine angle at the level of the porus acousticus?

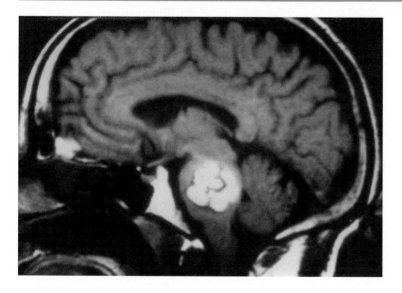
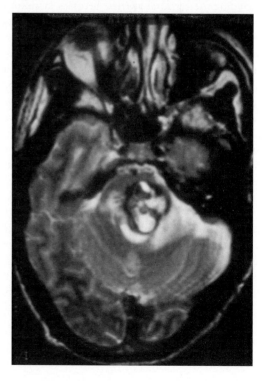

1. Where anatomically is the lesion located?

2. What is the differential diagnosis?

3. In what percentage of cases are cavernous malformations multiple?

4. De novo development of cavernomas has been reported in what subsets of patients?

Posterior Circulation Infarcts Due to Distal Vertebral and Basilar Artery Thrombosis

1. Diffusion imaging.

2. The first image shows an acute infarct in the posterior inferior cerebellar artery (PICA) territory, and the second image shows brainstem infarcts due to ischemia in the perforating arteries arising from the basilar artery.

3. The distal vertebral artery.

4. The anterior inferior cerebellar artery.

Reference

Johnson MH, Christman CW: Posterior circulation infarction: anatomy, pathophysiology, and clinical correlation, *Semin Ultrasound CT, MRI* 16:237-252, 1995.

Cross-Reference

Neuroradiology: THE REQUISITES, pp 59-60, 106-114.

Comment

This case illustrates acute infarctions in multiple vascular territories of the posterior circulation, namely the posteroinferior cerebellar artery and perforating branches of the basilar artery. In older patients (as in this case), the most common cause of posterior circulation ischemia is thromboembolic disease resulting from accelerated atheromatous disease or embolic disease from a cardiac source. However, in that the vasculature (including the vertebral arteries) becomes more tortuous as a patient ages, in the elderly population in the setting of embolic disease from a systemic source it is less common to have embolic disease isolated to the posterior fossa (usually patients also have embolic disease to the anterior circulation). In my experience, isolated posterior fossa embolic disease is more common in young patients in whom the vertebral arteries course vertically with little tortuosity. In young patients with posterior fossa ischemia, in addition to embolic disease the diagnosis of a dissection should also be considered. This can be evaluated with MRI and MRA. MRI should include unenhanced axial T1W images through the distal vertebral arteries with and without fat saturation when possible to look for clot in the vessel wall, which is hyperintense due to methemoglobin. In addition, the dissected vessel may be enlarged due to mural hematoma, and occlusion (absence of signal void) or luminal narrowing (reduced size of the signal void) may be seen. In this case, the patient's ischemic disease was related to thrombosis of the distal left vertebral artery and proximal basilar artery on the basis of severe atherosclerosis.

Notes

Acute and Subacute Hemorrhage in a Large Pontine Cavernous Malformation

1. The pons.

2. Hemorrhage into an underlying occult vascular malformation or hemorrhage into a brainstem neoplasm (glioma).

3. Approximately 25%.

4. Those with a familial history of cavernous malformations and those with previous radiation therapy to the brain.

Reference

Zimmerman RS, Spetzler RF, Lee KS, Zabramski JM, Hargraves RW: Cavernous malformations of the brain stem, *J Neurosurg* 75:32-39, 1991.

Cross-Reference

Neuroradiology: THE REQUISITES, pp 141-142.

Comment

The sagittal T1W image shows a lobular, hyperintense pontine mass. There is associated expansion of the brain stem and high signal intensity in the adjacent right pons and the left middle cerebellar peduncle on the axial T2W image. The mass extends to the posterior surface of the pons and extends into the fourth ventricle. Before MRI hemorrhagic cavernous malformations were often mistaken for neoplasms. Nonetheless the differentiation of a CM from a hemorrhagic neoplasm on MRI may still be difficult in the face of acute hemorrhage, particularly, in the presence of edema and mass effect. Several imaging features may help to distinguish these two lesions. Findings favoring a CM include focal heterogeneous high signal intensity representing methemoglobin, a complete hypointense peripheral ring representing hemosiderin, and the absence of enhancing solid tissue. When all else fails, follow-up imaging in 4 to 6 weeks may be performed to assess for the expected temporal evolution of hemorrhage when secondary to a CM. In this case, the central high signal intensity on the unenhanced T1W image and the surrounding rim of hypointensity on the T2W image are highly suggestive of hemorrhage into a CM.

Cavernous malformations may be present in as much as 5% of the population. The majority are located superficially in the cerebrum and are often closely associated with the adjacent subarachnoid space. They may occur deep within the cerebral hemispheres, although this is less common. Cavernous malformations occur less frequently in the infratentorial compartment. The most common brainstem location is the pons. Symptoms may be related to lesion location or acute hemorrhage. In the cerebrum the most common presentation is seizures. In the infratentorial compartment, neurologic deficits may occur on the basis of acute hemorrhage, thrombosis, or progressive enlargement of a CM related to recurrent hemorrhage.

Notes

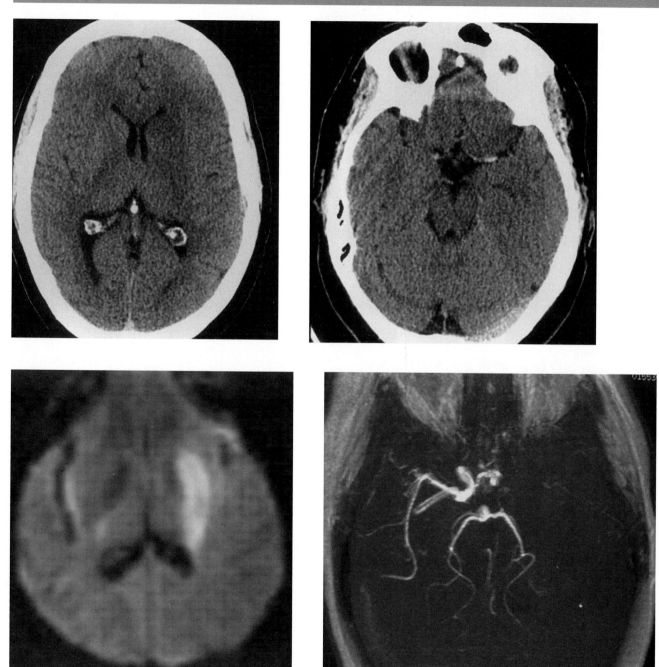

1. In this young patient, what is the most likely cause of the abnormality?

2. What are common causes of thromboembolic stroke?

3. What are hypercoagulable causes for stroke?

4. What are relative contraindications for intraarterial lytic therapy in the treatment of acute anterior circulation strokes?

Thromboembolic Stroke in the Middle Cerebral Artery and Lenticulostriate Territories

1. Embolic disease.

2. Atherosclerosis, cardiac lesions, dissection, pulmonary sources, and paradoxical embolus from the legs.

3. Oral contraceptives, sickle cell disease, antiphospholipid antibodies, and protein S or C deficiency.

4. CT evidence of acute intracranial hemorrhage or infarction, symptomatology that extends beyond the accepted time window (usually more than 6 hours from onset of symptoms), and contraindications to anticoagulation (recent major surgery, brain tumor).

Reference

Crain MR, Yuh WT, Greene GM, et al: Cerebral ischemia: evaluation with contrast-enhanced MR imaging, *AJNR Am J Neuroradiol* 12:631-639, 1991.

Cross-Reference

Neuroradiology: THE REQUISITES, pp 116-117.

Comment

The CT scan in this case reveals abnormal hypodensity in the left basal ganglia consistent with acute ischemia and infarction. In addition, a hyperdense proximal middle cerebral artery (MCA) is noted on the left, consistent with an embolus. Follow-up MRI and MRA performed within 6 hours of the CT show the acute stroke extending into the lenticulostriate territory as marked hyperintensity on diffusion imaging. The compressed image from the MRA confirms embolic disease with absence of filling of the left middle cerebral artery territory vasculature. Especially in a young patient with an acute stroke, causes for thromboembolic disease must be sought. Atherosclerosis, cardiac sources (endocarditis with valvular disease, mural thrombi in the setting of a recent myocardial infarction), vascular dissection (traumatic or nontraumatic such as seen in underlying dysplasias of the vascular wall), and pulmonary source AVM should be excluded. Some hypercoagulable causes for stroke include the use of oral contraceptives, pregnancy, sickle cell disease, hematologic malignancy, antiphospholipid antibodies (such as lupus anticoagulant in systemic lupus erythematosus), homocystinuria, L-asparaginase therapy, antithrombin III deficiency, and protein S or C deficiency (such as may occur in nephrotic syndrome). Diagnostic work up should include a detailed patient history, appropriate blood analysis, and imaging (echocardiography, chest radiography, carotid MRA, and conventional catheter angiography as necessary).

Notes

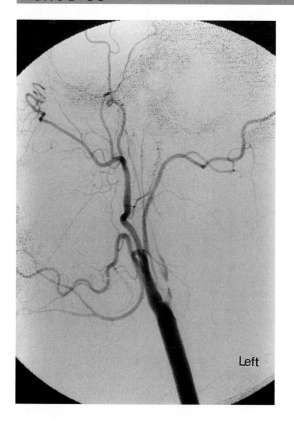

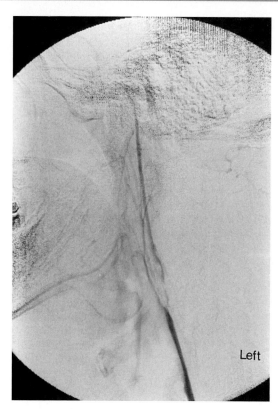

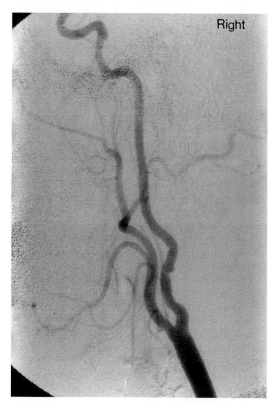

1. This is the angiogram of the same patient as case 82. What is the cause of the patient's stroke?

2. What is the most common location for an intracranial vascular dissection?

3. Of the vessels that supply the CNS, which is most commonly affected with fibromuscular dysplasia?

4. What systemic vessels are most commonly involved with fibromuscular dysplasia?

Fibromuscular Dysplasia (Same Patient as in Case 82)

1. Dissection of the cervical internal carotid artery with a distal embolus.

2. The supraclinoid internal carotid artery.

3. The cervical internal carotid artery.

4. The renal arteries.

Reference

Heiserman JE, Drayer BP, Fram EK, Keller PJ: MR angiography of cervical fibromuscular dysplasia, *AJNR Am J Neuroradiol* 13:1454-1457, 1992.

Cross-Reference

Neuroradiology: THE REQUISITES, pp 116-117.

Comment

Conventional catheter angiography demonstrates findings consistent with an extracranial dissection of the proximal internal carotid artery on the left, distal to the carotid bifurcation. There is marked narrowing and irregularity of the proximal internal carotid artery with poor distal filling and very slow antegrade flow seen on delayed images. An extracranial dissection may result from trauma or manipulation of the neck (such as chiropractic manipulation). Alternatively, extracranial dissection may result from an underlying vascular abnormality or dysplasia. In this case, injection of the right internal carotid artery demonstrates a normal appearance of the proximal internal carotid artery distal to the carotid bifurcation; however, there is irregularity with regions of narrowing alternating with dilation, producing a "string of beads" appearance that is commonly described in fibromuscular dysplasia. There are many subtypes (medial, intimal, and adventitial) of fibromuscular dysplasia in which one or all layers of the arterial wall may be involved; however, involvement of the media with hyperplasia/dysplasia is the most common variant, seen in up to 90% of cases. Thinning of the media is associated with abnormalities in the internal elastic lamina resulting in the dilation seen in this condition. The cervical internal carotid artery is most commonly affected and, importantly, the proximal 2 cm of the vessel is usually spared. The extracranial vertebral artery and external carotid arteries may be involved; however, intracranial fibromuscular dysplasia is relatively uncommon. The incidence of intracranial aneurysms is increased in patients with fibromuscular dysplasia.

Notes

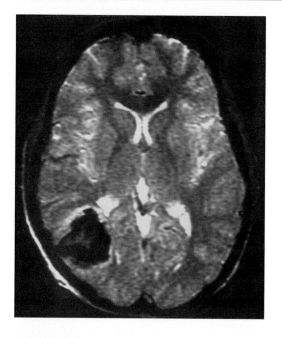
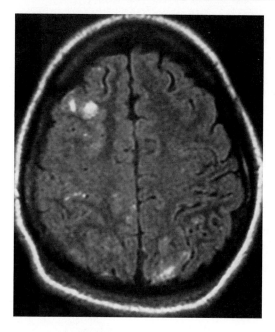
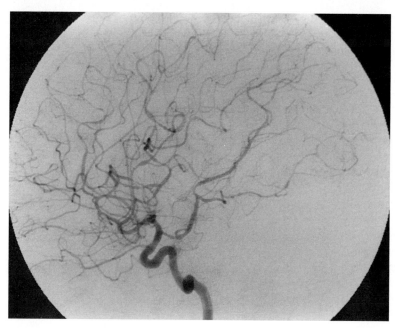

1. What are the imaging findings on the gradient echo MRI scan, FLAIR image, and digital subtraction angiogram?
2. Given all of the findings, what is the best diagnosis?
3. What is the differential diagnosis of segmental regions of narrowing of the cerebral vessels?
4. What systemic condition is often associated with antiphospholipid antibodies?

Vasculitis Presenting With Intraparenchymal Hemorrhage and Infarcts

1. Right parietal lobe hemorrhage, multifocal regions of increased signal intensity involving the cortex and gray-white matter interface consistent with ischemia, and diffuse segmental narrowing with alternating regions of dilation involving the cerebral vessels, respectively.

2. Vasculitis in this middle-aged woman.

3. Vasculitis, atherosclerosis, hypercoagulable states (antiphospholipid antibodies), and vasospasm. Neoplasms may cause focal regions of segmental narrowing due to encasement of the vessel by tumor; however, this tends to be more focal in distribution. Rarely, arterial lymphoma may simulate vasculitis.

4. Systemic lupus erythematosus.

Reference

Fauci AS, Haynes B, Katz P: The spectrum of vasculitis: clinical, pathologic, immunologic, and therapeutic considerations, *Ann Intern Med* 89:660-676, 1978.

Cross-Reference

Neuroradiology: THE REQUISITES, pp 114-116.

Comment

The vasculitides that can affect the cerebral arteries may be divided into infectious and noninfectious causes. Infectious etiologies include tuberculosis, which frequently involves the vessels around the basal cisterns. CNS neurosyphilis may cause a basilar meningitis and vasculitis; however, it may also affect more distal cerebral vessels, especially the middle cerebral arteries. There are several classifications of noninfectious vasculitis that result from inflammatory infiltrates both within and surrounding the vessel walls that lead to regions of segmental narrowing and dilation on catheter angiography. Among the noninfectious causes of vasculitis are the necrotizing vasculopathies such as primary angitis, periarteritis nodosa, sarcoidosis, and Wegener's granulomatosis. Vasculitis is occasionally associated with collagen vascular disease such as systemic lupus erythematosus and rheumatoid arthritis; however, this is probably less frequent than is commonly reported. More often, the cause of ischemic events in these patients is related to antiphospholipid antibodies (lupus anticoagulant and anticardiolipin antibodies). Certain recreational drugs have also been associated with vasculitis, including amphetamines, ecstasy, and cocaine. Clinical presentation can vary from headache, changes in mental status, and meningitis to stroke and intracranial hemorrhage.

A normal (negative) angiogram does not exclude CNS vasculitis. If vasculitis is highly suspect clinically, biopsy is indicated to make the diagnosis. Even in cases in which angiography is positive, biopsy may still be necessary to confirm the diagnosis.

Notes

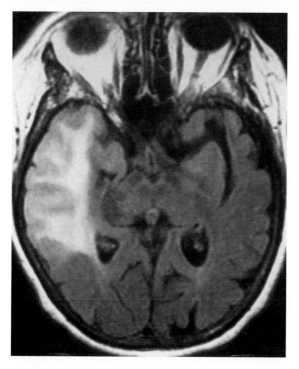 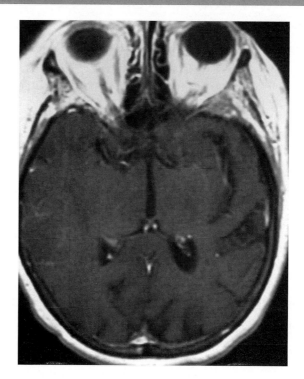

1. What is the differential diagnosis?
2. What imaging findings are atypical for herpes encephalitis?
3. What is the most common location for an anaplastic astrocytoma in children?
4. What clinical presentation would help differentiate an acute stroke from an infiltrating glioma?

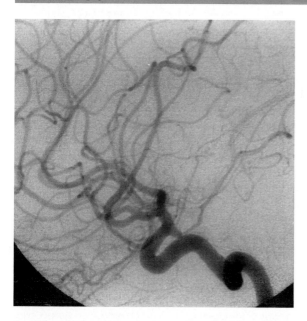

1. What is the most common site of origin of aneurysms from the internal carotid artery?
2. How does one differentiate an infundibulum from an aneurysm?
3. What percentage of patients with nontraumatic subarachnoid hemorrhage will have unrevealing angiograms?
4. What are some causes of angiographically negative subarachnoid hemorrhage?

Anaplastic Astrocytoma

1. Infiltrating glioma, cerebritis, and infarction.

2. Although herpes typically involves the temporal lobe(s), involvement of the medial temporal lobe is characteristic. In this case, signal abnormality and mass effect are localized laterally with relative sparing of the medial temporal lobe (which is atypical).

3. The pons.

4. In the setting of infarction, patients present with abrupt onset of symptoms. In comparison, infiltrating astrocytomas more often present with progressive chronic neurologic signs and symptoms.

Reference

Graif M, Bydder GM, Steiner RE, Niendorf P, Thomas DG, Young IR: Contrast-enhanced MR imaging of malignant brain tumors, *AJNR Am J Neuroradiol* 6:855-862, 1985.

Cross-Reference

Neuroradiology: THE REQUISITES, pp 87-92.

Comment

This case illustrates abnormal signal intensity involving both the superficial cortex and the subcortical white matter of the right temporal lobe. There is mild local mass effect manifest by sulcal effacement. No contrast enhancement was identified (not shown). The differential diagnosis includes neoplasia (infiltrating glioma), encephalitis, and infarction. Infarction can usually be distinguished from a neoplastic process based on clinical presentation. In addition, MRI may be able to distinguish acute infarction from neoplasm. Acute infarcts are markedly hyperintense (cytotoxic edema) on diffusion-weighted images, whereas neoplasms (vasogenic edema) are not. On proton MR spectroscopy, an increased choline peak is highly suggestive of neoplasm and is usually not seen with infarction or encephalitis. N-acetyl-aspartate is usually decreased with neoplasms but may also be decreased in infarction and encephalitis depending on the age of the lesions. Differentiating a neoplasm from encephalitis may be more difficult from a radiologic standpoint; however, correlation with history and laboratory analysis (CSF) may be useful. When all else fails, follow-up imaging usually differentiates neoplasm from encephalitis.

Histologically anaplastic astrocytomas have features that are between an astrocytoma and a GBM. On imaging they typically show heterogeneous enhancement; however, the enhancement pattern in anaplastic astrocytoma may vary from avid and nodular to minimal (as in this case). Necrosis, although more common than in diffuse astrocytomas, is much less common than that seen in the more malignant GBM. Anaplastic astrocytomas are highly malignant, with an average survival time of 2.5 years following diagnosis.

Notes

Posterior Communicating Artery Infundibulum

1. The origin of the posterior communicating artery.

2. An infundibulum should meet the following criteria: (1) it should measure ≤ 3 mm in size, (2) it should be triangular or funnel shaped, and (3) the posterior communicating artery should arise from its apex.

3. Approximately 10% to 15%.

4. Aneurysms may not be detected because of vasospasm that inhibits filling of the aneurysm, spontaneous thrombosis of the aneurysm, or misinterpretation of the images. Other causes of angiogram negative subarachnoid hemorrhage include perimesencephalic venous hemorrhages and spinal vascular malformations.

Reference

Bagley LJ, Hurst RW: Angiographic evaluation of aneurysms affecting the central nervous system, *Neuroimaging Clin North Am* 7:721-737, 1997.

Cross-Reference

Neuroradiology: THE REQUISITES, p 138.

Comment

These angiographic images demonstrate the typical appearance of a posterior communicating artery infundibulum, showing its funnel shape as well as the origin of the posterior communicating artery from the apex of the infundibulum. Because the management is dramatically different, angiographic images in anteroposterior, lateral, and oblique projections should be obtained in order to accurately differentiate an aneurysm from an infundibulum (infundibula are considered in many cases to represent a normal variation).

Conventional catheter angiography remains the standard in the diagnosis and evaluation of intracranial aneurysm. In the acute setting there are several indications for prompt angiography, including nontraumatic subarachnoid hemorrhage; acute onset third nerve palsy, which involves the pupil (to exclude a posterior communicating or superior cerebellar artery aneurysm); and in the postoperative setting to evaluate complications following placement of an aneurysm clip. In patients with angiogram-negative acute nontraumatic subarachnoid hemorrhage, follow-up angiography is usually indicated. It is important to remember that all potential sites of aneurysm formation must be assessed with conventional angiography. In the acute setting postoperative angiography is often indicated in the evaluation of perioperative ischemic sequelae (which may be due to embolic phenomena, vasospasm, or vascular occlusion). Postoperative or intraoperative angiography on an elective basis may be performed to assess for residual aneurysm following aneurysm clipping.

Notes

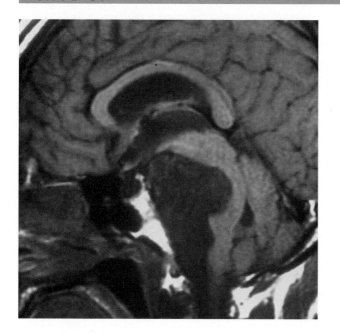
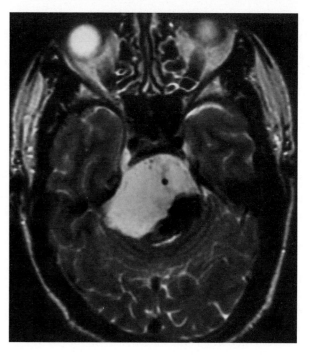
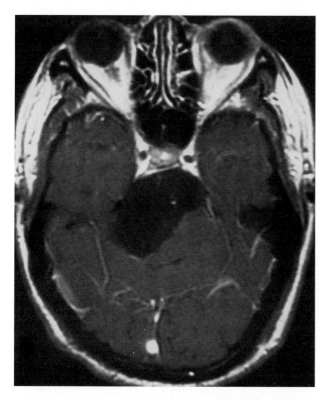

1. What is the enhancement pattern of epidermoid cysts?
2. What are the characteristic MRI findings of an arachnoid cyst?
3. What are common locations for intradural epidermoid cysts?
4. How do you suspect the patient in this case presented clinically?

Epidermoid Cyst—Cerebellopontine Cistern

1. On occasion, there may be minimal enhancement around the periphery of these lesions; like all other cysts, however, they should not enhance.

2. They tend to be circumscribed lesions that follow the signal characteristics of CSF on all pulse sequences (T1W, intermediate, FLAIR, and T2W images).

3. The cerebellopontine angle cistern, suprasellar cistern, cisterna magna, and peripenial region.

4. Given the location of the lesion in the cerebellopontine angle cistern around the brain stem, multiple cranial neuropathies (especially trigeminal neuralgia).

References

Tien RD, Felsberg GJ, Lirng JF: Variable bandwidth steady-state free-precession MR imaging: a technique for improving characterization of epidermoid tumor and arachnoid cyst, *AJR Am J Roentgenol* 164:689-692, 1995.

Tampieri D, Melanson, D, Ethier R: MR imaging of epidermoid cysts, *AJNR Am J Neuroradiol* 10:351-356, 1989.

Cross-Reference

Neuroradiology: THE REQUISITES, pp 76-77.

Comment

Epidermoid cysts are congenital lesions that result from incomplete separation of the neural and cutaneous ectoderm at the time of closure of the neural tube. They are lined by a single layer of stratified squamous epithelium. Within these cysts are desquamated epithelium, keratin, and cholesterol crystals. Many of these lesions are incidental findings, but when symptomatic epidermoid cysts typically present in the third or fourth decade of life.

This case illustrates the typical appearance of an epidermoid. On the unenhanced T1W image the mass in the cerebellopontine cistern is hypointense (although mildly hyperintense to CSF with a fine internal architecture). On the T2W image the lesion is isointense to CSF; however, heterogeneity within the cyst is noted. Unlike arachnoid cysts, which are typically isointense to CSF on intermediate and FLAIR images, the epidermoid is hyperintense relative to CSF on these pulse sequences. Following contrast, there is no enhancement. Other characteristic appearances of epidermoids that distinguish them from arachnoid cysts (the major differential consideration here) are also presented in this case, including the lobulated and scalloped borders of this lesion; the insinuating nature of this lesion, which fills and conforms to the shape of the space that it occupies; and the encasement of the basilar artery (compared with an arachnoid cyst, which tends to displace vessels).

Notes

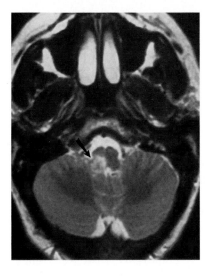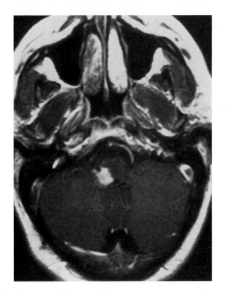

1. What part of the brain stem and which cerebellar peduncle are involved by this lesion?

2. What cranial nerves arise from the olivary sulcus *(arrow)*?

3. The posterior inferior cerebellar artery supplies perforating vessels to what part of the brain stem?

4. What imaging finding makes infarct an unlikely etiology for this lesion?

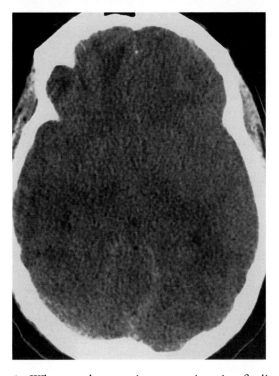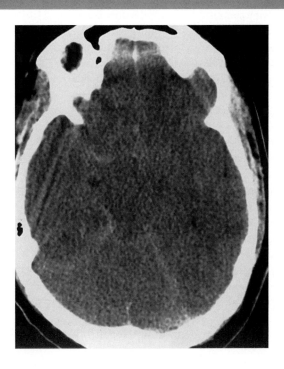

1. What are the most important imaging findings in this patient?

2. What are the imaging findings in subfalcine herniation?

3. What type of secondary hemorrhages may occur in the brain stem with transtentorial herniation?

4. What are causes of upward herniation (superior vermian herniation)?

Primary Lymphoma Involving the Brain Stem (Immunocompetent Patient)

1. The medulla and the inferior cerebellar peduncle.

2. IX and X.

3. The lateral and posterior medulla in the retroolivary region.

4. The avid homogeneous enhancement.

References

Johnson BA, Fram EK, Johnson PC, Jacobowitz R: The variable MR appearance of primary lymphoma of the central nervous system: comparison with histopathologic features, *AJNR Am J Neuroradiol* 18:563-572, 1997.

Nozaki M, Tada M, Mizugaki Y, et al: Expression of oncogenic molecules in primary central nervous system lymphomas in immunocompetent patients, *Acta Neuropathol* 95:505-510, 1998.

Cross-Reference

Neuroradiology: THE REQUISITES, pp 30-34, 59-60.

Comment

These images demonstrate abnormal signal intensity involving the posterior and lateral medulla on the right. There is associated mild mass effect. Following contrast administration there is avid homogeneous enhancement of the lesion. The imaging findings are not specific for a particular disease entity. Correlation with the patient's clinical history is necessary. Differential considerations include inflammatory disorders, demyelinating disease such as multiple sclerosis or acute disseminated encephalomyelitis, sarcoidosis, and infectious etiologies such as tuberculosis. Other considerations include neoplastic disorders such as lymphoma and astrocytoma; however, primary brainstem gliomas are uncommon in adults. Although primary lymphoma may involve the posterior fossa contents, it is much more common in the supratentorial compartment. The configuration of the lesion makes metastatic disease less likely. Although possible, brainstem metastases in the absence of other lesions in the supratentorial compartment are unusual. Finally, infarction in the posterior inferior cerebellar artery territory can produce the lateral medullary (Wallenberg's) syndrome, which causes loss of pain and temperature sensation on the contralateral side of the body and the ipsilateral side of the face. Other symptoms may include ataxia, IX and X cranial neuropathies, nystagmus, and vertigo. However, the extensive involvement of the posterior medulla, as well as the enhancement pattern, makes an ischemic etiology less likely. In this patient it is important to evaluate the remainder of the brain to assess for additional lesions. This patient had an isolated lesion, and biopsy revealed primary CNS lymphoma. Primary CNS lymphoma is most commonly seen in the immunocompromised host (especially HIV infection).

Notes

116

Transtentorial Herniation

1. Effacement of the cerebral sulci, basal cisterns, and ventricles, as well as loss of gray-white matter differentiation.

2. Herniation of the cingulate gyrus beneath the anterior free edge of the falx on coronal MRI. Secondary changes include ischemia in the anterior cerebral artery territory related to compression of these vessels.

3. Duret hemorrhages.

4. Rapid reduction of supratentorial increased intracranial pressure (such as in decompression of large extraaxial hematomas), or posterior fossa lesions resulting in cerebellar mass effect.

Reference

Reich JB, Sierra J, Camp W, Zanzonico P, Deck MD, Plum F: Magnetic resonance imaging measurements and clinical changes accompanying transtentorial and foramen magnum brain herniation, *Ann Neurol* 33:159-170, 1993.

Cross-Reference

Neuroradiology: THE REQUISITES, pp 161-162.

Comment

The brain is confined by the cranial vault and an inelastic dura. CSF surrounding the brain serves as a shock absorber. With increased intracranial pressure, herniation of brain from one compartment to another may occur. There are multiple patterns of herniation. In the posterior fossa, there may be inferior tonsillar and cerebellar herniation with displacement of these structures into the foramen magnum, or there may be upward herniation (superior vermian herniation) in which cerebellar tissue obliterates the quadrigeminal and superior vermian cisterns. Herniation syndromes in the supratentorial compartment include subfalcine, temporal lobe, and central transtentorial herniation. Transtentorial herniation is typically caused by mass lesions or global cerebral swelling in the supratentorial compartment resulting in vector forces that are directed both medially and inferiorly. There is resultant effacement of the basal cisterns and ventricles, as well as caudal displacement of the upper brain stem. In transtentorial herniation, the temporal lobe(s) shift(s) over the tentorium. Caudal displacement of the brain stem and effacement of the ambient cisterns may result in compression of the oculomotor nerve (resulting in ipsilateral pupillary dilation) and compression of the posterior cerebral arteries resulting in ischemic changes in the occipital lobes and brain stem/ diencephalon. There may be secondary small hemorrhages (Duret lesion), which are typically centrally located within the rostral pons and midbrain.

This case illustrates global cerebral swelling following resuscitation from a respiratory arrest resulting in transtentorial herniation. Hypodensity in the brain stem is consistent with ischemia from vascular compression within the basal cisterns.

Notes

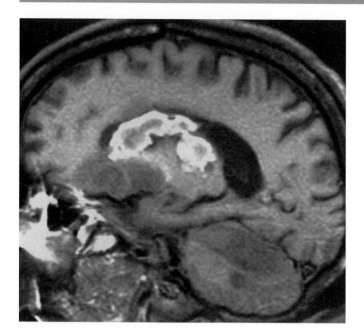

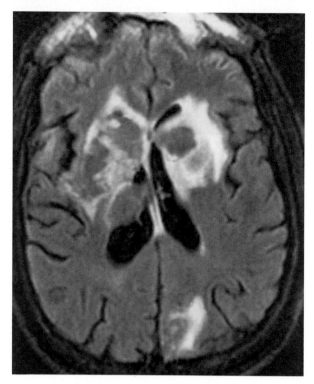

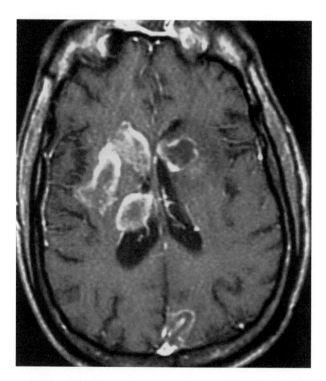

1. What is the most common opportunistic CNS infection in patients with AIDS?

2. In an immunocompromised patient, what is the differential diagnosis for this case?

3. In infants congenitally infected with toxoplasmosis, what are the typical neuroimaging findings?

4. In differentiating toxoplasmosis from primary CNS lymphoma, which demonstrates increased uptake on thallium-201 scintigraphy?

Toxoplasmosis Infection in a Patient With Acquired Immunodeficiency Syndrome

1. Toxoplasmosis.

2. Toxoplasmosis, primary CNS lymphoma, and other infectious agents (fungus, tuberculosis).

3. Multiple focal calcifications within the basal ganglia and cortex and hydrocephalus. Microcephaly may be present in severe cases.

4. Lymphoma. In ^{201}Th single photo emission CT, tissue that is metabolically active will show increased uptake relative to the adjacent brain parenchyma. Therefore tumors often show increased uptake, whereas infections do not.

References

Ernst TM, Chang L, Witt MD, et al: Cerebral toxoplasmosis and lymphoma in AIDS: perfusion MR imaging experience in 13 patients, *Radiology* 208:663-669, 1998.

Kessler LS, Ruiz A, Donovan Post MJ, Ganz WI, Brandon AH, Foss JN: Thallium-201 brain SPECT of lymphoma in AIDS patients: pitfalls and technique optimization, *AJNR Am J Neuroradiol* 19:1105-1109, 1998.

Cross-Reference

Neuroradiology: THE REQUISITES, pp 92, 193.

Comment

Central nervous system toxoplasmosis is caused by the intracellular protozoan *Toxoplasma gondii*. Toxoplasma encephalitis is most commonly seen in immunocompromised patients with impaired cellular immunity, especially in the setting of AIDS. Other immunodeficient conditions associated with increased infection include following organ transplantation, long-term steroid or chemotherapy, an underlying malignancy, and collagen vascular disease. Toxoplasma can be transmitted through raw meat, milk, blood products, and cat feces and by in utero exposure. Because a high percentage of the U.S. population is seropositive for toxoplasma, serologic testing may not be useful in establishing the diagnosis.

On CT CNS toxoplasmosis typically demonstrates multifocal areas of hypodensity. There is a predilection for the basal ganglia and the white matter at the corticomedullary junction. Lesions are often hyperintense on T2W imaging, but they may vary widely in their signal characteristics. Lesions may be hemorrhagic (as in this case) and may also be isointense to hypointense relative to gray matter with surrounding high signal intensity edema.

In the setting of AIDS, radiologic differentiation between toxoplasmosis and lymphoma is often difficult. Both entities frequently have multiple lesions, and both may have solid or ring enhancement. Distinguishing these two disease processes is important because they are treated differently, and they have different prognoses. Primary lymphoma responds to radiation therapy, which results in a severalfold increase in survival rates. However, the benefit of radiation therapy is diminished when treatment is delayed, such as in cases of patients first treated empirically for toxoplasmosis. Radiologic findings that favor lymphoma are hyperdense masses on unenhanced CT: the presence of ependymal spread on enhanced MRI seen in approximately one third of cases (but rare in toxoplasmosis); and a periventricular distribution. ^{201}Th SPECT can be effective (sensitive and specific) in distinguishing lymphoma from toxoplasmosis and other infections. Neoplasms take up significant amounts of thallium, whereas normal brain and infections generally do not. Recent investigations with perfusion MRI have suggested that it may play a role in differentiating toxoplasmosis and lymphoma. Quantification of regional blood volume using dynamic enhanced echo planar imaging has shown decreased regional blood volumes in toxoplasmosis lesions (attributed to the avascularity of abscesses) compared with increased blood volumes in lymphoma (attributed to increased vascularity in regions of metabolically active tumor).

Notes

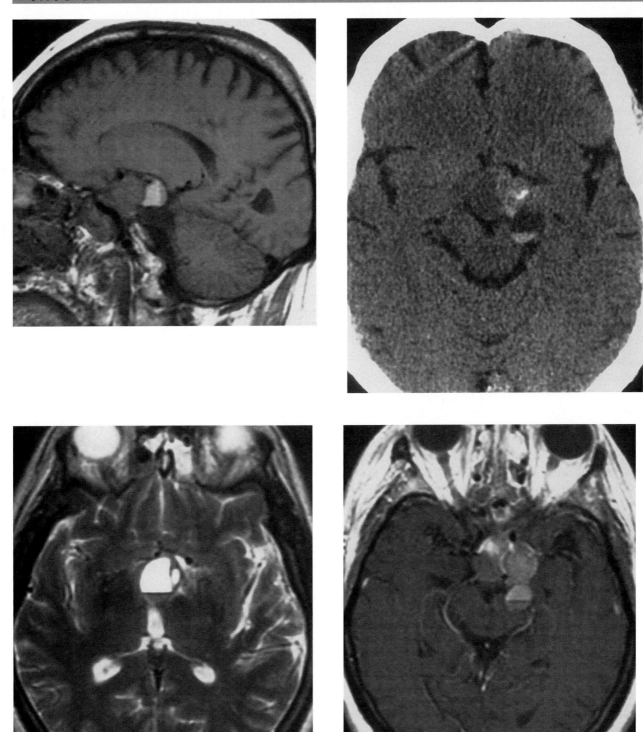

1. What is the differential diagnosis in this case?

2. What is the typical age of presentation of craniopharyngioma?

3. What are characteristic imaging findings seen with craniopharyngioma?

4. On imaging, how do squamous papillary craniopharyngiomas differ from adamantinomatous craniopharyngiomas?

Suprasellar Craniopharyngioma

1. Hemorrhagic pituitary adenoma and craniopharyngioma. The presence of solid enhancing tissue excludes a Rathke's cleft cyst.

2. They have a bimodal age distribution. Those in children between the ages of 5 and 10 years are of the adamantinomatous type. The second peak is in the fifth and sixth decades of life.

3. Cystic or cystic and solid mass, calcification, and enhancement.

4. Squamous papillary craniopharyngiomas are typically solid, do not calcify, are frequently present within the third ventricle rather than in the suprasellar cistern, and the majority are seen in adults.

Reference

Sartoretti-Schefer S, Wichmann W, Aguzzi A, Valavanis A: MR differentiation of adamantinous and squamous-papillary craniopharyngiomas, *AJNR Am J Neuroradiol* 18:77-87, 1997.

Cross-Reference

Neuroradiology: THE REQUISITES, pp 313, 320-325, 332.

Comment

Craniopharyngiomas arise from metaplastic squamous epithelial rests along the hypophysis. They account for 1% to 3% of all intracranial neoplasms and 10% to 15% of all supratentorial tumors. They are more common in males. The vast majority arise within the suprasellar cistern (80% to 90%); however, they may arise within the sella turcica and occasionally the third ventricle. Clinical presentation includes visual disturbances related to compression of the optic chiasm, pituitary hypofunction related to compression of the gland or hypothalamus, and/or symptoms of increased intracranial pressure.

Imaging findings typically include a cystic or a solid and cystic mass lesion. Approximately 80% to 90% of all craniopharyngiomas have a cystic component. Smaller lesions may be purely solid. The vast majority (90%) have calcification and/or enhance following the administration of intravenous contrast material. Because MRI is not sensitive in detecting the presence of calcification, CT may be quite useful in establishing the diagnosis of craniopharyngioma. On MRI, the signal characteristics may be quite variable, depending on the contents and viscosity within the cysts. Whereas the cystic portion is frequently hyperintense on T2W imaging, it may be hypointense, isointense, or hyperintense on T1W imaging. High signal intensity on T1W images may be due to high concentrations of protein or methemoglobin (rather than cholesterol or lipid products). Rim enhancement may be seen around the cystic portions of these tumors, and the solid portions typically demonstrate more avid, solid enhancement.

Notes

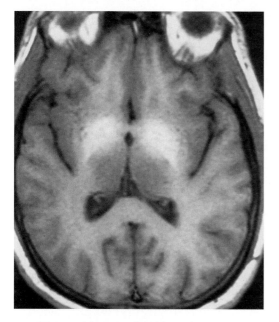 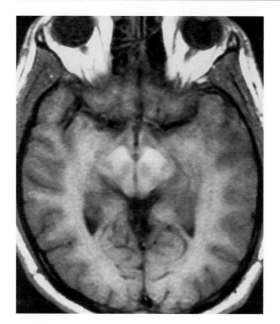

1. What is the pertinent finding?
2. What disorders of calcium and phosphate metabolism are associated with this finding?
3. What neurocutaneous syndrome is associated with high signal intensity foci in the brain on unenhanced T1W images?
4. What is the signal intensity of paramagnetic material on T2W images?

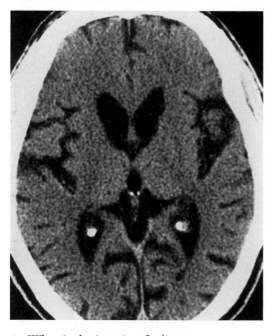 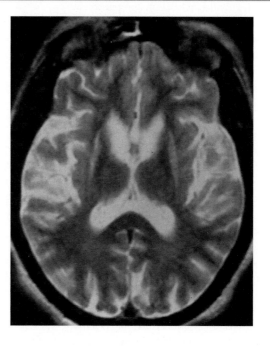

1. What is the imaging finding?
2. Lesions involving the extrapyramidal nuclei (deep gray matter) typically result in what type of neurologic disorders?
3. Hallervorden-Spatz syndrome is an autosomal recessive disorder that results in accumulation of iron products in which deep gray matter structures?
4. In Wilson's disease (hepatolenticular degeneration), abnormal copper deposition is caused by a deficiency of what serum transport protein?

Basal Ganglia T1W High Signal Intensity (Liver Failure)

1. Bilaterally symmetric high signal intensity in the basal ganglia.

2. Hyperparathyroidism and hypoparathyroidism (as well as every "pseudo" variety, including pseudohypoparathyroidism and pseudopseudohypoparathyroidism).

3. Neurofibromatosis type 1.

4. Low signal intensity.

References

Inoue E, Hori S, Narumi Y, et al: Portal-systemic encephalopathy: presence of basal ganglion lesions with high signal intensity on MR images, *Radiology* 179:551-555, 1991.

Terada H, Barkovich AJ, Edwards MS, Ciricillo SM: Evolution of high-intensity basal ganglia lesions on T1-weighted MR in neurofibromatosis type 1, *AJNR Am J Neuroradiol* 17:755-760, 1996.

Cross-Reference

Neuroradiology: THE REQUISITES, p 236.

Comment

This case illustrates bilaterally symmetric high signal intensity in the basal ganglia on unenhanced T1W images in a patient with chronic liver failure. High signal intensity in the basal ganglia on T1W images is also described in patients on hyperalimentation, portosystemic shunting, and abnormal calcium and phosphate metabolism. The high signal intensity is believed to be most likely related to deposition of paramagnetic ions, particularly manganese; however, other materials such as copper have been suggested. In the setting of liver failure, high signal intensity is frequently most pronounced in the globus pallidus; however, it may also be noted in the putamen, brain stem, and pituitary gland.

Neurofibromatosis type 1 is the most common neurocutaneous disorder. It is associated with a variety of intracranial lesions, the most common of which are foci of high signal intensity on long TR images within the brain parenchyma. The foci of high signal intensity are seen most commonly in the basal ganglia; however, they are frequently noted in the white matter tracts of the corpus striatum, in the brain stem, and in the cerebellum. The basal ganglia lesions may be hyperintense on unenhanced T1W images. It has been suggested that the pathologic basis of these foci in neurofibromatosis type 1 may be related to hypomyelination, migrational abnormalities, and nonneoplastic hamartomatous changes. A recent study, however, in which pathologic correlation was obtained suggests that the foci of signal abnormality may be related to vacuolar and/or spongiotic change.

Notes

Huntington's Disease

1. Bilateral caudate atrophy.

2. Motor dysfunction/movement disorders.

3. The globus pallidus and/or substantia nigra.

4. Ceruloplasmin.

Reference

Simmons JT, Pastakia B, Chase TN, Shults CW: Magnetic resonance imaging in Huntington disease, *AJNR Am J Neuroradiol* 7:25-28, 1986.

Cross-Reference

Neuroradiology: THE REQUISITES, pp 233-235.

Comment

A variety of disease processes affect the extrapyramidal nuclei (the basal ganglia, thalami) as well as the nuclei in the brain stem. These conditions are most commonly degenerative and/or metabolic (many are inherited) in nature. In addition, a second disease category, namely toxic exposures, may result in abnormalities of the deep gray matter. Lesions in these structures typically result in movement disorders that can occur in isolation or in combination and include the following subtypes: abnormalities in muscle tone, involuntary movements, abnormal postural reflexes, and the inability to carry out voluntary movements. Among the neurodegenerative processes that can affect the deep gray matter are Huntington's disease, Wilson's disease, and Hallervorden-Spatz syndrome. Toxic disorders that can affect the basal ganglia include carbon monoxide, cyanide, hydrogen sulfide, ethylene glycol, and toluene poisoning. Although there is a wide variation in the deep gray matter structures involved, many disease processes have characteristic involvement of specific structures.

Huntington's disease is inherited in an autosomal dominant manner. Clinical manifestations typically include involuntary movement (choreoathetosis), dementia, and rigidity. The disease typically presents in the fourth or fifth decades of life. The disease is progressive with death occurring 10 to 15 years following its onset. On imaging (as in this case), Huntington's disease is characterized by atrophy of the caudate nuclei, which results in ballooning of the frontal horns of the lateral ventricles ("boxcar" ventricles). There may also be involvement of the putamen, which undergo volume loss. MRI may show signal changes in these nuclei. These changes may be hyperintense on T2W images (as in this case) believed to be related to gliosis; other cases show T2W hypointensity, which is likely related to iron deposition. Other findings include cortical atrophy.

Notes

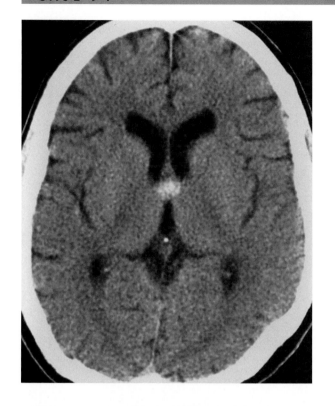

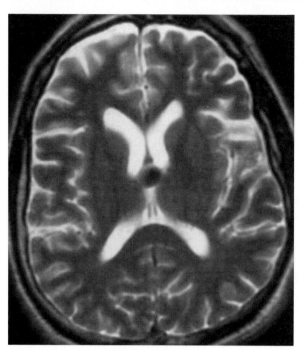

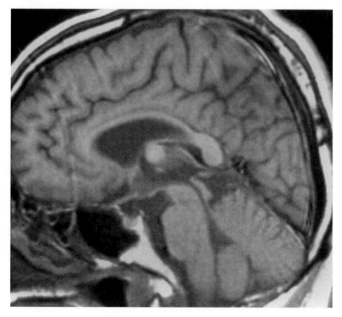

1. Where anatomically is this lesion located?
2. What is the enhancement pattern of these lesions?
3. What is the management of these lesions when they are symptomatic?
4. When symptomatic, what is a common clinical presentation?

Colloid Cyst

1. At the superior aspect of the anterior third ventricle, between the fornices.

2. With the exception of mild thin peripheral enhancement of the epithelial lining, these lesions should not demonstrate enhancement.

3. Stereotactic aspiration, surgical resection, and/or shunting.

4. Signs and symptoms of hydrocephalus (headache, nausea, vomiting) that may be positional and intermittent.

Reference

Waggenspack GA, Guinto FC Jr: MR and CT of masses of the anterosuperior third ventricle, *AJNR Am J Neuroradiol* 10: 105-110, 1989.

Cross-Reference

Neuroradiology: THE REQUISITES, pp 511-512.

Comment

Colloid cysts are benign masses typically located in the superior aspect of the anterior third ventricle in relation to the columns of the fornix. They are lined by a single layer of epithelium and represent the most common type of neuroepithelial cyst (although the origin of these cysts has been debated). Many of these lesions are incidental findings in patients being evaluated for other reasons. Alternatively, patients may present with hydrocephalus due to obstruction at the foramen of Monro. Although other mass lesions may occur in this region, including those related to the choroid plexus, gliomas, craniopharyngiomas, and occasionally meningiomas, it is not usually difficult to distinguish a colloid cyst because of its somewhat characteristic radiologic appearance.

Within colloid cysts is thick mucoid material, as well as a variety of other products including old blood, CSF, protein, and paramagnetic ions such as magnesium. The contents of these cysts result in their extremely variable signal characteristics on CT and MRI. Depending on the specific makeup of the individual cyst, on unenhanced CT these lesions may be anywhere from isodense to extremely hyperdense to the CSF and brain tissue. Colloid cysts also vary somewhat extensively in their signal characteristics on MRI, ranging from very high to low intensity on both unenhanced T1W and T2W images. A thin wall is usually seen that commonly enhances following contrast administration; however, a colloid cyst should never have solid enhancement.

Notes

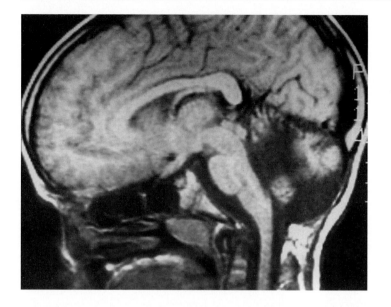
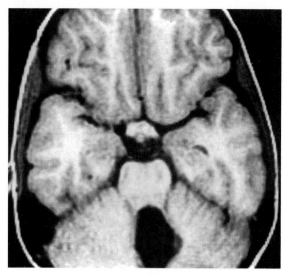
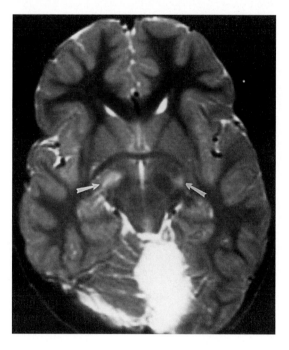
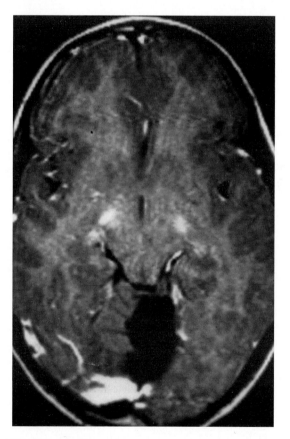

1. What anatomic structures *(arrows)* have abnormal T2W hyperintensity?
2. What imaging finding is diagnostic of neurofibromatosis type 2?
3. What is the usual histology of optic pathway gliomas in patients with neurofibromatosis type 1?
4. What neoplasms are seen with an increased incidence in patients with neurofibromatosis type 1?

Optic Pathway Glioma—Neurofibromatosis Type 1 (von Recklinghausen's Disease)

1. The posterior optic pathways (optic tracts and radiations).

2. Bilateral acoustic schwannoma.

3. Pilocytic astrocytoma.

4. Neurofibrosarcoma (malignant degeneration of a neurofibroma) in up to 5% of patients, pilocytic astrocytoma, leukemia, lymphoma, medullary thyroid carcinoma, pheochromocytoma, melanoma, and Wilms' tumor.

Reference

Pomeranz SJ, Shelton JJ, Tobias J, Soila K, Altman D, Viamonte M: MR of visual pathways in patients with neurofibromatosis, *AJNR Am J Neuroradiol* 8:831-836, 1987.

Cross-Reference

Neuroradiology: THE REQUISITES, pp 266-267.

Comment

The most common CNS tumor in neurofibromatosis type 1 is optic nerve glioma, reported in 15% to 28% of patients. These are benign, low grade neoplasms with pilocytic histology that involve one or both optic nerves and extend to the chiasm. Growth along the optic tract, the lateral geniculate, and the optic radiations may occur. MRI is the best imaging modality for assessing the extent of these tumors. Their signal intensity and enhancement patterns are variable. Typically when there is posterior extension along the optic tracts and radiations there is enhancement. In this case the optic chiasm is enlarged, with extension along the posterior optic pathways *(arrows)*.

Neurofibromatosis type 1 is caused by a mutation of chromosome 17. In half of the cases this mutation is transmitted by autosomal dominant inheritance; in the other half it is sporadic. Neurofibromatosis type 1 can be diagnosed when two or more of the following criteria are present: a first-degree relative with neurofibromatosis type 1, one plexiform neurofibroma or two or more neurofibromas of any type, six or more cafe-au-lait spots, two or more Lisch nodules (iris hamartomas), axillary or inguinal freckling, optic pathway glioma, and/or a characteristic bone abnormality (dysplasia of the greater wing of the sphenoid, overgrowth of a digit or limb, pseudarthrosis, lateral thoracic meningocele, dural ectasia with vertebral dysplasia).

Low grade astrocytic tumors in locations other than the optic pathways such as the brain stem are also seen with increased incidence in neurofibromatosis type 1. In this case the patient had prior resection of a cerebellar astrocytoma. Neurofibromatosis type 1 may be associated with nonneoplastic hyperintense lesions on T2W sequences within the basal ganglia, cerebellar peduncles, brain stem, and white matter.

Notes

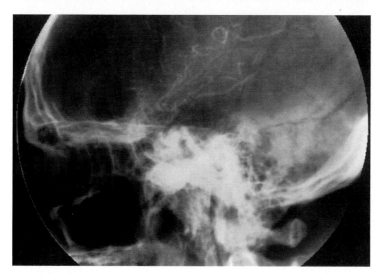
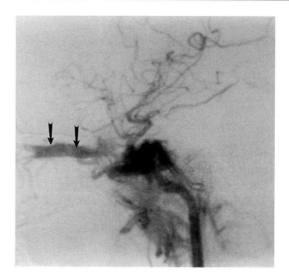

1. What is the most common cause of this lesion?
2. What is the structure labeled with arrows?
3. What is believed to be the cause of dural malformations involving the cavernous sinus?
4. In cases of high flow carotid-cavernous fistulas, filling of the contralateral venous system may occur through what communicating veins?

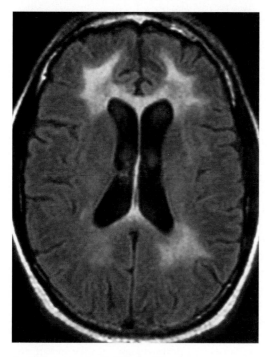
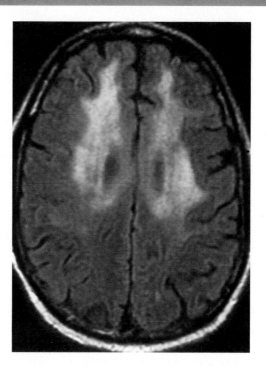

1. What are the MRI findings?
2. In a patient with HIV infection, what are the differential diagnostic considerations?
3. What MRI findings would favor neoplasm over encephalopathy or demyelinating disease (PML)?
4. What clinical presentation might help distinguish HIV encephalopathy from PML or primary CNS lymphoma?

Carotid-Cavernous Fistula

1. Trauma.

2. The superior ophthalmic vein.

3. Venous thrombosis.

4. The inferior petrosal venous plexus, as well as small veins bridging the right and left cavernous sinuses.

Reference

Elster AD, Chen MY, Richardson DN, Yeatts PR: Dilated intercavernous sinuses: an MR sign of carotid-cavernous and carotid-dural fistulas, *AJNR Am J Neuroradiol* 12:641-645, 1991.

Cross-Reference

Neuroradiology: THE REQUISITES, pp 294-296, 326-327.

Comment

There are two basic types of carotid-cavernous vascular malformations, "direct" and "indirect," each of which has a different etiology. Carotid-cavernous fistulas represent a "direct" communication between the intracavernous portion of the internal carotid artery and the cavernous venous sinus. The typical clinical presentation is that of proptosis, pain, chemosis, and orbital bruit. These symptoms are most commonly related to head trauma; however, carotid-cavernous fistulas may be seen in a spectrum of disorders, including atherosclerosis in the elderly, rupture of a cavernous-carotid aneurysm, or in association with underlying vascular dysplasias. An "indirect" carotid-cavernous vascular malformation, otherwise known as a dural arteriovenous fistula (AVF), is a shunt between meningeal branches of the internal and/or external carotid arteries and the cavernous sinus.

Management of these lesions in the majority of cases is usually with interventional neuroradiologic procedures. Treatment of direct and indirect fistulas may differ. Direct carotid-cavernous fistulas are usually treated transarterially with coil or balloon embolization. Complicated carotid-cavernous fistulas, residual carotid-cavernous fistulas following embolization from an arterial approach, and dural AVFs of the cavernous sinus may sometimes be treated transvenously. Gamma knife radiosurgery has also been shown to be effective in treating these dural AVFs.

The clinical presentation and imaging findings are normally diagnostic of a carotid-cavernous fistula. CT and MRI often demonstrate enlargement of the superior ophthalmic vein, cavernous sinus, and/or inferior petrosal sinus. Proptosis, periorbital soft tissue swelling, and diffuse enlargement of the extraocular muscles are commonly present. Catheter angiography demonstrates direct communication between the cavernous internal carotid artery and the cavernous sinus; and early filling of the ipsilateral cavernous sinus, superior and/or inferior ophthalmic veins, and petrosal venous complex. In very high flow lesions, the contralateral venous system may opacify.

Notes

Human Immunodeficiency Virus Encephalopathy

1. Bilateral increased signal intensity in the periventricular and deep white matter; global cortical atrophy.

2. HIV encephalopathy (direct infection with the retrovirus), CMV infection, demyelinating disease (PML), and neoplasm (lymphoma).

3. The presence of mass effect and/or enhancement associated with lesions other than PML.

4. HIV encephalopathy typically presents with progressive dementia and cognitive decline (in talking with the patient, the symptoms usually precede radiologic evidence of encephalopathy). In contrast, PML and lymphoma may present with focal neurologic symptoms.

Reference

Post MJ, Berger JR, Duncan R, Quencer RM, Pall L, Winfield D: Asymptomatic and neurologically symptomatic HIV-seropositive subjects: results of long-term MR imaging and clinical follow-up, *Radiology* 188:727-733, 1993.

Cross-Reference

Neuroradiology: THE REQUISITES, pp 185-186.

Comment

The main cells targeted for direct infection with HIV are macrophages and multinucleated giant cells. The HIV virus is in the CNS in up to 75% of AIDS patients undergoing pathologic evaluation. Clinical symptoms may be useful in differentiating HIV encephalopathy from other disorders. HIV encephalopathy presents with progressive cognitive decline and dementia. Unlike PML or primary CNS lymphoma, focal neurologic deficits are much less common. Although CMV may have a similar clinical and radiologic appearance as HIV encephalopathy, the majority of AIDS-related dementia cases are believed to be secondary to direct infection with HIV.

CT is insensitive to the findings of HIV encephalopathy. MRI may be normal. When abnormal, the most common MRI finding is global atrophy. Evaluation of T2W images may show hyperintense lesions within the periventricular white matter, including the centrum semiovale and corona radiata. There may be deep gray matter involvement. The lesion distribution may be quite variable. Although unilateral disease, multifocal disease, and bilateral asymmetric disease may be present, HIV encephalopathy and encephalitis are more commonly diffuse with confluent, symmetric periventricular T2W hyperintensity, as in this case. Lesions characteristically do not enhance and are not associated with mass effect. Serial MRI examinations have shown progression of atrophy and white matter changes (which become more diffuse and confluent). The extent of disease may parallel neurologic deterioration.

Notes

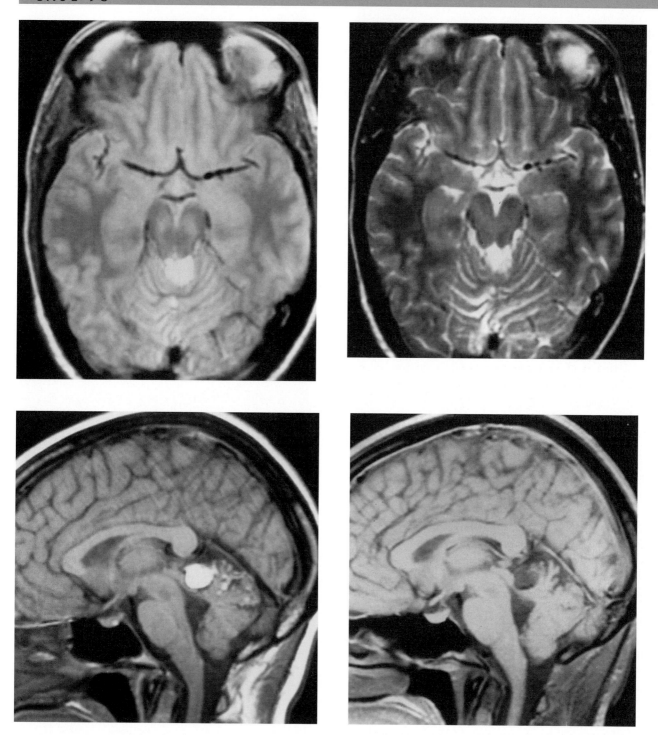

1. What substances are hyperintense on unenhanced T1W imaging?

2. On MRI, what other findings are indicative of the presence of fat?

3. Among epidermoid, dermoid, and teratomatous lesions, which is most likely to be associated with enhancement following the administration of intravenous contrast material?

4. What causes chemical shift artifact?

Ruptured Dermoid

1. Fat, proteinaceous material, methemoglobin (hemorrhage), manganese, some calcium, liquid cholesterol, pantopaque contrast, and melanin.

2. Chemical shift artifact. In addition, fat is hyperintense on fast spin echo T2W images and hypointense on conventional spin echo images. When there is a question, fat suppression with T1W imaging can be applied to confirm the presence of fat.

3. Teratoma.

4. Fat and water precess at slightly different Larmor frequencies (fat precesses more slowly). For correct spatial localization, the Larmor frequency must be uniform throughout the section. Therefore chemical shift artifact results because the position of fat protons relative to water is altered during frequency encoding because its signal is assumed to originate from an incorrect location.

Reference

Smith AS, Benson JE, Blaser SI, Mizushima A, Tarr RW, Bellon EM: Diagnosis of ruptured intracranial dermoid cysts: value of MR over CT, *AJNR Am J Neuroradiol* 12:175-180, 1991.

Cross-Reference

Neuroradiology: THE REQUISITES, pp 76-77, 320.

Comment

Epidermoid and dermoid lesions are developmental anomalies that may be considered congenital inclusions within the neural tube related to incomplete dysjunction of the neuroectoderm from the cutaneous ectoderm. Both lesions are of epidermal origin and may be associated with dermal sinuses or a bone defect. Dermoid lesions typically occur in or near the midline. In the intracranial compartment, they may be found in the parasellar, frontal, basal surface of the brain and in the posterior fossa. Within the posterior fossa, the superior cerebellar cistern and fourth ventricular regions are the most common locations.

On CT, dermoids are decreased in attenuation (less than −120 Hounsfield units) because of their fat content. Calcification may be seen in the periphery of the lesion. On MRI dermoids show the signal characteristics of fat, and chemical shift artifact is frequently seen. When necessary, fat suppression can be applied to confirm the diagnosis. Compare the third image in this case, which is an unenhanced T1W image, with the last image, which is an unenhanced T1W image with frequency selective fat saturation applied. Importantly, dermoid lesions (as in this case) have a tendency to rupture into the subarachnoid spaces and/or within the ventricles. It is important on imaging to check for fat droplets within these locations. When rupture occurs, an inflammatory chemical meningitis may occur. Dermoid cysts may contain dermal appendages, including sebaceous and sweat glands, as well as hair follicles.

Notes

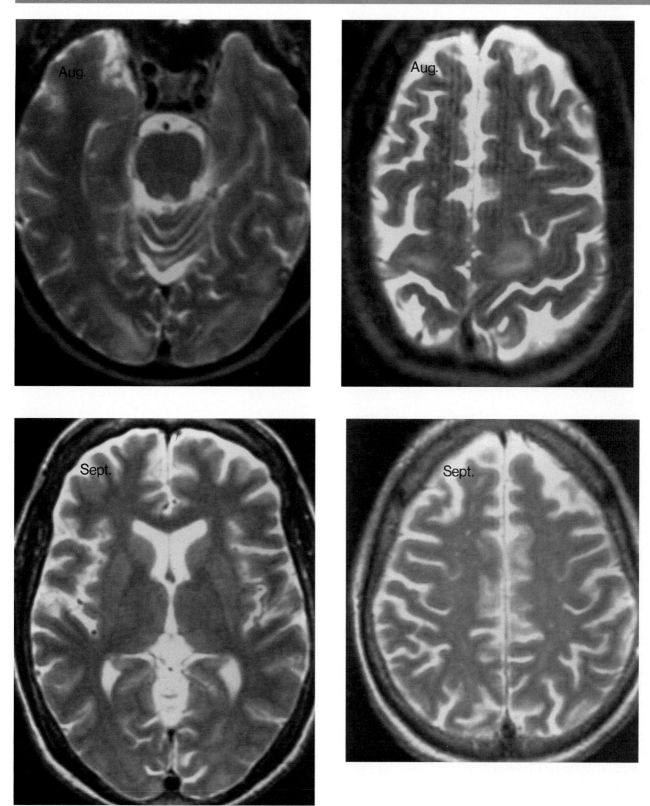

1. What is the most common cause of hypertensive encephalopathy in women?

2. What are some other causes of hypertensive encephalopathy?

3. What areas of the brain are particularly prone to the changes of hypertension?

4. What are the most common imaging findings in hypertensive encephalopathy?

Malignant Hypertension With Partial Resolution of the Imaging Findings Following Treatment

1. Pregnancy-related hypertension (toxemia/eclampsia).

2. Noncompliance with hypertensive medications, thrombotic thrombocytopenic purpura, hemolytic-uremic syndrome, renal dialysis, cyclosporine use.

3. The cerebellum and occipital lobes (the posterior circulation).

4. CT shows low attenuation in areas of involvement, whereas T2W images show foci of increased signal intensity within the cortex and subcortical white matter that is frequently bilateral and somewhat symmetric.

Reference

Schwartz RB, Jones KM, Kalina P, et al: Hypertensive encephalopathy: findings on CT, MR imaging and SPECT imaging in fourteen cases, *AJR Am J Roentgenol* 159:379-383, 1992.

Cross-Reference

Neuroradiology: THE REQUISITES, p 118.

Comment

The first two images (August; blood pressure 200/130) show foci of increased signal intensity within the subcortical white matter (and cortex) that is predominantly in the occipital lobes; however, regions of signal alteration are also present in the parietal lobes. Follow-up images (September) show significant partial resolution of the abnormalities following treatment of the patient's hypertension. This case illustrates many of the typical imaging manifestations of hypertensive encephalopathy. The posterior circulation is more sensitive to the changes of accelerated hypertension. This may be related to a difference in the sympathetic innervation. One theory is that the normal autoregulatory control of the cerebral vasculature that allows continuous perfusion over a range of blood pressures is exceeded. This may result in engorgement of distal cerebral vessels with breakdown of the blood-brain barrier. Signal abnormalities may represent reversible vasogenic edema. Although the radiologic findings are nonspecific (seen in a variety of disorders such as cyclosporine toxicity), the imaging findings in combination with the patient's clinical presentation (elevated blood pressure associated with progressive neurologic symptoms, including change in mental status, headache, blurred vision, seizures, and/or focal neurologic deficits) allow correct diagnosis. Both symptomatology and radiologic findings may be reversible with treatment of the blood pressure.

In addition to foci of abnormal signal intensity at the gray-white matter interface, the basal ganglia and white matter tracts of the corpus striatum may be involved. Enhancement in regions of signal abnormality may be observed. Acute hemorrhage may be present, although this is less common.

Notes

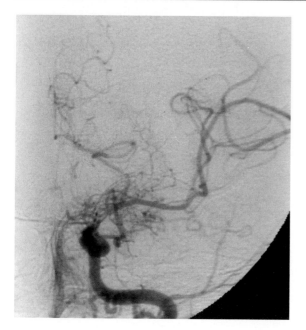 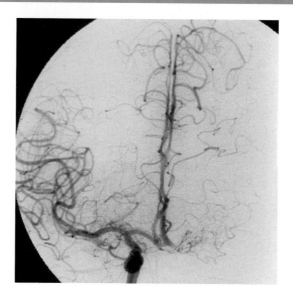

1. What are the pertinent angiographic findings?
2. What disorders have been associated with these angiographic findings?
3. What is the characteristic clinical presentation in children with this disorder?
4. This disorder in particular has a predilection for individuals of what nationality?

Moyamoya Disease

1. Marked narrowing of the left supraclinoid internal carotid artery, occlusion of the proximal left anterior cerebral artery, and collateral vessels from the external carotid circulation as well as the perforating vessels in the basal ganglia.

2. Sickle cell disease, neurofibromatosis type 1, atherosclerosis, and radiation therapy. However, in many cases these findings are idiopathic.

3. Transient ischemic attacks and/or strokes.

4. Japanese.

Reference

Yamada I, Matsushima Y, Suzuki S: Moyamoya disease: diagnosis with three-dimensional time-of-flight MR angiography, *Radiology* 184:773-778, 1992.

Cross-Reference

Neuroradiology: THE REQUISITES, p 117.

Comment

Moyamoya refers to slow, progressive occlusive disease of the distal intracranial internal carotid arteries and its proximal branches, including the anterior (A1) and middle (M1) cerebral arteries. There may also be involvement of the posterior cerebral arteries. Moyamoya disease is predominantly an idiopathic arteriopathy. However, a moyamoya pattern has been associated with a variety of conditions, including neurofibromatosis type 1, sickle cell disease, radiation therapy, chronic infection, and atherosclerosis. Because of the slowly progressive development of high grade stenoses and/or occlusions of the distal internal carotid arteries and/or its proximal branches, collateral circulation develops through a number of pathways, including leptomeningeal collaterals from the cerebral arteries; parenchymal collaterals through the perforating vessels (particularly the basal ganglia); and transdural collaterals, which most commonly arise from the external carotid artery (the ophthalmic artery and the middle meningeal artery).

Moyamoya disease is more symptomatic when it presents in childhood, typically with transient ischemic attacks and stroke. In adults the disease is less frequently symptomatic, but when it is it more commonly presents with intracranial hemorrhage. Catheter angiography shows narrowing and/or occlusion of the distal internal carotid artery and its proximal branches (as in this case). In addition, the late arterial phase in particular demonstrates the extensive collateral circulation. MRI may demonstrate occlusion of the distal internal carotid artery, and when the disease is severe enough multiple regions of hypointensity may be seen within the basal ganglia bilaterally, corresponding to the collateral network arising from the perforating arteries.

Notes

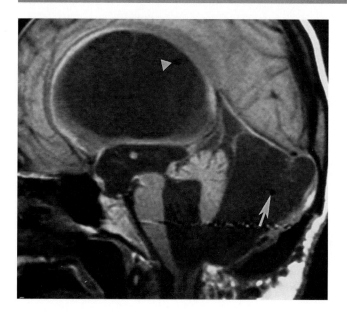
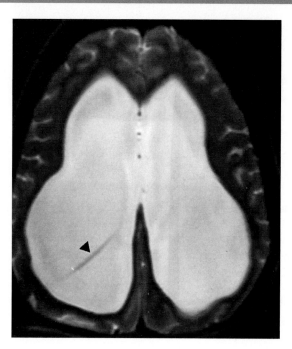

1. What are the major imaging findings?
2. What is the differential diagnosis of nonneoplastic posterior fossa cystlike masses?
3. Which of these lesions may be associated with enlargement of the posterior fossa?
4. Which of these cystlike masses is associated with supratentorial anomalies?

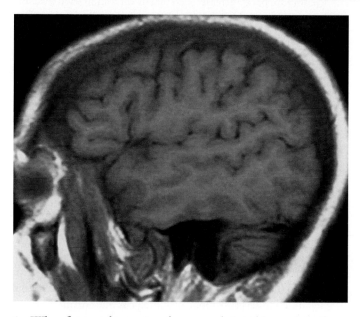

1. What factors determine the normal signal intensity of marrow?
2. What MRI pulse sequence is best for evaluating alterations of normal marrow signal intensity?
3. What is the normal T1W signal intensity of marrow in adults (after 21 years of age)?
4. What is the differential diagnosis for diffuse hypointensity of the calvarial marrow?

Dandy-Walker Malformation With Hydrocephalus

1. A cystic mass in the posterior fossa that is secondarily enlarged and hydrocephalus with dilation of the lateral and third ventricles.

2. Arachnoid cyst, Dandy-Walker malformation, and giant cisterna magna.

3. Dandy-Walker malformation and arachnoid cysts.

4. Dandy-Walker malformation.

Reference

Barkovich AJ, Kjos BO, Norman D, Edwards MS: Revised classification of posterior fossa cysts and cyst-like malformations based on the results of multiplanar MR imaging, *AJR Am J Roentgenol* 153:1289-1300, 1989.

Cross-Reference

Neuroradiology: THE REQUISITES, pp 259-261.

Comment

The Dandy-Walker complex (which includes Dandy-Walker malformation and its variants) is a congenital anomaly believed to be related to an in utero insult to the fourth ventricle leading to complete or partial outflow obstruction of CSF. As a result, there is cystlike dilation of the fourth ventricle, which protrudes up between the cerebellar hemispheres to prevent their fusion, and there is incomplete formation of all or part of the inferior vermis. The spectrum of Dandy-Walker variant depends on the time in utero at which the insult occurs, as well as the severity of the insult (the degree of fourth ventricular outflow obstruction). Dandy-Walker malformations are associated with hydrocephalus in approximately 75% of cases. In addition, a significant number of patients have associated supratentorial anomalies, including dysgenesis of the corpus callosum, migrational anomalies, and encephaloceles.

This case demonstrates a large retrocerebellar cyst (with a shunt; *arrow*) and enlargement of the posterior fossa with remodeling of the inner table of the occipital bone. In addition, there is hydrocephalus resulting in thinning of the corpus callosum, as well as balloon dilation and inferior displacement of the infundibular and chiasmatic recesses of the third ventricle. A shunt is present in the lateral ventricle *(arrowhead)*. The radiologic hallmark of Dandy-Walker malformation is communication of a retrocerebellar cyst with the fourth ventricle, which is readily appreciated on MRI. However, following shunting of a cyst the cerebellar hemispheres are often in apposition (without an intervening inferior vermis) such that the direct communication is not seen (as in this case).

Notes

Diffuse Replacement of the Fat in the Diploic Space of the Calvaria (Chronic Anemia)

1. Cellularity, fat, and water content.

2. T1W imaging. Short TI inversion recovery and fat-saturated enhanced images may also be useful.

3. Hyperintense (isointense or hyperintense to the white matter).

4. Infiltrative processes of the marrow (hematopoietic malignancies, granulomatous disorders such as sarcoid or tuberculosis, myelofibrosis, metastases), chronic anemia, and dysplasias (Paget's disease, fibrous dysplasia, osteopetrosis).

Reference

Ricci C, Cova M, Kang YS, et al: Normal age-related patterns of cellular and fatty bone marrow distribution in the axial skeleton: MR imaging study, *Radiology* 177:83-88, 1990.

Cross-Reference

Neuroradiology: THE REQUISITES, pp 481-482.

Comments

This case has two purposes. The first is to remind radiologists to look at the edges of the film (the skull base and calvaria should be assessed in all patients). It is equally important to understand that the normal signal intensity of marrow is dependent on the ratio of cells, fat, and water. In children, hematopoietic (red) marrow has a high cell:fat ratio and is hypointense. As we age, the amount of fat increases such that by early adulthood (usually by 21 years of age) the marrow has undergone fatty conversion (yellow marrow) and on T1W images is isointense to hyperintense to white matter. Unenhanced T1W imaging is probably the best way to assess for marrow abnormalities. In order to detect enhancing lesions, fat suppression should be applied. In addition, lesions that are hyperintense on unenhanced T1W images (e.g., hemangioma or melanoma) may be missed. In patients with known melanoma, assessment of all of the pulse sequences obtained, as well as acquisition of unenhanced T1W images with the application of fat saturation (to suppress the normal marrow and make the hyperintense melanoma lesions more conspicuous), are useful.

The differential diagnosis of diffuse replacement of the fatty marrow with hypointense tissue (cells and/or water) includes hematologic malignancies (lymphoma, leukemia, and myeloma), granulomatous disease (sarcoid and tuberculosis), chronic anemias such as thalassemia, sickle cell disease, or chronic blood loss; and AIDS (hypointense marrow has been attributed to several factors, including chronic anemia and low CD4 counts). Metastases may diffusely replace the marrow (in my experience this is most common with breast carcinoma in women and prostate carcinoma in men). More often, metastatic disease presents with multiple focal lesions.

Notes

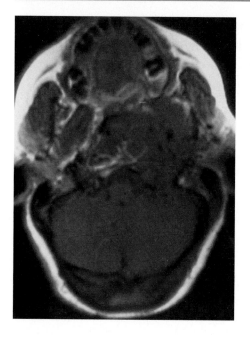
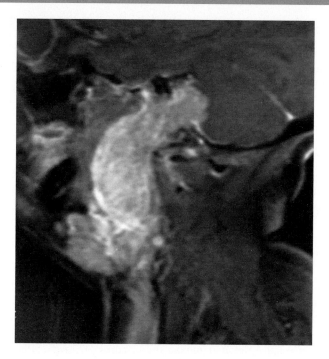

1. Where is the lesion located?

2. What is the differential diagnosis of an enhancing mass in this location?

3. What cranial nerves in the jugular foramen may give rise to nerve sheath tumors?

4. When this lesion arises in the middle ear along the cochlear promontory, what is it referred to as?

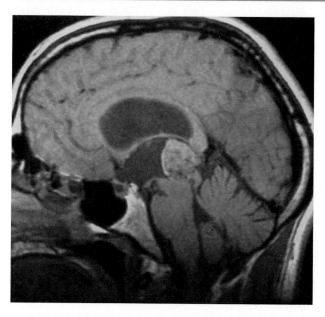
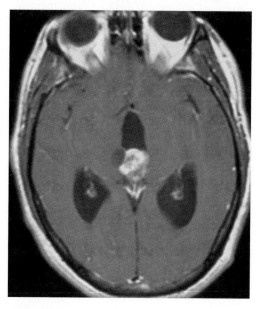

1. Based on the cells of origin, what are the two types of pineal tumors?

2. Which category of pineal tumors does not have a gender preference?

3. What is the most common germ cell tumor in the pineal region?

4. What is the typical imaging appearance of a germinoma on unenhanced CT?

Glomus Jugulare

1. The jugular foramen.

2. Glomus jugulare, metastatic disease, schwannoma, naso-pharyngeal carcinoma, and meningioma.

3. IX, X, and XI.

4. Glomus tympanicum.

Reference

Olsen WL, Dillon WP, Kelly WM, Norman D, Brant-Zawadzki M, Newton TH: MR imaging of paragangliomas, *AJR Am J Roentgenol* 148:201-204, 1987.

Cross-Reference

Neuroradiology: THE REQUISITES, pp 332, 346.

Comment

Glomus jugulare tumors (paragangliomas) are typically centered within the jugular foramen; however, they often extend superiorly into the middle ear cavity and inferiorly below the skull base. The exact origin of glomus tumors from cranial nerves IX and X is controversial. Glomus jugulare tumors arise from Arnold's nerve (auricular branches of the vagus nerve), whereas glomus tympanicum tumors arise from the auricular branch of the glossopharyngeal nerve (Jacobson's nerve). Glomus jugulare tumors arise in the lateral portion of the jugular foramen from the pars vascularis and on MRI frequently have a typical "salt and pepper" appearance related to enhancing tumor with extensive vascularity seen as multiple flow voids. Although this appearance is somewhat characteristic of paraganglioma, vascular metastases such as renal cell or thyroid carcinoma may have a similar imaging appearance. In addition to metastases, other enhancing mass lesions in this location include schwannomas and occasionally meningiomas. Schwannomas typically arise from the pars nervosa in the medial portion of the jugular foramen (although the pars vascularis contains cranial nerves X and XI, and so schwannomas may occur here also) and may displace the jugular vein. In contrast, glomus jugulare tumors almost always involve the jugular vein, which may be filled with tumor. In addition, metastases and glomus tumors often result in bony erosion of the jugular foramen and temporal bone, whereas schwannomas tend to result in smooth remodeling. Finally, chordomas and chondroid lesions may arise in this location; however, they are usually readily distinguished due to typical imaging characteristics (such as the presence of stippled calcification).

Notes

Pineal Germinoma

1. Germ cell origin and pineal cell origin.

2. Those of pineal cell origin (pineoblastoma, pineocytoma).

3. Germinoma (also referred to as seminoma or dysgerminoma).

4. A hyperdense mass.

Reference

Kilgore DP, Strother CM, Strashak RJ, Haughton VM: Pineal germinoma: MR imaging, *Radiology* 158:435-438, 1986.

Cross-Reference

Neuroradiology: THE REQUISITES, pp 95-96.

Comment

The majority of pineal tumors are of germ cell origin. There are a variety of histologies of germ cell tumors; however, germinoma accounts for the majority of these lesions, comprising 65% of all pineal germ cell neoplasms and approximately 40% of all pineal region tumors. Other germ cell tumors that occur in the pineal region include teratoma, embryonal carcinoma, and choriocarcinoma. This case demonstrates a pineal region mass that is heterogeneous on the unenhanced T1W image. The small regions of hypointensity represent calcification on CT. There is controversy as to whether germinomas calcify because the normal pineal gland is calcified and the degree of calcification increases with age. Therefore, it is uncertain whether the calcification seen in these lesions represents tumor engulfing normal pineal gland calcification or calcification within tumor matrix. Due to their marked cellularity, germinomas are typically hyperdense on unenhanced CT and isointense to brain on T2W MRI. Cystic change is uncommon (although a cyst is seen in this case), and following contrast these lesions typically demonstrate prominent enhancement. Teratomas may be distinguished from other germ cell tumors due to the presence of fat, calcification, and cyst formation (the fat and calcification/bone may have characteristic appearances on imaging). Choriocarcinomas may be differentiated due to the high incidence of hemorrhage within these tumors. In addition, β-human chorionic-gonadotropin is a good serum marker for choriocarcinoma. Less common germ cell tumors, including embryonal cell carcinoma, endodermal sinus (yolk sac) tumors, and teratomas, may have hormonal markers such as β-human chorionic-gonadotropin and AFP.

Notes

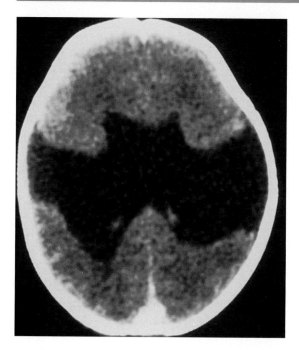

1. This lesion is classified as what type of abnormality?

2. This finding in combination with absence of the septum pellucidum and optic nerve hypoplasia is consistent with what diagnosis?

3. What associated migrational abnormality is typically seen in the adjacent cortex?

4. Porencephalic cysts are lined by what type of tissue?

Schizencephaly*

1. Migrational anomaly.

2. Septo-optic dysplasia.

3. Polymicrogyria.

4. White matter.

References

Barkovich AJ, Kjos BO: Schizencephaly: correlation of clinical findings with MR characteristics, *AJNR Am J Neuroradiol* 13:85-94, 1992.

Barkovich AJ, Norman D: MR imaging of schizencephaly, *AJR Am J Roentgenol* 150:1391-1396, 1988.

Cross-Reference

Neuroradiology: THE REQUISITES, pp 253-254.

Comment

Schizencephaly is a migrational abnormality that result from an insult to the germinal matrix and causes failure of normal migration and neuronal differentiation. Specifically, this anomaly is believed to be related to an in utero watershed ischemic event leading to damage not only to the germinal matrix but also to the radial glial fibers along which the neurons normally migrate to their final destination in the cortex. As a result, schizencephaly extends from the ventricular surface to the subarachnoid surface of the brain and is lined by dysplastic gray matter. Usually there is a CSF cleft between the layers of gray matter. When the CSF cleft is large and gaping it is referred to as "open-lip" schizencephaly. When the layers of gray matter are in apposition or there is only a thin layer of CSF between them, the condition is referred to as "closed-lip" schizencephaly.

Up to 25% to 50% of patients with schizencephaly have septo-optic dysplasia. Patients with migrational anomalies usually present with a seizure disorder. Depending on the size of the migrational abnormality, there may also be focal neurologic deficits such as hemiparesis. MRI is the imaging modality of choice to assess these abnormalities. Closed-lip schizencephaly, when the gray matter layers are apposed, may be difficult to detect. A small ventricular "dimple" or diverticulum may be a tip-off to the diagnosis and should prompt a close search for closed-lip schizencephaly. Other conditions that may cause dimpling of the ventricle are prior insults such as periventricular ischemia or infection.

Notes

---

*Figure for Case 105 courtesy Jill Langer, MD.

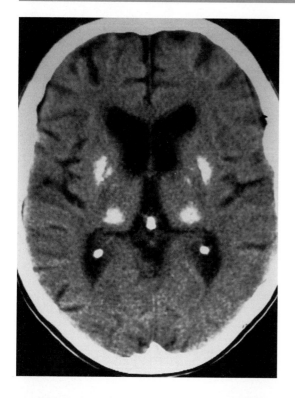

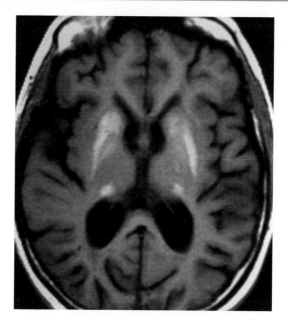

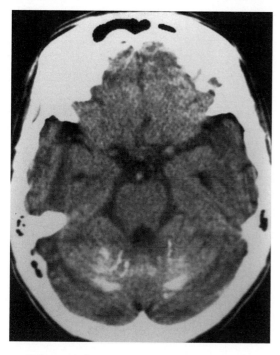

1. What are the pertinent imaging findings?
2. What toxic exposure classically causes abnormal hypodensity in the globus pallidus bilaterally?
3. What toxic exposure has been associated with calcification of the basal ganglia?
4. In Hallervorden-Spatz syndrome there is accelerated iron deposition in what structures?

Fahr Disease (Familial Cerebrovascular Ferrocalcinosis)

1. Bilaterally symmetric calcification within the basal ganglia, thalami, and dentate nuclei of the cerebellum.

2. Carbon monoxide poisoning.

3. Lead toxicity.

4. The globus pallidus, substantia nigra, and red nuclei.

Reference

Wolpert SM, Anderson ML, Kaye EM: Metabolic and degenerative disorders. In Wolpert SM, Barnes PD, editors: *MRI in pediatric neuroradiology,* St Louis, 1992, Mosby, pp 121-150.

Cross-Reference

Neuroradiology: THE REQUISITES, pp 236-237.

Comment

This case shows bilateral, symmetric calcification within the basal ganglia (including the caudate and lentiform nuclei), thalami, and dentate nuclei of the cerebellum. Calcification is also seen along the cerebellum. Fahr disease represents a variety of disorders characterized by extensive bilateral basal ganglia calcifications, as well as variable neurologic manifestations, including movement disorders and psychologic impairment. Calcification may also be seen in the dentate nuclei (as in this case), as well as within the white matter, including the centrum semiovale, corona radiata, and subcortical white matter. Familial patterns of Fahr disease have been noted. In addition, hypoparathyroidism has not infrequently been identified. Symptomatic patients may respond to correction of serum calcium phosphate abnormalities.

The differential diagnosis of calcification within the deep gray matter of the cerebral hemispheres, particularly the basal ganglia, is extensive. Probably the most common cause is idiopathic. Calcification in the globus pallidus bilaterally may be noted as a normal finding representing senescent calcification in the elderly. A variety of endocrine disorders, including abnormalities in phosphate and calcium metabolism, may result in calcification in these locations. Another common cause of calcification is in the postinflammatory setting. Specifically, calcification may be seen in such infections as tuberculosis and cysticercosis. In recent years, calcification within the basal ganglia has been described in in utero HIV infection.

Notes

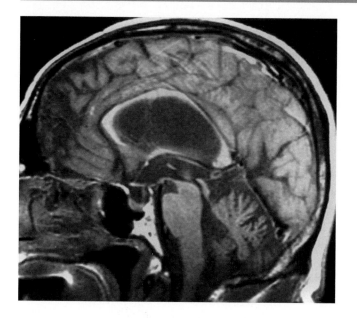

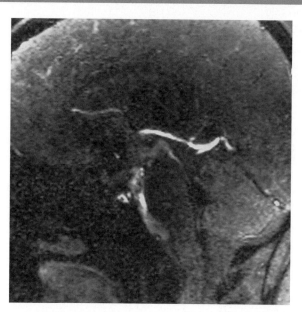

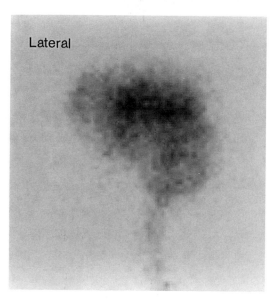

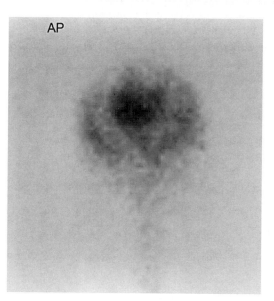

1. What is the diagnosis?

2. What clinical triad may be present in this elderly patient?

3. In normal-pressure hydrocephalus (NPH), what are the imaging findings in a positive isotope (indium-DTPA) cisternogram?

4. Who gets external hydrocephalus, and what are the radiologic findings?

Normal-Pressure Hydrocephalus

1. Communicating hydrocephalus.

2. Gait disturbance, urinary incontinence, and dementia.

3. Reflux of isotope into the ventricular system and to a lesser extent the sylvian cisterns, and no ascent of the radiotracer over the cerebral convexities at 24 hours.

4. Typically it is seen in children younger than 2 years of age and results from decreased resorption of CSF at the arachnoid villi. Imaging typically shows enlargement of the cerebral sulci (especially in the frontal region and along the interhemispheric fissure). In contrast to NPH and other types of communicating hydrocephalus, the ventricles are relatively normal in size; this may be because the cranial sutures are still open (instead there may be mild enlargement of the head circumference).

Reference

Bradley WG Jr, Scalzo D, Queralt J, Nitz WN, Atkinson DJ, Wong P: Normal-pressure hydrocephalus: evaluation with cerebrospinal fluid flow measurements at MR imaging, *Radiology* 198:523-529, 1996.

Cross-Reference

Neuroradiology: THE REQUISITES, pp 240-241.

Comment

In NPH the lateral ventricles (particularly the temporal horns) and third ventricle are enlarged in comparison with the fourth ventricle. Distention of the lateral ventricles may result in thinning and elevation of the corpus callosum, whereas enlargement of the third ventricle may result in dilation of the infundibular and optic recesses, which may be displaced inferiorly. Patients typically have accentuation of the flow void in the aqueduct of Sylvius on spin echo images, and CSF flow in the aqueduct may be demonstrated on flow-sensitive gradient echo imaging. Transependymal CSF spread may be present.

Although the cause of NPH is still debated, it is believed to result most often from remote intracranial hemorrhage or infection (meningeal). Others have suggested that ischemic injury or edema in the periventricular white matter reduces the tensile strength of the ventricles, resulting in their enlargement. Some patients with NPH have marked improvement of their symptomatology following shunting. Response to shunting is most favorable when ataxia is the predominant symptom, the patient has had symptoms for only a short time, isotope cisternography is positive, the patient has a known history of prior intracranial hemorrhage or infection, MRI shows a prominent CSF flow void in the aqueduct, and there is relative absence of deep periventricular white matter atrophy. Lumbar puncture with removal of 15 to 30 ml of CSF and subsequent improvement of clinical symptoms may also indicate a patient who might respond to shunting.

Notes

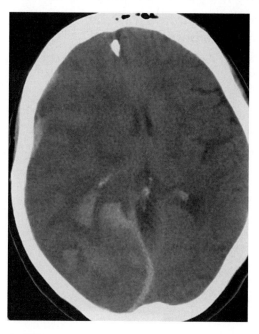
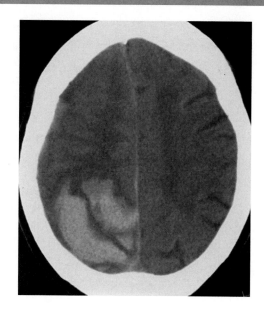

1. What are some common causes of nontraumatic intracranial hemorrhage?
2. What is the major risk factor for amyloid angiopathy?
3. What regions of the brain are typically spared in amyloid angiopathy?
4. What MRI findings suggest the diagnosis of amyloid angiopathy?

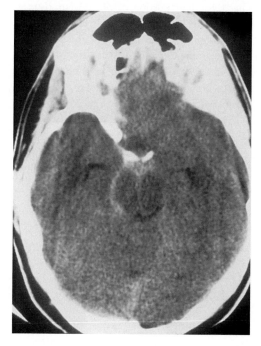

1. What is the pertinent radiologic finding?
2. What is the probability that an aneurysm will be found on conventional catheter angiography?
3. What is believed to be the cause of nontraumatic, nonaneurysmal subarachnoid hemorrhages?
4. In the posterior circulation, what is the most common location for a saccular aneurysm?

Amyloid Angiopathy

1. The causes are numerous, and some may be separated by age of presentation. Common etiologies include hypertension, underlying vascular malformations, hemorrhagic stroke, coagulopathies, blood dyscrasias, recreational drug use (cocaine), pregnancy (eclampsia), vasculitis, amyloid angiopathy, and infection (e.g., aspergillus).

2. Age.

3. The basal ganglia, brain stem, and cerebellum.

4. Multiple, peripherally located hemorrhages of different ages.

Reference

Awasthi D, Voorhies RM, Eick J, Mitchell WT: Cerebral amyloid angiopathy presenting as multiple intracranial lesions on magnetic resonance imaging, *J Neurosurg* 75:458-460, 1991.

Cross-Reference

Neuroradiology: THE REQUISITES, pp 132-133.

Comment

Central nervous system amyloid angiopathy results from deposition of β-pleated proteins within the walls of small- and medium-sized vessels of the cortex and leptomeninges. Amyloid deposition increases with age and results in loss of elasticity of involved vessels. On pathologic examination microaneurysms are often present. Amyloid stains intensely with Congo red dye (previously referred to as "congophilic angiopathy") and demonstrates yellow-green birefringence under polarized light.

On CT and MRI hemorrhages are characteristically lobar in location. Multiple hemorrhages of different ages, as well as multiple simultaneous hemorrhages, are often present. Subarachnoid and subdural blood may be present due to perforation of blood through the piaarachnoid or involvement of superficial blood vessels with amyloid deposition. MRI, including gradient echo images, may be especially useful for demonstrating the full extent of intracranial involvement (CT readily reveals acute hemorrhages; however, regions of old blood products are often occult). Patients may have numerous small subcortical regions of focal hypointensity (multiple hypointense foci may also be related to cavernomas and/or microhemorrhages such as is seen in hypertension). Importantly, there is no association of hypertension in the development of amyloid angiopathy.

Notes

Nonaneurysmal Perimesencephalic Subarachnoid Hemorrhage

1. Acute subarachnoid hemorrhage localized in the cisterns anterior to the brain stem, the interpeduncular cistern, and the ambient cisterns.

2. Very low.

3. Rupture of small veins and/or capillaries.

4. The basilar artery tip.

Reference

Rinkel GJE, Wijdicks EFM, Vermeulen M, et al: Nonaneurysmal perimesencephalic subarachnoid hemorrhage: CT and MR patterns that differ from aneurysmal rupture, *AJNR Am J Neuroradiol* 12:829-834, 1991.

Cross-Reference

Neuroradiology: THE REQUISITES, pp 139-140.

Comment

Nonaneurysmal perimesencephalic subarachnoid hemorrhage is an increasingly recognized cause of nontraumatic subarachnoid hemorrhage. These patients typically present in adulthood with an acute headache. On CT acute subarachnoid hemorrhage is present and has a somewhat characteristic location. Specifically, hemorrhage is noted predominantly in the cisterns around the brain stem, including the prepontine, interpeduncular, and ambient cisterns. A small amount of hemorrhage may be present in the dependent portion of the sylvian cisterns. Significant intraventricular hemorrhage should not be present, and blood is not usually localized in the anterior interhemispheric fissure. Catheter angiography (which currently should still be performed even in the presence of a characteristic localization of subarachnoid hemorrhage) reveals no aneurysm. Subarachnoid hemorrhage in nonaneurysmal bleeds is believed to be related to venous or capillary rupture. In the presence of a characteristic pattern of subarachnoid hemorrhage and a negative high quality conventional angiogram, follow-up angiography may not be necessary. Patients with this type of subarachnoid hemorrhage generally have an excellent prognosis.

Notes

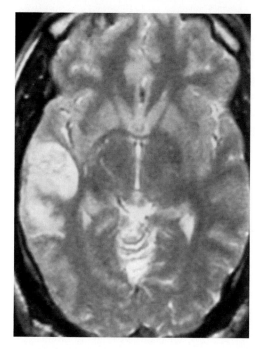 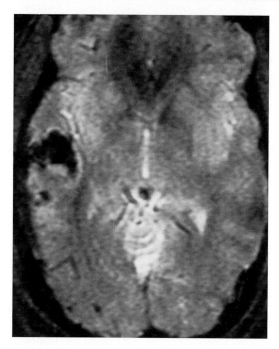

1. What are the two common types of antiphospholipid antibodies?

2. In hypercoagulable states related to antiphospholipids antibodies, which is more common in the cerebrovascular circulation, arterial or venous infarcts?

3. What particular group of patients has a high incidence of circulating antiphospholipid antibodies?

4. What kidney disorder is associated with a hypercoagulable state?

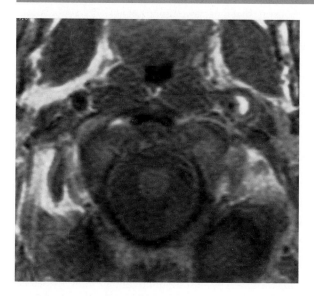

1. What structure is abnormal?

2. What is the cause of the high signal intensity around the vessel?

3. What is the advantage of acquiring fat-suppressed unenhanced T1W images?

4. How might this patient have presented clinically?

CASE 110

Hemorrhagic Venous Infarction

1. Lupus anticoagulant and anticardiolipin.

2. Arterial.

3. Those with systemic lupus erythematosus.

4. Nephrotic syndrome.

References

Provenzale JM, Heinz ER, Ortel TL, Macik BG, Charles LA, Alberts MJ: Antiphospholipid antibodies in patients without systemic lupus erythematosus: neuroradiologic findings, *Radiology* 192:531-537, 1994.

Provenzale JM, Loganbill HA: Dural sinus thrombosis and venous infarction associated with antiphospholipid antibodies: MR findings, *J Comput Assist Tomogr* 18:719-723, 1994.

Cross-Reference

Neuroradiology: THE REQUISITES, pp 131-132.

Comment

This case illustrates a hemorrhagic venous infarction in the right temporal lobe. Unlike arterial infarctions, the anatomic territories for venous occlusive disease are less consistent than with the territory supplied by arteries. Several findings should at least raise suspicion of a venous infarct: (1) the presence of hemorrhage, especially in the white matter or at the gray-white matter interface; (2) the presence of an abnormality that is not in a single arterial distribution; and (3) an infarct in a young patient. This patient had acute thrombosis of the superior sagittal sinus (note the hyperdense clot in the superior sagittal sinus as well as the right transverse sinus). The hemorrhagic infarct in the right temporal lobe is in the territory drained by vein of Labbé. Because of the network of venous collaterals in the brain, a patient with a venous occlusive process that is slow enough to allow time to develop collateral circulation may remain asymptomatic. However, in the setting of acute occlusion of a large vein or dural venous sinus, venous congestion will result in back pressure that extends to the capillary bed where the flow will be diminished such that there is ischemia and, if extensive enough, infarction.

Before MRI, the diagnosis of venous occlusive disease was difficult. Many CT findings have been described; however, they are highly inconsistent (including the delta sign, in which there is enhancement around the clot in the sinus, and the cord sign, in which high density is seen in a venous sinus or vein). Symptoms of venous occlusion are related to the rate at which collateral venous drainage is established, the location of the clot, and the rate of clot formation.

Notes

CASE 111

Internal Carotid Artery Dissection

1. The left internal carotid artery.

2. Intramural hematoma (methemoglobin).

3. With fat suppression vascular mural blood products (which remain hyperintense) can be distinguished from perivascular fat (which saturates out).

4. With neck pain, Horner's syndrome, and/or transient ischemic attack or stroke.

Reference

Ozdoba C, Sturzenegger M, Schroth G: Internal carotid artery dissection: MR imaging features and clinical-radiologic correlation, *Radiology* 199:191-198, 1996.

Cross-Reference

Neuroradiology: THE REQUISITES, pp 133-135, 162-164.

Comment

This case illustrates the characteristic appearance of a dissection of the internal carotid artery. MRI demonstrates overall enlargement of the left internal carotid artery when compared with the right due to extensive intramural hematoma (methemoglobin) that is hyperintense on unenhanced T1W images. Narrowing of the arterial lumen, which is still patent as signal void consistent with flow, can also be seen. MRI combined with MRA is probably more sensitive for detecting vascular dissections because they allow evaluation of both the vascular lumen (like angiography) and the vessel wall and the tissues around the vascular structures. An occluded vessel can usually be differentiated from one that is narrowed but patent using a combination of conventional spin echo MRI and MRA. It is important to acquire a phase contrast MRA because with this sequence the high signal intensity mural hematoma is nulled. One may be "burned" if only time-of-flight MRA is used in which mural hematoma may be mistaken for flow because it remains hyperintense on this sequence.

Vascular dissections may result from trauma or neck manipulation (watch out for the chiropractors) and are more common in patients with underlying vascular dysplasias (fibromuscular dysplasia, Marfan syndrome, Ehlers-Danlos syndrome, and cystic medial necrosis). Treatment in uncomplicated cases usually includes anticoagulation therapy and aspirin. It is important to obtain follow-up MRI in these patients to assess for recanalization of the vascular lumen or progressive stenosis. In addition, these patients are at increased risk for development of pseudoaneurysms, which can be catastrophic if they go undetected and rupture. The most common complication of vascular dissection is probably thromboembolic disease (transient ischemic attack and stroke).

Notes

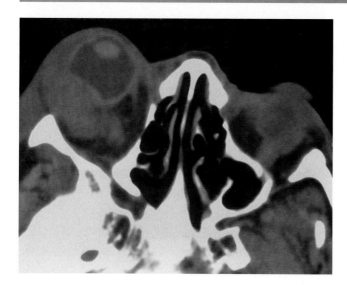 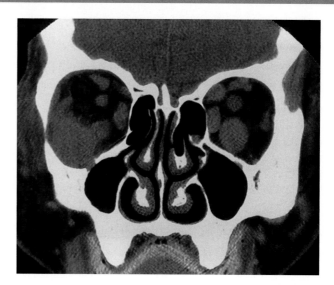

1. Between what anatomic structures does the superior ophthalmic vein course?
2. Regarding orbital metastases, what structure is most commonly involved?
3. What is the most common cause of orbital metastases in children?
4. What characteristic imaging finding, when present, is highly suggestive of metastatic breast carcinoma to the orbit?

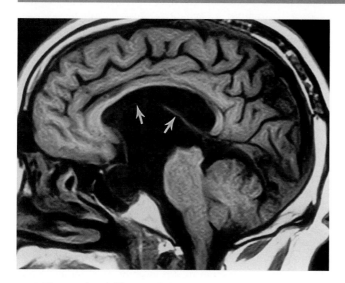

1. What is the differential diagnosis of a cyst within the third ventricle?
2. What suprasellar lesions may mimic dilation of the third ventricle?
3. What percentage of intracranial arachnoid cysts arise in the suprasellar region?
4. When symptomatic, what is the most common clinical presentation of arachnoid cysts in the quadrigeminal cistern?

Orbital Metastases—Carcinoid

1. The superior rectus muscle and the optic nerve.

2. The globe.

3. Neuroblastoma.

4. Enophthalmos. Inward retraction of the globe (just like the skin of the breast involved) is characteristic of metastatic scirrhous breast carcinoma.

Reference

Gunalp I, Gunduz K: Metastatic orbital tumors, *Jpn J Ophthalmol* 39:65-70, 1995.

Cross-Reference

Neuroradiology: THE REQUISITES, pp 284-287.

Comment

Metastatic disease to the orbits is quite common. The imaging diagnosis of orbital metastases as the first manifestation of metastatic disease is not uncommon in radiology. For every case of orbital metastases that are clinically evident, there are several asymptomatic cases that go unrecognized. In autopsy series, as many as 7% of patients with known systemic carcinoma have metastases involving the orbit. By far the most common location for orbital metastases is the globe, usually involving the region of the choroid and retina. Ocular metastases characteristically involve the uveoscleral region, resulting in thickening in this location on imaging. Ocular metastases are often associated with retrobulbar extension. The most common tumors to metastasize to the globe are breast and lung carcinoma in adults. In general, outside of the globe orbital metastases most often are extraconal and are usually related to bone metastases. When extraosseous spread from a bone metastasis is large enough, there may be direct invasion of the adjacent extraocular muscles. Occasionally sinonasal metastases may extend secondarily into the orbit. The most common neoplasm to metastasize to the sinuses is renal cell carcinoma. Intraconal metastatic disease, specifically retrobulbar metastasis, is usually related to direct extension of an ocular metastasis.

Clinical manifestations of ocular metastases may be quite variable, ranging from asymptomatic to proptosis, blurred vision, pain, and ophthalmoplegia, depending on the site of involvement.

Notes

Suprasellar Arachnoid Cyst

1. Ependymal cyst, arachnoid cyst, colloid cyst, cysticercosis (or other parasitic cyst), and epidermoid cyst. Cystic neoplasms such as craniopharyngioma may occasionally occur here also.

2. Suprasellar arachnoid cyst, cystic craniopharyngioma, and occasionally a cyst of the septum pellucidum.

3. Approximately 10%.

4. Obstructive hydrocephalus related to compression of the aqueduct.

References

Ide C, De Coene B, Gilliard C, et al: Hemorrhagic arachnoid cyst with third nerve paresis: CT and MR findings, *AJNR Am J Neuroradiol* 18:1407-1410, 1997.

Wiener SN, Pearlstein AE, Eiber A: MR imaging of intracranial arachnoid cysts, *J Comput Assist Tomogr* 11:236-241, 1987.

Cross-Reference

Neuroradiology: THE REQUISITES, pp 247-249, 319-320.

Comment

Arachnoid cysts are common and frequently asymptomatic, especially when located in the middle cranial fossa or over the cerebral convexities. Arachnoid cysts positioned in strategic locations may be symptomatic. Large cysts in the posterior fossa may present with ataxia or other symptoms of mass effect related to hydrocephalus. Similarly, cysts in the quadrigeminal cistern when large enough may cause hydrocephalus by compressing the aqueduct of Sylvius. As in this case, arachnoid cysts in the region of the suprasellar cistern or third ventricle may cause headache, visual symptoms (related to compression of the optic chiasm), or symptoms related to mass effect and hydrocephalus. Arachnoid cysts of the suprasellar cistern may be mistaken for cystic third ventricular masses such as seen with parasitic infection (cysticercosis), ependymal cysts, or epidermoid cysts.

Usually arachnoid cysts follow the signal characteristics of CSF on all MRI pulse sequences and are isodense to CSF on CT. Occasionally CSF stasis or protein within the cyst may result in different intensities on MRI and different densities on CT. When looking at a lesion in this location, localization to the suprasellar cistern rather than the third ventricle may be determined by looking for elevation of the floor of the third ventricle *(arrows)*. Arachnoid cysts should have smooth margins, and calcification is rarely present. On cisternography following intrathecal administration of contrast material, arachnoid cysts on immediate scanning will not take up contrast; however, a CSF contrast level may be present in the cyst on delayed imaging. Most asymptomatic arachnoid cysts are left alone. In cases of cysts strategically positioned resulting in symptomatology, shunting and/or surgical resection may be necessary.

Notes

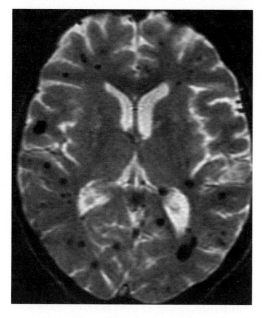
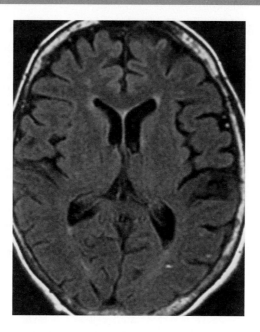

1. What is the differential diagnosis?
2. The higher sensitivity to susceptibility of gradient echo imaging is due to what feature of the pulse sequence?
3. In gradient echo imaging, what factors contribute to T1 and T2 weighting?
4. Gradient echo imaging for detection of blood products is achieved by using what type of flip angles and TEs?

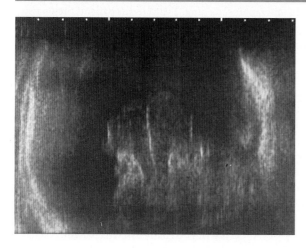
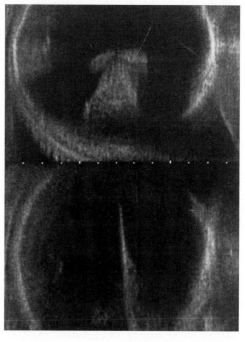

1. What congenital abnormalities may have markedly enlarged supratentorial CSF spaces and associated decreased brain parenchyma?
2. What structure is uniformly absent in all types of holoprosencephaly but is present in maximal-pressure hydrocephalus and hydranencephaly?
3. The large CSF cyst in holoprosencephaly represents what structure?
4. What structures are typically spared in hydranencephaly?

Multiple Cavernous Malformations—Familial Pattern

1. Multiple cavernous malformations, hemorrhagic metastases, metastatic melanoma, amyloid angiopathy, and hypertension.

2. Gradient echo imaging is more sensitive to magnetic field inhomogeneities and susceptibility due to lack of a 180-degree rephasing pulse.

3. The flip angle and the time to echo (TE).

4. The lower the flip angle and the longer the TE, the greater the sensitivity will be to susceptibility effects.

Reference

Rigamonti D, Hadley MN, Drayer BP, et al: Cerebral cavernous malformations: incidence and familial occurrence, *N Engl J Med* 319:343-347, 1988.

Cross-Reference

Neuroradiology: THE REQUISITES, pp 8-9, 141-142.

Comment

Cavernous malformations have a characteristic appearance on MRI. Specifically, they have central high signal intensity on unenhanced T1W and T2W imaging and are surrounded by a rim of hemosiderin that is hypointense on T2W and gradient echo imaging. In approximately 25% of cases these lesions are multiple, and in a small percentage there is a familial pattern. Many patients with multiple cavernomas have lesions too numerous to count. As in this case, many of the lesions may be quite small and only identifiable on gradient echo susceptibility images. Although cavernomas are believed to be congenital lesions, de novo development has been described in patients with a familial pattern of multiple lesions, as well as following radiation therapy and in association with developmental venous anomalies (venous angiomas).

Gradient echo imaging has increased sensitivity to magnetic susceptibility due to the lack of a 180-degree rephasing pulse. Therefore, blood products (hemosiderin), calcium, iron, and other ions are more readily seen on this sequence as areas of marked hypointensity. The T1 or T2 weighting of a gradient echo scan may be determined by selection of the flip angle and the TE. Small flip angles and long TEs result in more T2 weighting. Similarly, a lower flip angle and longer TE will result in greater sensitivity to susceptibility effects. In addition to increased sensitivity to magnetic field inhomogeneities, gradient echo scanning has several other useful features. It is generally faster than conventional spin echo imaging. In addition, flow-related enhancement (bright blood) may be attained and is the basis of MRA. Another advantage of gradient echo scanning is that three-dimensional imaging allows for very thin slices (1.0 mm). Such thin sections may also be acquired with three-dimensional fast spin echo imaging.

Notes

Hydranencephaly*

1. Holoprosencephaly, maximal hydrocephalus, and hydranencephaly.

2. The septum pellucidum (and other midline structures).

3. The monoventricle.

4. The diencephalon and posterior fossa contents (however, the thalami may be involved in rare cases).

Reference

Sutton LN, Bruce DA, Schut L: Hydranencephaly versus maximal hydrocephalus: an important clinical distinction, *Neurosurg* 6:34-38, 1980.

Cross-Reference

Neuroradiology: THE REQUISITES, pp 250-251.

Comment

Hydranencephaly represents a congenital anomaly manifest by destruction of normally developed brain tissue (as opposed to abnormal brain development). Although the exact etiology has not been clearly delineated, it is believed to represent sequelae of an in utero ischemic event. Hydranencephaly has the appearance of large bilateral internal carotid artery infarcts/occlusions (however, some autopsy series in patients with hydranencephaly show that the vessels are patent). Most cases of hydranencephaly are now detected during pregnancy as a result of the increased use of sonographic screening. Typically the patients present with a large supratentorial CSF space with sparse cerebral tissue. Pathologically in hydranencephaly the cerebral hemispheres to a large extent are replaced by cystic cavitation and are covered by the leptomeninges. Hydranencephaly has an extremely poor prognosis because most of the cerebrum is destroyed.

The differential diagnosis of hydranencephaly includes alobar holoprosencephaly, maximal hydrocephalus, and bilateral open-lip schizencephaly. Alobar holoprosencephaly can usually be readily identified because of the absence of the midline structures (the interhemispheric fissure and septum pellucidum), as well as fusion of the thalami and basal ganglia. Patients with open-lip schizencephaly often have septooptic dysplasia, and these patient will also have absence of the septum pellucidum; however, the interhemispheric fissure is present. Maximal hydrocephalus and hydranencephaly have preservation of the midline structures. Although hydranencephaly essentially has absence of the cortical tissue in the distribution of the anterior and middle cerebral arteries (although this is not always the case), maximal-pressure hydrocephalus normally has thinned but present cortical brain tissue that forms a mantle around the lateral ventricles.

Notes

---

*Figures for Case 115 courtesy Jill Langer, MD.

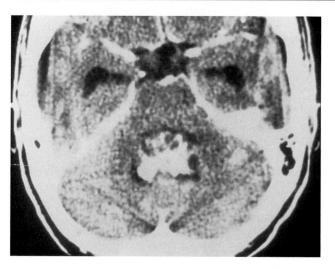
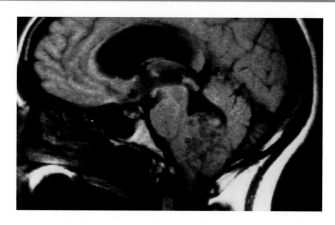

1. Where is the lesion arising?
2. What is the differential diagnosis of a midline posterior fossa mass in a child?
3. What primary neoplasm in the posterior fossa has the highest incidence of calcification in children?
4. What is the typical growth pattern of this entity?

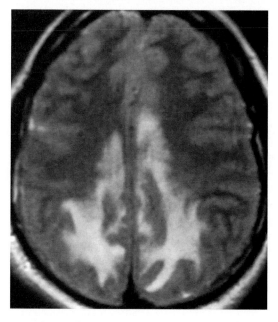

1. What infectious agent has been implicated in the development of progressive multifocal leukoencephalopathy?
2. What is the classic clinical presentation of Guillain-Barré syndrome?
3. What is the pathophysiology of acute disseminated encephalomyelitis (ADEM)?
4. What region of the white matter is most commonly affected in ADEM?

Fourth Ventricle Ependymoma

1. The fourth ventricle.

2. Primitive neuroectodermal tumor (medulloblastoma), ependymoma, and, less often, cerebellar astrocytoma or oligodendroglioma.

3. Ependymoma, with approximately 40% showing calcification on imaging.

4. Through the foramina of Magendie and Luschka.

Reference

Spoto GP, Press GA, Hesselink JR, Solomon M: Intracranial ependymoma and subependymoma: MR manifestations, *AJNR Am J Neuroradiol* 11:83-91, 1990.

Cross-Reference

Neuroradiology: THE REQUISITES, pp 85-86.

Comment

This case demonstrates the typical appearance of a posterior fossa ependymoma, the third most common cause of infratentorial tumors in children after cystic astrocytoma and medulloblastoma (primitive neuroectodermal tumors). Ependymomas account for approximately 9% of primary brain tumors in children and 15% of posterior fossa neoplasms. As in this case, ependymomas typically are midline masses that arise from the ependymal lining of the fourth ventricle. As a result, the lesions tend to fill the fourth ventricle, which is secondarily expanded (on close observation of multiplanar MRI a CSF cleft can often be seen around some portions of the mass). The major differential consideration of a midline posterior fossa mass in a child is medulloblastoma (and, less commonly, astrocytoma). Ependymomas can usually be distinguished from medulloblastomas by their imaging appearance (but again, I wouldn't bet my house on it). There are several differentiating features. Whereas ependymomas tend to fill, expand, and conform to the shape of the fourth ventricle, medulloblastomas tend to compress and displace it. In addition, calcification (present in 30% to 40% at imaging) and hemorrhage are much more common in ependymomas (CT is frequently complimentary to MRI). Finally, the growth pattern of these two neoplasms is different. Ependymomas tend to spread through the foramen of Luschka into the cerebellopontine angle and through the foramen of Magendie into the cisterna magna (40% to 60%) as well as the foramen magnum, resulting in compression of the upper cervical spinal cord and medulla. Growth of medulloblastomas through these foramina is atypical.

Notes

Acute Disseminated Encephalomyelitis

1. Papovavirus (JC virus).

2. Ascending paralysis/peripheral neuropathy.

3. Autoimmune (cell mediated).

4. The subcortical white matter.

Reference

Mader I, Stock KW, Ettlin T, Probst A: Acute disseminated encephalomyelitis: MR and CT features, *AJNR Am J Neuroradiol* 17:104-109, 1996.

Cross-Reference

Neuroradiology: THE REQUISITES, pp 212-213.

Comment

Acute disseminated encephalomyelitis is an immune-mediated demyelinating disease related to an antecedent viral infection or vaccination. The cause is believed to be an allergic or autoimmune (cell-mediated) response against the myelin basic protein due to cross-reaction with viral proteins. ADEM has most commonly been associated with the measles; however, it has also been associated with antecedent chickenpox, rubella, mumps, and other viral agents. Both clinically and on MRI, ADEM may appear identical to the initial presentation of multiple sclerosis. Patients may present with symptoms and focal neurologic deficits typically within 2 to 3 weeks following a viral illness. In addition to focal neurologic deficits, unlike multiple sclerosis, ADEM is not infrequently associated with seizures.

Although ADEM more commonly involves the white matter, especially in the subcortical region, the gray matter may also be involved. On MRI patients typically present with multiple foci of hyperintensity on T2W images. These lesions may or may not be associated with enhancement. In that ADEM is a monophasic process, no new lesions should develop after 6 months following clinical presentation. The diagnosis of ADEM can usually be made by clinical history and CSF analysis, which frequently shows an inflammatory reaction with lymphocytes, as well as elevated myelin basic protein. Follow-up MRI is also helpful in distinguishing multiple sclerosis from ADEM.

Notes

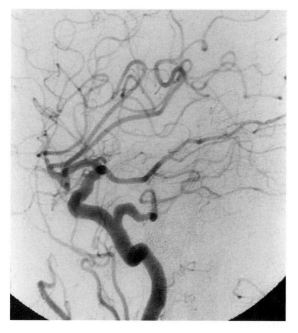
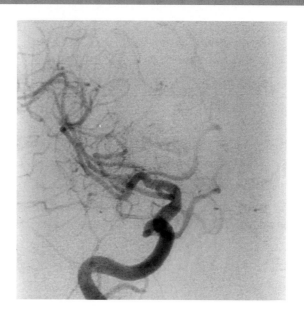

1. What is the anatomic variant in this case?

2. What are the three intracranial embryologic anastomoses between the carotid (anterior) and vertebrobasilar (posterior) circulations?

3. What other intracranial vascular abnormalities have been associated with persistent trigeminal arteries?

4. What percentage of cerebral arteriograms reveal a persistent trigeminal artery?

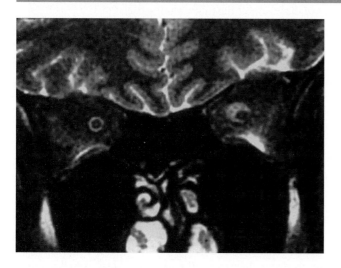
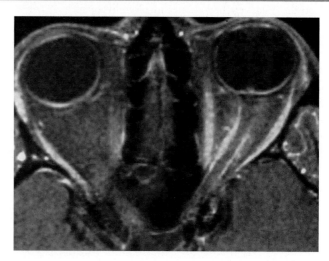

1. In what condition can this lesion be present bilaterally?

2. When this lesion involves the optic nerve sheath complex bilaterally, from what area does it usually arise?

3. How often is calcification present in these lesions on CT?

4. What is the differential diagnosis of this enhancement pattern?

CASE 118

Persistent Trigeminal Artery

1. Persistent trigeminal artery.

2. The trigeminal, otic, and hypoglossal arteries.

3. Aneurysms and arteriovenous malformations.

4. Approximately 0.1% to 0.5%.

References

Piotin M, Miralbes S, Cattin F, et al: MRI and MR angiography of persistent trigeminal artery, *Neuroradiology* 38: 730-733, 1996.

Boyko OB, Curnes JT, Blatter DD, Parker DL: MRI of basilar artery hypoplasia associated with persistent primitive trigeminal artery, *Neuroradiology* 38:11-14, 1996.

Cross-Reference

Neuroradiology: THE REQUISITES, pp 55, 317.

Comment

The trigeminal, otic, and hypoglossal arteries (named after the cranial nerves with which they course) are the three embryologic anastomoses between the internal carotid artery and the vertebrobasilar circulations. The persistent trigeminal artery is the most common embryonic carotid-vertebrobasilar anastomosis to persist into adulthood, reported in as many as 0.1% to 0.5% of cerebral arteriograms. Persistence of a trigeminal artery may be associated with hypoplasia or absence of the ipsilateral posterior communicating artery or hypoplasia of both posterior communicating arteries. In addition, the proximal basilar artery and the distal vertebral arteries are often hypoplastic. A persistent trigeminal artery usually arises from the precavernous internal carotid artery; however, origin from the intracavernous internal carotid artery has been reported. In some cases, trigeminal arteries may course through the sella turcica before joining the basilar artery (knowledge of this variant is critical in patients before transsphenoidal surgery). Persistent trigeminal arteries are associated with a variety of intracranial vascular abnormalities, including aneurysms and AVMs, as well as a spectrum of clinical syndromes such as tic douloureux (cranial nerve V), other cranial neuropathies, and vertebrobasilar insufficiency. Aneurysms arising from the trigeminal artery itself have been reported. Correct identification and an understanding of this anatomic variation is important because interventional neuroradiologic and neurosurgical procedures (often performed to treat an associated vascular abnormality) may need to be modified appropriately.

Notes

CASE 119

Optic Nerve Meningioma

1. Neurofibromatosis.

2. The tuberculum sellae or planum sphenoidale.

3. In 25% to 50% of cases.

4. Meningioma, sarcoid, lymphoma, metastatic disease, and pseudotumor may result in this "tram-track" enhancement pattern.

Reference

Atlas SW, Bilaniuk LT, Zimmerman RA, Hackney DB, Goldberg HI, Grossman RI: Orbit: initial experience with surface coil spin-echo MR imaging at 1.5 T, *Radiology* 164:501-509, 1987.

Cross-Reference

Neuroradiology: THE REQUISITES, pp 293-294.

Comment

Optic nerve sheath meningiomas typically present first with vision loss followed by proptosis as the tumor enlarges. They most commonly present in middle-aged women; however, they may also be present in children with neurofibromatosis in whom they are also frequently bilateral. The other situation in which bilateral orbital meningiomas may occur is when they arise from the tuberculum sellae or planum sphenoidale. In this situation, meningiomas normally grow anteriorly along the optic nerves from the optic canal into the orbit. In every patient with suspected optic meningioma it is important to assess both eyes and the region of the tuberculum sellae.

On imaging, "tram-tracking" has been used to describe both the patterns of enhancement and calcification. On CT, up to 50% of optic nerve meningiomas have calcification along the nerve sheath, with the optic nerve sandwiched between the "tracks" of calcification. Linear enhancement may be seen on both sides of the optic nerve. Other findings to assess on CT include secondary bony changes (erosion and/or hyperostosis) of the optic canal, sphenoid sinus, and planum sphenoidale. There may be enlargement of the optic canal. A major advantage of MRI is its ability to evaluate the optic nerve separately from the surrounding nerve sheath. This is extremely helpful in differentiating lesions arising from the optic nerve itself (gliomas, optic neuritis) from those arising from the nerve sheath (meningiomas, metastases, and granulomatosis disorders). In addition, because of artifact arising from the bones, MRI is better than CT in evaluating the nerve within the optic canal, as well as spread into the intracranial compartment. It is important when performing orbital MRI to use fat suppression so that the full extent of the tumor around the optic nerve can be assessed. Limitations of MRI include its inability to detect small calcifications, as well as artifacts (chemical shift or susceptibility from the aerated paranasal sinuses) in the orbit that may obscure small lesions.

Notes

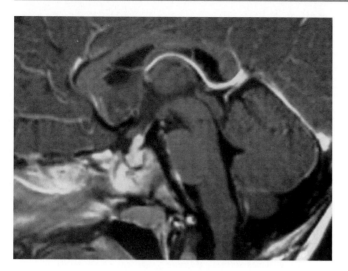 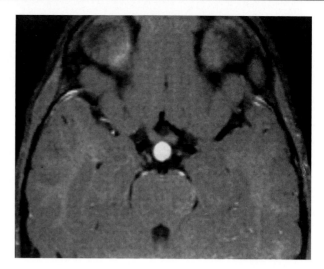

1. What structure is abnormal in this case?

2. What is a common clinical presentation of lesions involving this region?

3. What is the differential diagnosis of a mass in this location in children?

4. Is the infundibular stalk normally wider at the median eminence or inferiorly along its insertion with the pituitary gland?

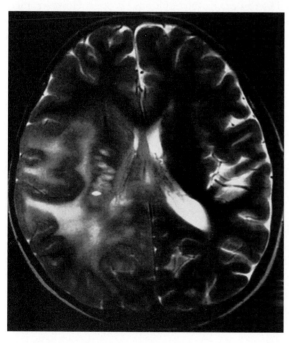

1. Histopathologically, what is meant by *gliomatosis cerebri*?

2. What is the most common age group of patients affected with this entity?

3. What are the three major types of noninfiltrating astrocytic tumors?

4. What is the most common location of pleomorphic xanthoastrocytoma, and what is its typical imaging appearance?

Eosinophilic Granuloma of the Pituitary Stalk (Langerhans' Cell Histiocytosis)*

1. There is thickening of the pituitary stalk.

2. Diabetes insipidus.

3. Langerhans' cell histiocytosis, germinoma, infection (meningitis, tuberculosis), lymphoproliferative disorders, and occasionally sarcoidosis.

4. The pituitary stalk is normally widest at the median eminence and should taper as it extends inferiorly to its insertion at the pituitary gland.

Reference

Maghnie M, Arico M, Villa A, et al: MR of the hypothalamic-pituitary axis in Langerhans cell histiocytosis, *AJNR* 13:1365-1371, 1992.

Cross-Reference

Neuroradiology: THE REQUISITES, pp 318-319.

Comment

This patient presented with diabetes insipidus. The MRI demonstrates abnormal thickening and enhancement along the pituitary stalk that lacks the normal tapering as it extends inferiorly toward the pituitary gland. In this young patient, this represents Langerhans' cell histiocytosis. The differential diagnosis for an infundibular mass in children includes germinoma, infection (sequelae of meningitis or tuberculosis), and, less likely, lymphoma/leukemia and glioma involving the hypothalamic region. Another finding on MRI that may be noted in patients with Langerhans' cell histiocytosis is the absence of the normal "bright spot" of the posterior pituitary gland in the sella on unenhanced T1W images. Langerhans' cell histiocytosis uncommonly affects the CNS. It is a disorder of the reticuloendothelial system. The most common cranial abnormality is a lytic, circumscribed, enhancing mass of the calvaria or skull base. In the cranium, it most commonly involves the temporal bone along the mastoid segment.

The differential diagnosis of an infundibular lesion in adults includes granulomatous disease (sarcoid or tuberculosis), metastasis, and germinoma. Less commonly, lymphoma or a hypothalamic glioma may present like this. Lymphocytic adenohypophysitis is a unique condition that almost always affects women. It is most common in the postpartum period or in the late stages (third trimester) of pregnancy. It is characterized by lymphocytic infiltration of the adenohypophysis and is usually self-limited.

Notes

Gliomatosis Cerebri

1. The term is used with glial neoplasms in which the amount of brain and the extensive infiltrative nature of the lesion is disproportionate to the other histologic features (cellularity, anaplasia, necrosis).

2. Young adults (third and fourth decades of life), although it can occur at any age.

3. Subependymal giant cell astrocytoma, juvenile pilocytic astrocytoma, and pleomorphic xanthoastrocytoma.

4. The temporal lobe and a solid and cystic mass, respectively.

Reference

del Carpio-O'Donovan R, Korah I, Salazar A, Melancon D: Gliomatosis cerebri, *Radiology* 198:831-835, 1996.

Cross-Reference

Neuroradiology: THE REQUISITES, pp 87-92.

Comment

This case illustrates the typical radiologic appearance of gliomatosis cerebri. Namely, there is extensive abnormality within the brain that particularly affects the white matter; however, the gray matter is also involved. A large portion of the brain is affected by this extensively infiltrative process. However, there are no regions of necrosis, there is no circumscribed mass, and in general the lesion demonstrates little enhancement. Gliomatosis cerebri is characterized by the fact that its extensive infiltrative pattern throughout the involved portions of the brain is relatively disproportionate to the remainder of the histologic findings, including a relative paucity of cellularity, anaplasia, and necrosis. In addition to the disproportionate histologic findings relative to the degree of infiltration, the clinical symptomatology is out of proportion to the degree of brain involvement. Patients often present only with a change in mental status or personality. Although this tumor may affect patients of any age, it is most common from young adulthood to the age of 40 years. In addition to the extensive parenchymal involvement and the signal alteration seen on MRI, other findings that may suggest the diagnosis include mild diffuse sulcal and ventricular effacement. Not uncommonly, a large resection or lobectomy is necessary to make the diagnosis pathologically because biopsy may provide insufficient material. Therefore recognition of the imaging findings in combination with the patient's history are important in diagnosing this neoplasm.

Notes

---

*Figures for Case 120 courtesy Robert A. Zimmerman, MD.

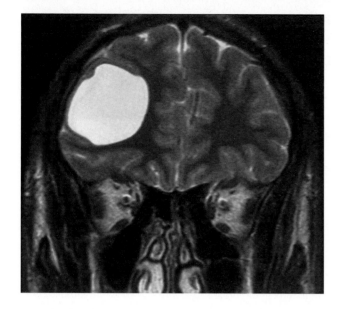
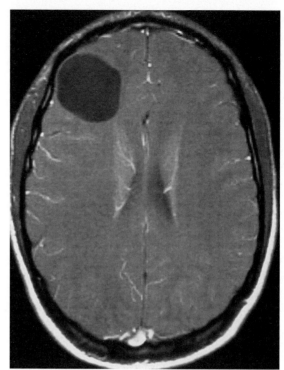

1. What are the causes of this entity?
2. What tissue lines the CSF-filled open-lip schizencephaly?
3. What lines the cystic cavity in this entity?
4. What particular type of infection is associated with this entity?

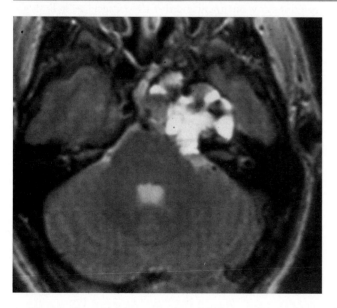
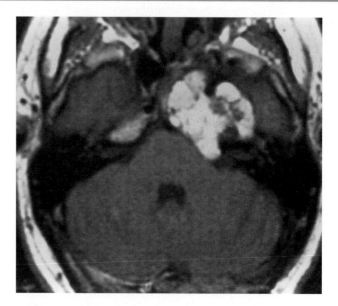

1. From where is this mass arising (what is the epicenter of the lesion)?
2. What is the differential diagnosis of an expansile mass of the petrous apex?
3. What is the etiology of cholesterol granulomas?
4. What is the typical appearance of a cholesterol granuloma on MRI?

CASE 122

Porencephalic Cyst*

1. An old insult usually related to infarction, infection, or trauma.

2. Gray matter.

3. White matter (which is frequently gliotic).

4. Viral.

Reference

Van Tassel P, Cure JK: Nonneoplastic intracranial cysts and cystic lesions, *Semin Ultrasound CT MRI* 16:186-211, 1995.

Cross-Reference

Neuroradiology: THE REQUISITES, p 233.

Comment

Porencephalic cysts occur in regions of encephalomalacic brain. Insults (usually in utero following development of the brain, postnatally, or in childhood) such as infarction, trauma, or infection (especially viral agents such as herpes and CMV) involving the cerebral cortex and underlying subcortical white matter typically predispose to this entity. The porencephalic cyst often communicates with the ventricles and extends to the surface of the brain. However, in some instances intervening tissue between the ventricle and cyst may be present. Transmission of CSF pulsations from the ventricles into the cyst or development of adhesions within the cyst resulting in a ball valve mechanism lead to ventricular and cystic enlargement, which may result in remodeling of the inner table of the calvaria or expansion of the calvaria such as is seen with superficial arachnoid cysts.

Another entity that extends from the superficial surface of the cerebrum to the ventricular margin is open-lip schizencephaly, which may appear like a porencephalic cyst (on initial observation). Schizencephaly is a developmental migrational abnormality (unlike a porencephalic cyst, which is destruction of normally developed brain). Schizencephaly can be distinguished from porencephaly in that the schizencephalic CSF cleft is lined by gray matter, whereas the porencephalic cyst is lined by white matter.

Notes

CASE 123

Petrous Apex Cholesterol Granuloma

1. The petrous apex.

2. Mucocele, cholesterol granuloma, multiple myeloma, metastasis, schwannoma of cranial nerve V, chondrosarcoma.

3. Recurrent rupture of small blood vessels within the petrous air cells due to negative pressures.

4. Hyperintense on all pulse sequences.

Reference

Isaacson JE, Sismanis A: Cholesterol granuloma cyst of the petrous apex, *Ear Nose Throat J* 75:425-429, 1996.

Cross-Reference

Neuroradiology: THE REQUISITES, p 353.

Comment

Cholesterol granulomas (otherwise known as blue-domed cysts, chocolate cysts, and epidermoids) typically occur in the petrous apex. They are believed to be due to chronic obstruction of the petrous air cells, resulting in negative pressures within them. As a result there are recurrent microhemorrhages from rupture of small blood vessels. Then a foreign body reaction by the mucosal lining of the petrous air cells occurs, with giant cell proliferation and a fibroblastic reaction, as well as deposition of cholesterol crystals within the cyst. On CT these lesions typically have a more benign appearance that is manifest by an expansile mass lesion with well-demarcated margins. There is usually bowing and thinning of the cortex with large lesions; however, there is no bony destruction. On MRI cholesterol granulomas are hyperintense on all pulse sequences. In particular, the marked hyperintensity on unenhanced T1W images, as well as the presence of hemorrhage-fluid levels within these lesions, is highly characteristic. Normal fat may occur in the petrous apex and, because it is hyperintense on both T1W and fast spin echo (FSE) T2W imaging, may be mistaken for a cholesterol granuloma. This problem can be avoided by obtaining fat-saturated T1W images in which fat will lose signal but the cholesterol granuloma will keep on shining!

The differential diagnosis of an expansile petrous apex mass includes a mucocele, petrous apicitis, an epidermoid, and hemorrhagic metastases (such as renal or thyroid carcinoma). Mucoceles are frequently unilocular (compared with cholesterol granulomas, which when large enough may be multilobular in appearance) and demonstrate rim enhancement. Their signal characteristics will vary depending on the protein content and viscosity within them.

Notes

---

*Figures for Case 122 courtesy Robert A. Zimmerman, MD.

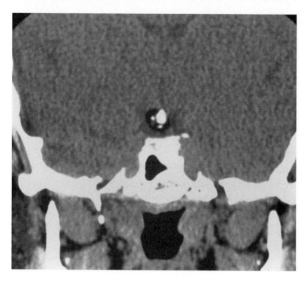
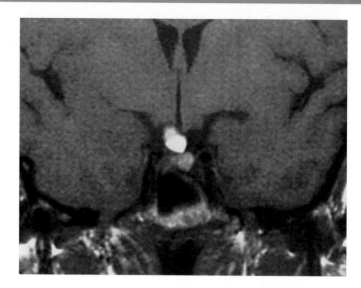

1. In what space is the lesion located?
2. What lesions on imaging may contain both fat and calcium?
3. In fat-containing lesions, chemical shift artifact is most pronounced on what pulse sequence?
4. What is the most serious complication of dermoid cysts?

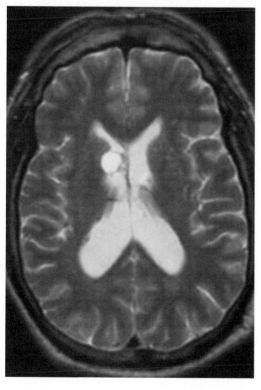
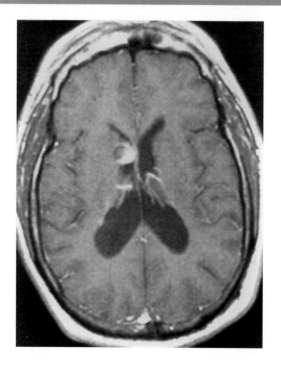

1. With what condition is this neoplasm characteristically associated?
2. This neoplasm typically arises at what level of the ventricle?
3. Are these lesions associated with subarachnoid seeding?
4. Central neurocytomas are typically attached to what structure of the lateral ventricle?

Suprasellar Dermoid

1. The suprasellar cistern.

2. Dermoid cysts and teratomas. Lipomas may also occasionally be associated with calcification; however, this is less common than with teratomas and dermoid cysts. When present, calcification is often seen in association with "tumefactive" lipomas in the interhemispheric fissure that are usually associated with dysgenesis of the corpus callosum, allowing differentiation from dermoid cysts and teratomas.

3. Long TR sequences.

4. Rupture into the subarachnoid space resulting in chemical meningitis.

Reference

Harrison MJ, Morgello S, Post KD: Epithelial cystic lesions of the sellar and parasellar region: a continuum of ectodermal derivatives? *J Neurosurg* 80:1018-1025, 1994.

Cross-Reference

Neuroradiology: THE REQUISITES, pp 320-512.

Comment

Fat-containing lesions may be readily identified both on CT and MRI. On CT fat is hypodense to the CSF and may be present in lipomas, dermoid cysts, and teratomas. On MRI fat-containing lesions (and, in this case, dermoid cysts) are typically markedly hyperintense on unenhanced T1W images and the fatty components are hypointense on conventional T2W images (long TR/long TE). Other common MRI findings in these relatively uncommon lesions include the presence of fat-fluid levels within the cyst, chemical shift artifact on long TR images (identified by the presence of a hyperintense and a hypointense rim at opposite borders of the lesion in the frequency encoding direction), and peripheral enhancement. CT is more sensitive than is MRI in the detection of calcification, and the combination of CT and MRI may be quite helpful in suggesting the diagnosis of a dermoid cyst or teratoma in the suprasellar cistern. Dermoid cysts and teratomas are typically midline lesions, and both occur more commonly in men. Dermoid cysts are often asymptomatic but may enlarge over time due to recurrent glandular secretions and/or recurrent desquamation of the epithelial lining of the cyst. When symptomatic, patients may have headaches. A serious complication of dermoid cysts is their propensity to rupture into the subarachnoid space, which may result in chemical meningitis, vasospasm with ischemia, and even death.

Notes

Subependymal Giant Cell Astrocytoma

1. Tuberous sclerosis.

2. The foramen of Monro.

3. No. They are subependymal in location, precluding such spread.

4. The septum pellucidum.

Reference

McMurdo SK Jr, Moore SG, Brant-Zawadzki M, et al: MR imaging of intracranial tuberous sclerosis, *AJR Am J Roentgenol* 148:791-796, 1987.

Cross-Reference

Neuroradiology: THE REQUISITES, pp 90, 269.

Comment

Subependymal giant cell astrocytomas are very low grade glial neoplasms that characteristically arise in patients with tuberous sclerosis. Approximately 15% of patients with tuberous sclerosis have giant cell astrocytomas. The occurrence of this neoplasm in the absence of tuberous sclerosis has been reported but is extremely rare. The primary means of differentiating this neoplasm from other intraventricular neoplasms that occur in this location (astrocytomas, ependymomas, oligodendrogliomas, central neurocytomas) is in identifying the other CNS manifestations of tuberous sclerosis (cortical tubers, subependymal nodules, and white matter dysplasia). On CT approximately 50% of subependymal giant cell astrocytomas are associated with calcification. Typically these circumscribed, solid masses are centered at the level of the foramen of Monro; however, these tumors are actually parenchymal in origin, arising from the subependyma. As a result, subarachnoid seeding of tumor does not occur. Typically these tumors protrude into the frontal horn of the lateral ventricle and may displace the septum pellucidum. On MRI the signal intensity characteristics of these lesions are variable and are affected by the presence and the degree of calcification. Enhancement is usually solid (unlike subependymal tubers, although in a small percentage of patients these too may enhance); however, there may be relative absence of enhancement in regions of calcification (and rarely cystic degeneration).

These are often incidental asymptomatic lesions; however, when symptomatic they typically present with obstructive hydrocephalus due to blockage of outflow of CSF from the lateral ventricles. Treatment is usually surgical resection with a subsequent excellent prognosis.

Notes

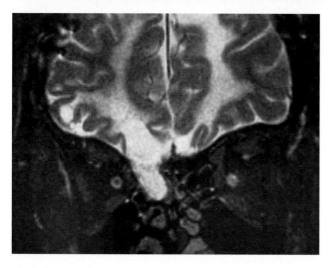
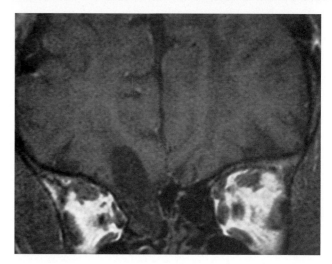

1. What are the most common causes of acquired meningo(encephalo)celes?

2. Congenital sinonasal encephaloceles have an increased incidence in what ethnic group?

3. What is a nasal glioma?

4. In the postoperative setting, what is the most common presentation of an encephalocele?

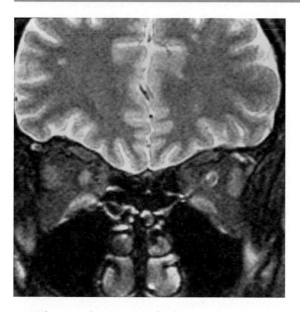
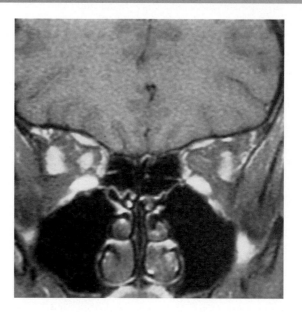

1. What are the imaging findings?

2. What are diagnostic considerations of enhancement of the optic nerve sheath complex?

3. What is the most common cause of optic neuritis?

4. What is Devic's disease?

Encephalocele Complicating Sinonasal Surgery

1. Trauma or iatrogenic (postoperative) causes.

2. Southeastern Asian women.

3. A misnomer in that the benign mass is composed of heterotopic glial tissue. Unlike meningo(encephalo)celes, nasal gliomas do not have CSF spaces that communicate with the intracranial subarachnoid spaces or ventricles. In 15% of cases, nasal gliomas are connected with the intracranial compartment via fibrous or glial bands.

4. Rhinorrhea.

Reference

Hudgins PA, Browning DG, Gallups J, et al: Endoscopic paranasal sinus surgery: radiographic evaluation of severe complications, *AJNR Am J Neuroradiol* 13:1161-1167, 1992.

Cross-Reference

Neuroradiology: THE REQUISITES, pp 368-369.

Comment

This case shows a posttraumatic, postoperative nasofrontal encephalocele. Encephalomalacia and high signal intensity related to prior trauma are noted in the frontal lobes. Meningo(encephalo)cele refers to herniation of the meninges, CSF, and/or brain through an osseous defect in the cranium. Meningoencephaloceles are more common than are meningoceles. In the setting of trauma or surgery, most meningoencephaloceles involve the nasal cavity and paranasal sinuses or the temporal bone. Patients may present with rhinorrhea.

A combination of imaging modalities, including nuclear scintigraphy, CT, and/or MRI, is complementary in evaluating this surgical complication. In a patient who presents with rhinorrhea, it is important to determine whether the CSF leak is due to a dural laceration or a meningo(encephalo)cele. Following the placement of pledgets in the nares, intrathecal instillation of indium-diethylene triamine pentaacetic acid (DTPA) may be used to confirm and localize the presence of a CSF leak. Counts from the pledgets placed in the nose are recorded. Once a leak is established, coronal CT may be performed for anatomic localization. Alternatively, cisternography may be performed in which iodinated contrast material is injected intrathecally, and subsequently CT is performed in the coronal plane. It is best to scan these patients in the prone position so as not to inhibit an active leak. If an encephalocele is suspected, MRI in the sagittal and coronal planes is most useful in establishing this diagnosis by showing direct continuity of the tissue in the sinonasal cavity with the intracranial brain. MRI is also best for establishing the type of tissue in the sac (CSF, brain). Although imaging may be useful in detecting CSF leaks, fluorescein injected intrathecally followed by endoscopic evaluation may allow direct visualization of an active leak.

Notes

Optic Neuritis (Multiple Sclerosis Plaque)

1. High signal intensity within the right optic nerve associated with avid enhancement.

2. Optic neuritis (demyelinating disease), sarcoid, infection, primary tumor (glioma and meningioma), and metastatic disease.

3. Demyelinating disease (multiple sclerosis).

4. Acute multiple sclerosis presenting with transverse myelitis and optic neuritis.

Reference

Beck RW, Cleary PA, Trobe JD, et al: The effect of corticosteroids for acute optic neuritis on the subsequent development of multiple sclerosis, *N Engl J Med* 329:1764-1769, 1993.

Cross-Reference

Neuroradiology: THE REQUISITES, pp 290-292.

Comment

Optic neuritis represents inflammation of the optic nerve with clinical manifestations that include decreased visual acuity, pain, and afferent pupillary defect. A wide spectrum of disease processes may be associated with optic neuritis, most commonly demyelinating disease followed by idiopathic disease. Approximately 50% of patients with optic neuritis develop multiple sclerosis, and about 15% of patients with multiple sclerosis have optic neuritis as their initial clinical presentation. Devic's disease (neuromyelitis optica) represents a specific syndrome of multiple sclerosis in which patients have isolated transverse myelitis and optic neuritis. These two may present simultaneously or on separate occasions. In older patients, vasculopathies and ischemia are more common causes of optic neuritis.

Evaluation of patients presenting with optic neuritis can be assessed using high resolution fat-suppressed fast spin echo T2W and enhanced T1W images. Imaging in the coronal plane is particularly useful. Imaging may demonstrate increased T2W signal intensity within the nerve itself, and postcontrast images may demonstrate enhancement of the nerve, as well as the nerve sheath due to perivenous inflammation (as in this case). In cases of clinically diagnosed optic neuritis, MRI of the brain is especially useful and is recommended because it may help to establish the diagnosis of demyelinating disease. In addition, several investigators have shown that the presence of brain lesions on MRI in patients with optic neuritis may be important in determining prognosis and outcome.

Notes

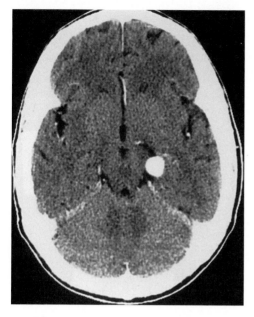
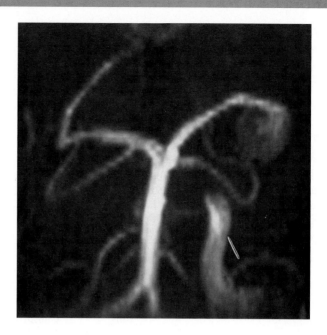

1. What are the CT imaging findings?
2. What is the differential diagnosis?
3. What imaging study could be done next to definitively establish the diagnosis?
4. Why are meningiomas frequently isodense or hyperdense to brain on unenhanced CT?

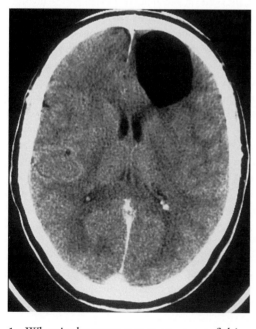
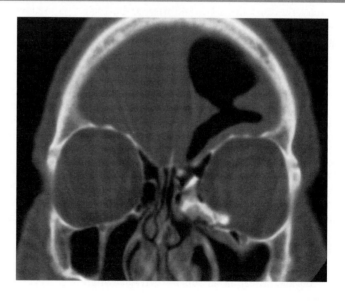

1. What is the most common cause of this entity?
2. This entity is most commonly described in association with what tumor of the paranasal sinuses?
3. Intracranial air is designated as "tension pneumocephalus" under what clinical circumstance?
4. What is the imaging modality of choice when there is clinical suspicion of tension pneumocephalus?

Aneurysm Arising From the Left Posterior Cerebral Artery

1. A well-demarcated, avidly enhancing mass in the left peri-mesencephalic cistern. There is no associated abnormality of the adjacent brain parenchyma.

2. Meningioma or an aneurysm arising from the posterior cerebral artery.

3. Spin-echo MR images should demonstrate the flow void associated with large aneurysms. MRA not only demonstrates the large posterior cerebral artery aneurysm but also evaluates the remainder of the circle of Willis for coexistent aneurysms. Catheter angiography remains the standard for complete evaluation of intracranial aneurysms.

4. Due to dense cellularity and/or calcification.

Reference

Setton A, Davis AJ, Bose A, et al: Angiography of cerebral aneurysms, *Neuroimag Clin North Am* 6:705-738, 1996.

Cross-Reference

Neuroradiology: THE REQUISITES, pp 136-138.

Comment

The majority of intracranial aneurysms arise from the supraclinoid segment of the internal carotid artery and its branches. Over 80% of saccular aneurysms arise from the anterior communicating artery, the distal internal carotid artery at the origin of the posterior communicating artery, the bifurcation of the supraclinoid internal carotid artery, and the middle cerebral artery bifurcation. Intracranial aneurysms are multiple in approximately 20% of cases. Aneurysms arising from the distal internal carotid artery at the origin of the ophthalmic artery account for 5% of intracranial aneurysms and have interesting features including a preponderance in women, multiplicity in 10% to 20% of cases, and bilaterality in up to 20% of cases.

Aneurysms arising from the posterior circulation are not uncommon; however, they occur much less frequently than do their anterior counterparts. Most originate from the tip of the basilar artery. Basilar tip aneurysms may become quite large in size, and not uncommonly the origins of one or both posterior cerebral arteries may be incorporated into the aneurysm. The next most common site for aneurysms in the posterior circulation is the origin of the posterior inferior cerebellar artery. Rarely, aneurysms may arise from the superior cerebellar artery or the anteroinferior cerebellar artery.

Aneurysms arising from distal arterial branches are usually acquired rather than congenital. They are frequently secondary to infection of the arterial wall (mycotic), trauma (aneurysms arising from the posterior circulation may be related to compression along the tentorium), and occasionally they may be related to tumor.

Notes

Tension Pneumocephalus

1. Trauma resulting in fractures of the paranasal sinuses.

2. Osteoma of the frontal sinuses and ethmoid air cells.

3. Tension pneumocephalus implies the presence of neurologic symptoms due to intracranial air leading to increased intracranial pressure.

4. CT.

Reference

Tobey JD, Loevner LA, Yousem DM, Lanza DC: Tension pneumocephalus: a complication of invasive ossifying fibroma of the paranasal sinuses, *AJR Am J Roentgenol* 166: 711-713, 1996.

Cross-Reference

Neuroradiology: THE REQUISITES, p 168.

Comment

Tension pneumocephalus is used to describe the situation in which there are neurologic symptoms due to intracranial air resulting in increased intracranial pressure. Symptoms are similar to those of other space-occupying lesions. Tension pneumocephalus can develop when there is communication between the extracranial and intracranial compartments (usually through a bony defect that is accompanied by a dural defect). When the intracranial pressure is lower such that the ingress of air into the intracranial compartment is favored, tension pneumocephalus may result. The most common cause of tension pneumocephalus is trauma resulting in fractures of the frontal sinuses and ethmoid air cells. It may also occur as a result of craniofacial surgery or tumors of the paranasal sinuses (most commonly described with osteomas). The pathogenesis of tension pneumocephalus is ascribed to a ball-valve mechanism. For instance, in the presence of a bony defect resulting in communication between the paranasal sinuses and anterior cranial fossa, pressure within the sinuses may transiently be increased with coughing or sneezing. In this situation air flows from the sinuses into the lower-pressure intracranial compartment until there is equilibration of pressure. Less commonly, a negative intracranial pressure gradient, such as might be seen with a large CSF leak, may draw air into the cranial compartment.

The diagnosis of pneumocephalus is readily established with CT, which can detect very small volumes of air (reportedly as small as 0.5 ml). CT also establishes the presence of mass effect and is useful in identifying osseous defects in the cranium.

Notes

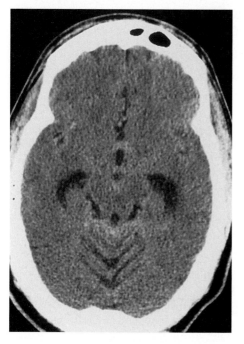 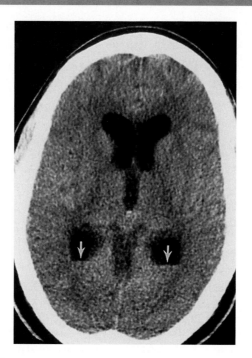

1. What are the pertinent imaging findings?
2. What infectious agents have a propensity to cause choroid plexitis?
3. What are the typical MRI findings of ventriculitis/ependymitis?
4. Periventricular calcification following neonatal ventriculitis is typically associated with what infectious agent?

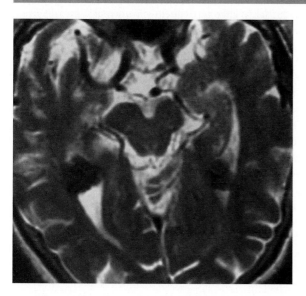

1. What is the most common location of choroid plexus papillomas in children?
2. What neurocutaneous syndrome may be associated with prominent calcification of the choroid plexus?
3. What benign lesion of the choroid plexus has been associated with chromosomal abnormalities?
4. What neoplasms may arise from the choroid plexus?

ANSWERS

CASE 130

Ventriculitis With Acute Hydrocephalus—*Streptococcus viridans*

1. Acute hydrocephalus and fluid-fluid levels layering in the lateral ventricles *(arrows)*.

2. *Cryptococcus* and *Nocardia*.

3. Ventricular enlargement, periventricular hyperintensity on FLAIR images, proton density, and T2W images.

4. CMV.

References

Goeser CD, McLeary MS, Young LW: Diagnostic imaging of ventriculoperitoneal shunt malfunctions and complications, *RadioGraphics* 18:635-651, 1998.

Bakshi R, Kinkel PR, Mechtler LL, Bates VE: Cerebral ventricular empyema associated with severe adult pyogenic meningitis: computed tomography findings, *Clin Neurol Neurosurg* 99:252-255, 1997.

Cross-Reference

Neuroradiology: THE REQUISITES, pp 174-175, 180.

Comment

This case demonstrates acute hydrocephalus and fluid-fluid levels *(arrows)* within the occipital horns of the lateral ventricles consistent with ventriculitis complicating pyogenic meningitis. Lumbar puncture yielded pus. Ventriculitis is due to the introduction of infectious organisms into the ependyma/ventricles and may be secondary to bacteremia, extension of an intraparenchymal abscess, trauma, or surgical instrumentation (especially placement of ventricular shunts). In addition to ventriculitis, other complications of ventriculoperitoneal shunts include overdrainage resulting in slit ventricle syndrome, subdural hematomas (which are frequently bilateral), shunt malfunction, surgery-related complications, and metastases in the setting of neoplasm (such as primitive neuroectodermal tumor).

Approximately 20% of patients with pyogenic bacterial meningitis will have complications necessitating neurosurgical intervention (surgery or a ventriculostomy) even after antibiotic therapy. Such complications include subdural empyema, parenchymal brain abscess, ventriculitis with hydrocephalus, and/or encephalitis. The development of such complications may correlate with inadequate treatment, as well as the duration of meningitis before the initiation of therapy.

Cytomegalovirus ventriculitis is unusual but may occur in patients with HIV infection. Most HIV-infected patients with CMV ventriculitis have already been diagnosed with an AIDS-defining condition. Pathologic findings include inflammation of the ependyma and periventricular structures, as well as ependymal necrosis with CMV intranuclear inclusion bodies. The differential diagnosis in this patient population is non-Hodgkin's lymphoma.

Notes

168

CASE 131

Xanthogranuloma of the Choroid Plexus

1. The atrium of the lateral ventricle.

2. Neurofibromatosis type 2.

3. Choroid plexus cyst.

4. Papilloma, carcinoma, meningioma, and hemangioma.

Reference

Gaskill SJ, Salvidor V, Rutman J, Marlin AE: Giant bilateral xanthogranulomas in a child: case report, *Neurosurg* 31:114-117, 1992.

Cross-Reference

Neuroradiology: THE REQUISITES, pp 78-79.

Comment

The most common neoplasm arising from the choroid plexus in children is the papilloma, which usually occurs in the trigone/atrium of the lateral ventricle. In adults they occur most commonly in the fourth ventricle. Choroid plexus carcinomas are rare lesions that also arise in the lateral ventricles of children. The majority also have seeding of the subarachnoid spaces at presentation. Meningiomas occur most commonly in the trigone of the lateral ventricle (they have been reported more commonly on the left side) and are seen in adults (except in patients with neurofibromatosis type 2). When large enough, intraventricular meningiomas may undergo spontaneous hemorrhage or may invade the brain parenchyma. Choroid plexus hemangiomas are benign neoplasms most commonly seen in the lateral ventricles. They are frequently incidental lesions detected on studies being performed for other reasons.

In addition to neoplasms, a spectrum of benign lesions occurs in the choroid plexus. Choroid plexus cysts are nonneoplastic lesions lined by epithelium that usually occur within the glomus. They are often bilateral. In a small percentage of cases, these cysts may be associated with chromosomal abnormalities (trisomies). Most choroid plexus cysts are identified on in utero ultrasound, in neonates, or in elderly patients. Xanthogranulomas are benign masses arising from the glomus of the choroid plexus in the lateral ventricles, which histologically have lymphocytes and macrophages incorporated within them. They represent a degenerative process, are most commonly seen in older patients, and are usually bilateral. They may become quite large and are occasionally confused with a tumor. Although uncommon, xanthogranulomas may be seen in children. On imaging they may have calcium, cystic change, and fat density/intensity within them.

Notes

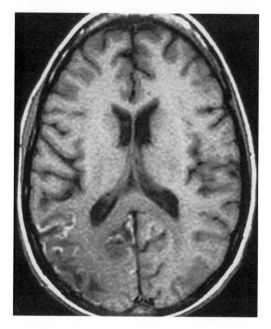 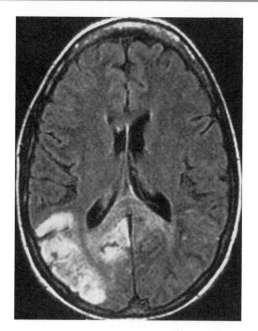

1. What are common causes of high signal intensity within the cerebral cortex on unenhanced T1W images?
2. What is the differential diagnosis in this case?
3. How can stroke, encephalitis, and neoplasm be differentiated clinically?
4. Subacute sclerosing panencephalitis typically occurs as a result of what previous infection?

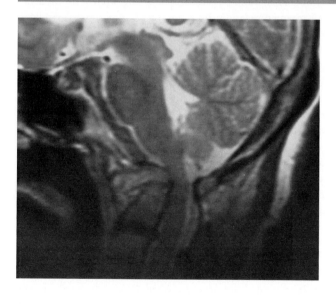 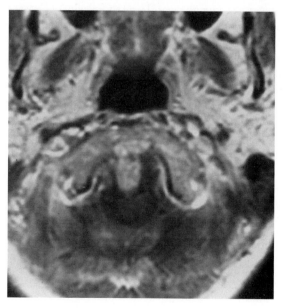

1. Does the patient in this case have platybasia or basilar invagination?
2. Define basilar invagination.
3. What is the basal angle?
4. What lines are used to define basilar invagination?

Viral Encephalitis

1. Petechial hemorrhage and calcification.

2. Ischemia, encephalitis, or primary neoplasm.

3. Stroke and encephalitis typically present with acute symptomatology compared with neoplasms, which have a more prolonged presentation. In the acute setting, focal motor deficits are more common with strokes than with encephalitis.

4. Measles. Subacute sclerosing panencephalitis typically occurs in children (boys more often than girls by a ratio of 2:1) and usually presents within 5 years following measles infection.

Reference

Jubelt B: Enterovirus and mumps virus infections of the nervous system, *Neurol Clin* 2:187-207, 1984.

Cross-Reference

Neuroradiology: THE REQUISITES, pp 181-185.

Comment

Encephalitis refers to an inflammatory process of the brain that manifests pathologically by an inflammatory infiltrate in the acute setting. Other pathologic findings include vascular congestion, edema, neuronal degeneration, hemorrhage, and/or necrosis. Viral encephalitis may result from an acute or latent (herpesvirus) infection. In the United States, arboviruses are probably the most common cause of viral encephalitis. They are frequently transmitted by insect bite (ticks and mosquitoes). Aseptic meningitis most commonly occurs with enteroviruses, although it is seen less often with mumps or herpes infection. Enteroviruses most commonly affect infants and children, and infection may occur through fecal-oral contamination, pets, or insects. Although aseptic meningitis is the most common presentation, meningoencephalitis may occur.

Subacute sclerosing panencephalitis (SSPE) occurs most commonly following a measles infection in children. The risk of SSPE is particularly increased when a child is infected with measles before 1.5 to 2 years of age. Children may present with cognitive decline, behavioral disorders, and problems with language. SSPE may have a slow, progressive course or may be rapidly progressive in some cases. Imaging findings include abnormalities in the periventricular white matter, the basal ganglia, and the posterior fossa (cerebellum and brain stem). Enhancement is not usually present. In the late stages of infection, diffuse cortical atrophy may be present.

Notes

Basilar Invagination—Rheumatoid Arthritis

1. Basilar invagination.

2. Implies superior migration of the odontoid process of the dens through the foramen magnum and into the intracranial compartment.

3. It is formed at the intersection of a line drawn from the tuberculum along the clivus to the anterior aspect of the foramen magnum and a line drawn from the nasion to the tuberculum sellae.

4. McGregor's, Chamberlain's, and digastric lines.

Reference

Goel A, Bhatjiwale M, Desai K: Basilar invagination: a study based on 190 surgically treated patients, *J Neurosurg* 88:962-968, 1998.

Cross-Reference

Neuroradiology: THE REQUISITES, pp 264-265.

Comment

Basilar invagination occurs when there is superior migration of the odontoid process of the dens into the foramen magnum. Two lines are used to define basilar invagination: (1) McGregor's line, which extends from the hard palate to the undersurface of the occiput, and (2) Chamberlain's line, which extends from the hard palate to the posterior margin of the foramen magnum. If there is superior migration of the dens into the foramen magnum by more than 5 mm above these lines, basilar invagination is present. Basilar invagination is more common than is platybasia. Platybasia, or flattening of the skull base, occurs when the basal angle is larger than 143 degrees. Platybasia may be seen with a variety of bone disorders, including those associated with achondroplasia, osteogenesis imperfecta, renal osteodystrophy, Paget's disease, cleidocranial dysplasia, and Down syndrome.

Symptoms associated with disorders of the craniovertebral junction are usually related to compression of the brain stem and/or cervical spinal cord. Symptoms may be related to myelopathy, gait disturbance, and/or cranial neuropathies. Basilar invagination may occur with inflammatory arthropathies, especially rheumatoid arthritis, and is also associated with a variety of metabolic disorders and bone dysplasias. Such disorders include fibrous dysplasia, Paget's disease, renal osteodystrophy, osteomalacia, and cleidocranial dysplasia. Chiari I malformations have been described with both platybasia and basilar invagination. Surgical decompression is performed in patients with severe symptomatology.

Notes

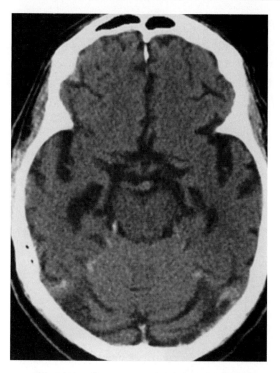 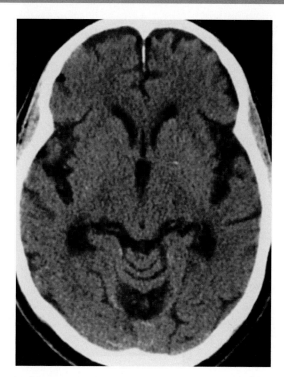

1. What are the pertinent imaging findings in this case?
2. This pattern of atrophy is characteristic of what neurodegenerative disorder?
3. What areas of the cerebrum are typically involved in Pick's disease?
4. Parkinson's disease is caused by an abnormality of the dopaminergic cells in what anatomic structure?

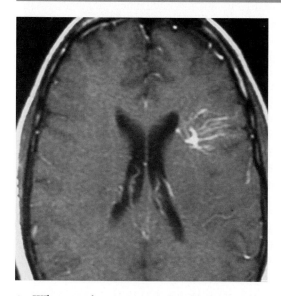

1. What are the most common locations of these lesions?
2. These lesions may be associated with what other vascular malformation?
3. What is the treatment of this lesion?
4. What neurocutaneous syndrome is associated with a diffuse venous malformation?

Alzheimer's Disease

1. Global cortical atrophy, with enlargement of the basal cisterns, the sylvian cisterns, and dilation of the choroidal-hippocampal fissure.

2. Alzheimer's disease.

3. The anterior frontal and temporal lobes.

4. The pars compacta of the substantia nigra.

References

Kitagaki H, Mori E, Yamaji S, et al: Frontotemporal dementia and Alzheimer disease: evaluation of cortical atrophy with automated hemispheric surface display generated with MR images, *Radiology* 208:431-439, 1998.

De Leon MJ, George AE, Golomb J, et al: Frequency of hippocampal formation atrophy in normal aging and Alzheimer's disease, *Neurobiol Aging* 18:1-11, 1997.

Cross-Reference

Neuroradiology: THE REQUISITES, p 230.

Comment

Each year approximately 1 in 500 people is diagnosed with dementia. Approximately 66% of these cases result from Alzheimer's disease. Alzheimer's disease is characterized clinically by progressive memory loss and cognitive decline. As the disease progresses, it is often difficult for patients to carry out the daily tasks of living. Not uncommonly depression accompanies Alzheimer's disease.

The most common imaging finding in Alzheimer's disease is diffuse cortical atrophy, which is often most pronounced in the temporal lobes. Approximately 70% of patients with Alzheimer's disease have dilation of the temporal horns. This is frequently accompanied by asymmetric dilation of the choroidal-hippocampal fissure (a response to medial temporal/hippocampal atrophy). Other imaging findings when compared with age-matched controls include an increase in the total CSF volume, enlargement of the sylvian cisterns, and an increase in ventricular size. In addition, longitudinal studies in patients with Alzheimer's disease compared with normal controls have demonstrated that atrophy progresses much more rapidly in patients with Alzheimer's disease. Deep white matter and periventricular regions of T2W hyperintensity are common in Alzheimer's disease. The literature suggests that there is no statistically significant difference in the extent of white matter disease between individuals with Alzheimer's disease and normal controls. Despite the radiologic findings in Alzheimer's disease, the findings are nonspecific and may be seen in a variety of other neurodegenerative processes. The major role of imaging in patients with dementia is to exclude underlying abnormalities such as tumors that may be amenable to therapy.

Notes

Venous Angioma

1. The frontal and parietal lobes.

2. CM.

3. None. Most venous angiomas are incidental findings that represent a compensatory venous drainage route for normal brain. Sacrifice of these lesions could result in venous infarction of the normal brain that they drain.

4. Sturge-Weber syndrome.

Reference

Lee C, Pennington MA, Kennedy CM III: MR evaluation of developmental venous anomalies: medullary venous anatomy of venous angiomas, *AJNR Am J Neuroradiol* 17:61-70, 1996.

Cross-Reference

Neuroradiology: THE REQUISITES, p 142.

Comment

Venous malformations (also referred to as venous angiomas, developmental venous anomalies, and medullary venous malformations) likely occur late in the first trimester and early in the second trimester of gestation when the medullary veins are developing. Insults leading to failure in the development of the normal venous structures are believed to be the cause of venous angiomas. Instead of the normal parallel appearance of the medullary veins as they drain into subependymal or superficial cortical veins, a disorganized network of dilated medullary veins converge in a "caput medusa" appearance and drain into an enlarged venous channel that subsequently drains into either the superficial or deep venous system. Simultaneous drainage into the superficial and deep venous systems is unusual. The brain parenchyma surrounding a venous angioma is typically normal. Although the incidence of venous angiomas has been reported to be approximately 3%, in my experience incidental venous angiomas are likely detected in a larger percentage of cases. Venous angiomas most commonly occur in the periventricular region (52%), although they may also occur in cortical (23%) and subcortical (17%) locations. Venous malformations are found most commonly in the frontal lobes; however, they also occur in the parietal and temporal lobes, the brain stem/brachium pontis, and the cerebellum. Sturge-Weber syndrome represents a more extensive venous malformation that results from failure of development of the normal venous system, often covering a large portion of a cerebral hemisphere. Large cerebral malformations may also be seen in Klippel-Trénaunay-Weber syndrome. Over 98% of venous angiomas are asymptomatic; however, rarely these lesions may hemorrhage (more commonly associated with cerebellar venous angiomas). Such patients may present with headache or focal neurologic symptoms.

Notes

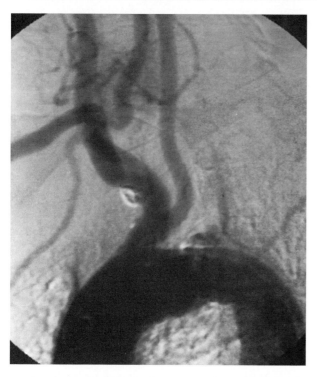
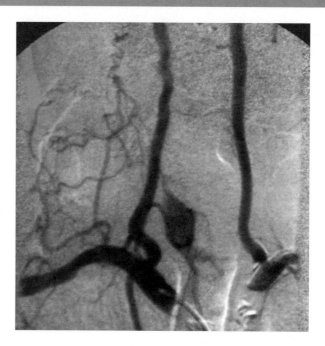

1. On the second image provided, what is the pertinent finding?

2. What is the name of this entity, and does it occur more frequently on the left or the right?

3. On physical examination, what might the findings be?

4. To confirm the diagnosis of "subclavian steal" on two-dimensional time-of-flight MRA, where would one position the stationary saturation pulse?

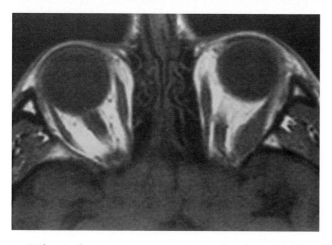
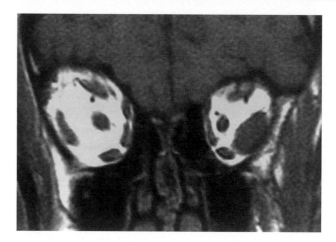

1. What is the most common cause of unilateral or bilateral proptosis?

2. What is the most common pattern of extraocular muscle involvement in thyroid ophthalmopathy?

3. What is the typical clinical presentation of orbital pseudotumor?

4. What structure runs between the superior rectus muscle and the optic nerve?

Subclavian Steal

1. Retrograde flow down the left vertebral artery.

2. "Subclavian steal"; on the left.

3. Differential blood pressures between the right and left arms (the left being lower), left supraclavicular bruit, and decreased pulses in the left arm.

4. In standard two-dimensional time-of-flight MRA, there is usually a stationary superior saturation pulse that is used to suppress the signal from the neck veins. Because in subclavian steal there is retrograde flow in the involved vertebral artery, this saturation pulse has to be removed or an inferior saturation pulse should be applied.

Reference

Turjman F, Tournut P, Baldy-Porcher C, et al: Demonstration of subclavian steal by MR angiography, *J Comput Assist Tomogr* 16:756-759, 1992.

Cross-Reference

Neuroradiology: THE REQUISITES, p 109.

Comment

Subclavian steal results from occlusion or a hemodynamically significant stenosis of the proximal subclavian or brachiocephalic artery. Subclavian steal occurs much more commonly on the left than on the right. As a result, there is a retrograde flow of blood down the ipsilateral vertebral artery in order to provide collateral blood supply to the arm (bypassing the occlusion/stenosis of the proximal subclavian artery).

In patients with subclavian steal, symptoms and signs may be related to decreased blood flow to the arm (decreased pulse, reduced blood pressure, decreased temperature, or claudication) or neurologic symptoms as a result of periodic ischemia in the posterior circulation. Neurologic symptoms include transient attacks, dizziness, and visual symptoms. Similar neurologic symptoms may occur with high grade stenoses or occlusions of the proximal vertebral artery (however, the arm is not symptomatic). Subclavian stenosis can often be diagnosed on physical examination. Imaging studies that may help confirm the diagnosis include Doppler and MRA studies, which may correctly demonstrate retrograde flow down the involved vertebral artery. On arch aortography, early arterial films show occlusion or stenosis of the proximal subclavian artery, whereas delayed films demonstrate retrograde flow. Neurointerventional techniques may be used to treat symptomatic patients and include percutaneous transluminal angioplasty or positioning of stents.

Notes

Orbital Pseudotumor

1. Thyroid ophthalmopathy.

2. Diffuse enlargement of all rectus muscles.

3. Pain, decreased ocular motility, and proptosis.

4. The superior ophthalmic vein.

Reference

Atlas SW, Grossman RI, Savino PJ, et al: Surface-coil MR of orbital pseudotumor, *AJR Am J Roentgenol* 148:804-808, 1987.

Cross-Reference

Neuroradiology: THE REQUISITES, pp 296-297.

Comment

Pseudotumor is a nonspecific inflammation of unknown etiology that involves the contents of the orbit. Typical clinical manifestations include proptosis, pain, and decreased ocular motility. Although the disorder is usually unilateral, it may be bilateral in less than 10% of patients. Underlying systemic disorders should be considered in cases of bilateral disease, including sarcoid, lymphoma, connective tissue disease, Wegener's granulomatosis, and autoimmune disorders. In the early stages of orbital pseudotumor, pathology is characterized by inflammation and edema. Histology shows an abundance of lymphocytes, plasma cells, and giant cells. In the late stages of disease, fibrosis may be abundant. Orbital pseudotumor may present with a spectrum of manifestations, including myositis (as in this case), dacryoadenitis (lacrimal gland involvement), periscleritis (uveal and scleral thickening), or retrobulbar soft tissue abnormality. In myositis, pseudotumor may involve one or more muscles and unlike thyroid ophthalmopathy often involves the tendinous insertion of the muscle as well as the muscle bellies. When idiopathic inflammation primarily involves the cavernous sinus and the orbital apex, it is referred to as *Tolosa-Hunt syndrome.* Ophthalmoplegia is secondary to involvement of cranial nerves III through VI in the cavernous sinus.

Because orbital pseudotumor radiologically may appear similar to a variety of disease processes, patient history is important (pseudotumor is classically associated with pain and acute onset). Importantly, there is usually a dramatic response to steroids that may be useful in confirming the diagnosis of pseudotumor. A small percentage of patients with pseudotumor do not respond to steroids and may require radiation and/or chemotherapy.

Notes

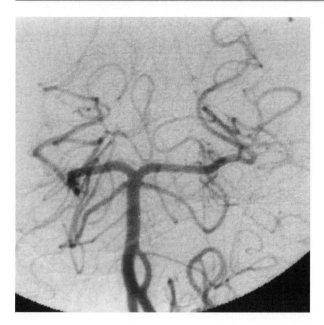

1. What branch of the basilar artery may extend into the IAC?
2. What arteries of the posterior circulation give rise to midbrain perforating arteries?
3. The basilar artery is formed by the fusion of what primitive vessels?
4. Do aneurysms arising from a fenestrated basilar artery more commonly arise from the proximal or distal end of the fenestration?

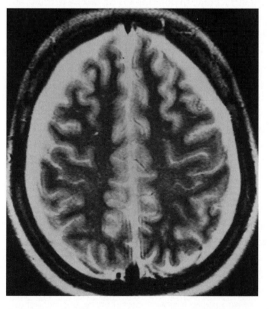 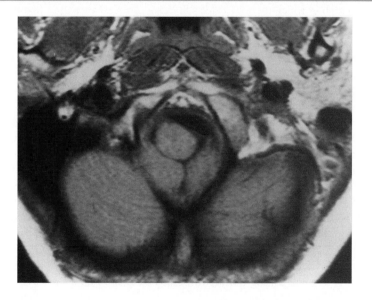

1. What are the pertinent imaging findings in this case?
2. What is the differential diagnosis of diffuse dural enhancement?
3. What is the typical clinical presentation of patients with spontaneous intracranial hypotension?
4. What are causes of intracranial hypotension?

Fenestrated Basilar Artery

1. The anterior inferior cerebellar artery.

2. The basilar and proximal posterior cerebral arteries.

3. The longitudinal neural arteries.

4. The proximal end.

References

Fujimura M, Sugawara P, Higuchi H, Oku P, Seki H: A ruptured aneurysm at the distal end of a basilar artery fenestration associated with multiple fenestrations of the vertebral basilar system: case report, *Surg Neurol* 47: 469-472, 1997.

Sanders WP, Sorek PA, Mehta BA: Fenestration of intracranial arteries with special attention to associated aneurysms and other anomalies, *AJNR Am J Neuroradiol* 14:675-680, 1993.

Cross-Reference

Neuroradiology: THE REQUISITES, pp 60-62.

Comment

Fenestration of a cerebral artery is defined as a division of the vessel lumen that results in two separate vascular channels that are frequently not equal in size. Each of the channels is lined by endothelium. Pathologic evaluation of basilar artery fenestrations has shown that the vascular channels may or may not share a common adventitial layer. Histologically there are short segmental regions at both the proximal and distal ends of the fenestration in which there are defects in the media, similar to bifurcations of cerebral arteries.

Fenestrations are more common in the posterior circulation, reported in up to 0.6% of cerebral angiograms. In comparison, the angiographic incidence of fenestrations in the anterior circulation has been reported in up to 0.2% of cases. On postmortem examination, fenestrations in the posterior and anterior circulation have been reported in 6% to 7% of cases. The discrepancy between pathologic and angiographic incidence is likely due to the increased sensitivity at pathology. The basilar artery is formed by fusion of bilateral longitudinal neural arteries early. Fenestrations occur along regions where there is failure of complete fusion of the medial aspects of these longitudinal arteries. Aneurysms may arise from a fenestration; however, when considering all fenestrations (anterior and posterior circulation) the incidence is approximately 3%, not significantly different from aneurysms arising at the circle of Willis. Aneurysms arising from fenestrations of the posterior circulation may occur more frequently (in up to 7% of cases).

The vertebral arteries are formed by fusion of primitive cervical segmental arteries and basivertebral anastomotic vessels. Extracranial duplications of a vertebral artery are most likely related to failure of regression of cervical segmental arteries, whereas intracranial duplications likely arise as a result of persistence of basivertebral anastomoses.

Notes

Spontaneous Intracranial Hypotension

1. Bilateral subdural effusions and low-lying cerebellar tonsils.

2. Metastatic disease (breast and prostate carcinoma), lymphoma/leukemia, granulomatous disease (tuberculosis, sarcoidosis, Wegener's granulomatosis, Erdheim Chester disease, lipid granulomatosis), spontaneous intracranial hypotension, and idiopathic hypertrophic pachymeningitis.

3. Postural headaches.

4. Thoracic diverticula due to focal thinning in the dura (postmyelography CT is useful in detecting these) and spontaneous, posttraumatic, and iatrogenic (after lumbar puncture or spinal surgery) causes.

References

Moayeri NN, Henson JW, Schaefer PW, Zervas NT: Spinal dural enhancement on magnetic resonance imaging associated with spontaneous intracranial hypotension, *J Neurosurg* 88:912-918, 1998.

Sishman RA, Dillon WP: Dural enhancement and cerebral displacement secondary to intracranial hypotension, *Neuroradiology* 43:609-611, 1993.

Cross-Reference

Neuroradiology: THE REQUISITES, pp 479-480.

Comment

Spontaneous intracranial hypotension is caused by chronic, and often intermittent, leakage of CSF from the subarachnoid space. This CSF leakage results in low intracranial pressure. Symptomatic patients typically present with headaches that are frequently postural in nature (exacerbated in the upright position). Trauma, spontaneous (rupture of Tarlov's cyst), or iatrogenic (after lumbar puncture or spine surgery) causes result in CSF leakage, which typically occurs somewhere along the spinal column. Imaging findings may be subtle and nonspecific such that in the absence of providing a history of postural headaches, the diagnosis of intracranial hypotension is frequently overlooked. Imaging findings include sagging of the posterior fossa contents with low-lying cerebellar tonsils, elongation of the fourth ventricle, bilateral subdural effusions, and/or diffuse dural enhancement. In addition, prominent dural veins have been reported. Symptoms of intracranial hypotension may resolve spontaneously; however, further workup, including myelography or nuclear scintigraphy, is often necessary to identify the source of the CSF leak. If a source can be identified, positioning of an epidural blood patch can be performed and typically results in resolution of symptoms.

Notes

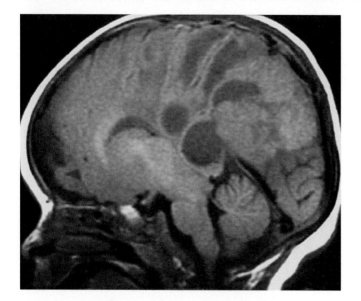

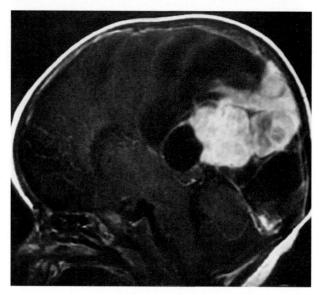

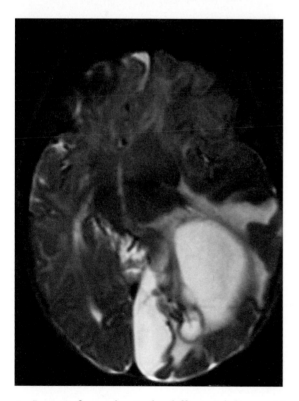

1. In an infant, what is the differential diagnosis?

2. What is the typical age of presentation of desmoplastic infantile gangliogliomas?

3. Pathologic evaluation with immunocytochemical stains demonstrates what type of cells within desmoplastic gangliogliomas?

4. What was the clinical presentation of this patient?

Desmoplastic Infantile Ganglioglioma*

1. Ependymoma, primitive neuroectodermal tumor, astrocytoma, and desmoplastic infantile ganglioglioma.

2. Most present before 1.5 years of age.

3. Glial and neuronal cell lines.

4. Enlarging head circumference and seizures.

Reference

Tenreiro-Picon OR, Kamath SV, Knorr JR, Ragland RL, Smith TW, Lau KY: Desmoplastic infantile ganglioglioma: CT and MRI features, *Pediatr Radiol* 25:540-543, 1995.

Cross-Reference

Neuroradiology THE REQUISITES, p 95.

Comment

Desmoplastic infantile gangliogliomas (DIGs) are clinically different from the typical ganglioglioma. Whereas gangliogliomas typically present in young adults (approximately 70% in patients younger than 30 years of age), the majority of DIGs present before 18 months of age. Whereas gangliogliomas most commonly occur in the temporal lobes, DIGs characteristically present in the frontal and parietal lobes (although temporal lobe lesions may occur). DIGs also differ from classic gangliogliomas pathologically in that they contain immature neuroepithelial cells and a dense desmoplastic reaction.

Desmoplastic infantile gangliogliomas typically present with seizures; however, enlarging head circumference and progressive hemiparesis are common. Unlike classic gangliogliomas, DIGs have been reported more often in males. These neoplasms have a distinct appearance on CT and MRI. They are typically large, with both a cystic and an avidly enhancing solid component that represents the desmoplastic reaction. The solid component is located superficially along the cortex abutting the meninges and dura. Although rare, because teratomas and sarcomas have their highest incidence in infancy, these should also be considered; from an imaging standpoint, however, their appearance is not similar to DIGs. The pathologic and histologic findings of DIGs is that of a cellular spindle cell neoplasm. Hypertrophic astrocytes typically have eosinophilic cytoplasm and eccentric nuclei. In addition, larger neurons with eccentric nuclei, as well as cytoplasm containing Nissl bodies, are noted. Ganglion cells are common. Immunocytochemical staining for glial fibrillary acidic protein is markedly positive for astrocytes, and immunostaining for synaptophysin or neurofilament protein is positive, consistent with the presence of neuronal differentiation.

Notes

---

*Figures for Case 140 courtesy David M. Yousem, MD.

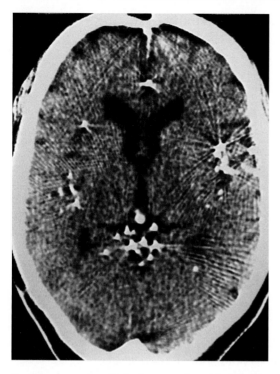

1. What neuroradiologic procedure(s) did this patient undergo many years ago?
2. What contrast agent did this patient receive during that procedure?
3. What complication is frequently associated with myelography performed with pantopaque?
4. What is the signal intensity of pantopaque on unenhanced T1W imaging?

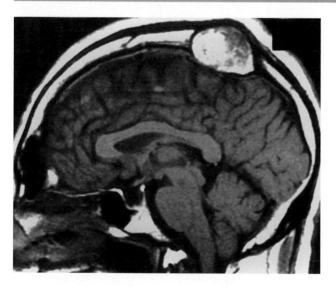 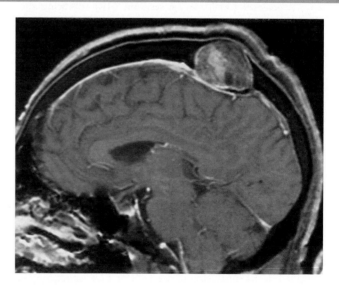

1. How would this lesion appear on plain film radiographs of the skull?
2. Osseous hemangiomas occur most frequently in what part of the skeleton?
3. What is the classic plain film appearance of a calvarial hemangioma?
4. What are the proposed causes of epidermoid cysts of the skull?

CASE 141

Subarachnoid Pantopaque

1. Myelography and/or cisternography.

2. Pantopaque (iophendylate).

3. Arachnoiditis.

4. Hyperintense because pantopaque is an oil-based contrast agent.

Reference

Lidov MW, Silvers AR, Mosesson RE, Stollman AL, Som PM: Pantopaque simulating thrombosed intracranial aneurysms on MRI, *J Comput Assist Tomogr* 20:225-227, 1996.

Cross-Reference

Neuroradiology: THE REQUISITES, pp 17-19, 455-457, 472-474.

Comment

This case shows punctate foci of high density throughout the intracranial subarachnoid spaces. This appearance is due to the radiopaque oil-based contrast agent pantopaque (a mixture of iodinated esters), which used to be used routinely to perform myelography. The use of intrathecal pantopaque, particularly in combination with hemorrhage such as might occur following surgery or lumbar puncture to perform a myelogram or cisternogram, was often complicated by arachnoiditis. MRI and postmyelography CT findings in arachnoiditis include clumping of nerve roots centrally within the thecal sac and/or adhesions of the nerve roots peripherally along the dura, resulting in an "empty sac" appearance. Enhancement of the nerve roots may sometimes be seen on MRI following the administration of intravenous gadolinium.

The advent of nonionic water-soluble contrast media has dramatically reduced the incidence of arachnoiditis. There is an approximate 3-g limit of iodinated contrast material that can be instilled into the thecal sac for myelography. Nonionic contrast agents are preferable in the CNS. Patients who have been taking medications that may lower seizure threshold should stop taking them 24 to 48 hours before myelography. Such medications include phenothiazines, tricyclic antidepressants, antipsychotics, monoamine oxidase inhibitors, and a variety of other medications such as lithium and isoniazid.

Although oil-based contrast agents such as pantopaque are no longer used for myelography, one can expect to see residua of this material in the subarachnoid space of the CNS for years to come. On plain film radiography, pantopaque is radiopaque. On MRI it is hyperintense on unenhanced T1W imaging, identified in the subarachnoid spaces. The T1W shortening is related to the fat within the contrast.

Notes

CASE 142

Intradiploic Epidermoid Cyst

1. As a well-circumscribed, lytic lesion.

2. The vertebral column.

3. A radiating sunburst or honeycomb pattern.

4. Inclusion of ectodermal cells rests during embryonic development; less commonly, it has been suggested that they may be acquired by traumatic implantation of ectodermal tissue into the bone.

References

Ochi M, Hayashi K, Hayashi T, et al: Unusual CT and MR appearance of an epidermoid tumor of the cerebellopontine angle, *AJNR Am J Neuroradiol* 19:1113-1115, 1998.

Arana E, Latorre FF, Revert A, et al: Intradiploic epidermoid cysts, *Neuroradiology* 38:306-311, 1996.

Gormley WB, Tomecek FJ, Qureshi N, Malik GM: Craniocerebral epidermoid and dermoid tumours: a review of 32 cases, *Acta Neurochir* 128:115-121, 1994.

Cross-Reference

Neuroradiology: THE REQUISITES, pp 76-77.

Comment

Epidermoid and dermoid cysts of the skull are rare. Both are proposed to occur as a result of inclusion of epithelial cells during closure of the neural tube between the third and fifth weeks of gestation. However, development of epidermoid cysts secondary to implantation of epithelial cells following trauma has been suggested as the cause in approximately 25% of cases. Epidermoid cysts account for less than 2% of intracranial/cranial tumors. Approximately 25% occur in the skull, whereas the remaining 75% are intradural. Dermoid cysts are even less common. Epidermoid cysts tend to present in young adults, whereas dermoids present in children and young adolescents. Approximately 10% of calvarial epidermoids are incidental lesions; the remaining 90% are symptomatic. The most common presentation is an enlarging scalp mass; however, pain and/or headache is present in approximately 20% of cases. The most common location of these cysts is the parietal bone, followed by the frontal and temporal bones. Approximately 70% of these lesions involve both the inner and outer tables of the skull. Involvement of only the outer cortical table or, less commonly, the inner table may occur. On plain films, epidermoid cysts typically appear as lytic lesions with sclerotic borders. The differential diagnosis includes hemangioma, eosinophilic granuloma, and leptomeningeal cysts, especially in childhood. Other lytic lesions, particularly in adults, cannot be definitively differentiated from plain films alone. These lesions are typically hyperintense on T2W imaging; however, on unenhanced T1W imaging their signal characteristics are variable. High T1W signal intensity may be due to the presence of blood products, protein, and/or fat.

Notes

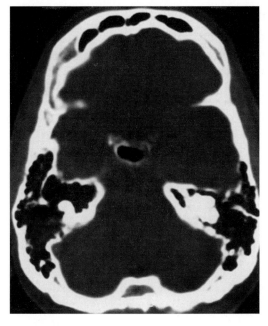
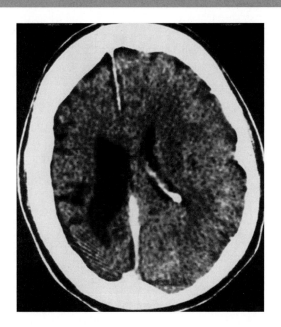

1. What are the pertinent imaging findings?

2. What neurocutaneous syndrome is associated with this entity?

3. What cerebral insult is most commonly implicated in this entity?

4. What syndrome associated with a hyperfunctioning pituitary adenoma may result in enlargement of the paranasal sinuses?

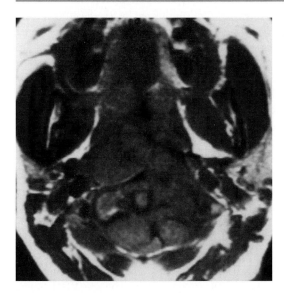
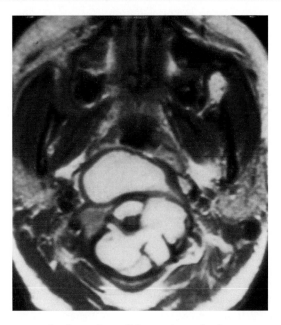

1. One may determine that the lesion arises in the prevertebral portion of the perivertebral compartment based on anterior displacement of what structures?

2. What primary skull base lesions arising from the clivus or craniovertebral junction are commonly associated with calcification and/or bony destruction?

3. Notochordal remnants give rise to what type of tumor?

4. Chordomas are most frequently found in what location?

CASE 143

Dyke-Davidoff-Masson Syndrome

1. Atrophy of the right cerebral hemisphere with compensatory enlargement of the right hemicranium.

2. Sturge-Weber syndrome.

3. A vascular insult (ischemia).

4. Acromegaly due to a growth hormone-secreting pituitary adenoma.

Reference

Sener RN, Jinkins JR: MR of craniocerebral hemiatrophy, *Clin Imaging* 16:93-97, 1992.

Cross-Reference

Neuroradiology: THE REQUISITES, pp 232-233.

Comment

The skull is composed of three distinct anatomic parts; the cranium, the face, and the skull base. The cranium may further be subdivided into the outer table, the diploic space, and the inner table. The outer table of the skull is structured to provide support for the attachments of numerous muscles and their ligaments. The diploic space contains hematopoietic tissue, fat, vessels, and water. The ratio of the cellular component relative to fat is determined by age. Red or hematopoietic marrow is seen in children. By 21 years of age the marrow in most people has undergone fatty conversion (yellow marrow). Abnormalities affecting the diploic space are usually related to hematopoietic marrow in the setting of chronic anemia, infiltrative processes (granulomatous disease, neoplasm), and myelofibrosis.

The inner table of the cranium is quite responsive to, and reflective of, the growth of the intracranial contents. Focal mass effect on the inner table such as may be seen with arachnoid cysts, meningiomas, and other neoplasms may cause thinning or remodeling of it. Conversely, with cerebral insults in utero or in early life that result in atrophy, there may be compensatory ipsilateral thickening of the inner table in response to the reduction in cerebral volume. Dyke-Davidoff-Masson syndrome refers to ipsilateral hypertrophy of the cranium from cerebral hemiatrophy. There is thickening of the ipsilateral cranium that may be recognized on imaging as thickening of the cortex (particularly the inner cortical table) as well as the diploic space. In addition, there is usually lack of calvarial digital markings. Elevation of the sphenoidal and petrous ridges, ipsilateral enlargement of the orbit, and enlargement of the paranasal sinuses (especially the frontal sinuses), as well as the mastoid air cells, may accompany these changes. Dyke-Davidoff-Masson syndrome is most commonly associated with vascular/ischemic insults. It may also be seen in Sturge-Weber syndrome in which there is frequently cerebral hemiatrophy related to a large pial venous malformation.

Notes

CASE 144

Chordoma

1. The longus colli muscle complex.

2. Chondrosarcoma, chordoma, plasmacytoma, lymphoma, and giant cell tumor.

3. Chordoma.

4. The sacrum.

Reference

Meyers SP, Hirsch WJ Jr, Curtin HD, Barnes L, Sekhar LN, Sen C: Chordomas of the skull base: MR features, *AJNR Am J Neuroradiol* 13:1627-1636, 1992.

Cross-Reference

Neuroradiology: THE REQUISITES, pp 331-332, 436-437.

Comment

Chordomas arise in locations where notochordal remnants are found. They occur most commonly in the sacrum, although not infrequently they are found at the clivus or at the upper cervical spine (C1-2). Although chordomas are considered benign neoplasms, they may grow quite invasively, particularly at the skull base where they can invade the neural foramen or the cavernous sinus and/or extend into the posterior and middle cranial fossa. Like giant cell tumors, chordomas (although considered benign based on their histologic appearance) may metastasize in a small percentage of patients. CT and MRI play complementary roles in assessing these tumors. On CT calcified matrix may be present and regions of bony erosion or destruction are best delineated. Multiplanar MRI allows complete identification of the extent of the lesion. On MRI the signal characteristics of chordomas are variable. These tumors are typically hypointense on T1W imaging and hyperintense on T2W imaging (although there may be marked heterogeneity due to cellularity, vascularity, and/or calcified matrix). Most chordomas enhance, although some tumors have minimal enhancement. In my experience, tumors arising at the C1-2 region have been associated with less enhancement and more cystic type changes. The differential diagnosis includes chondroid lesions (chondrosarcoma), metastatic disease, multiple myeloma, and lymphoma. The presence of calcified matrix usually limits the differential diagnosis to chordoma versus chondrosarcoma. In my experience and as the literature indicates, it may be difficult to distinguish these two entities. In addition, clinical symptoms of chordomas and chondrosarcomas may be quite similar at the skull base, including headache and cranial neuropathies (frequently cranial nerve VI). Clinical presentation is usually in the second through fourth decades of life.

Notes

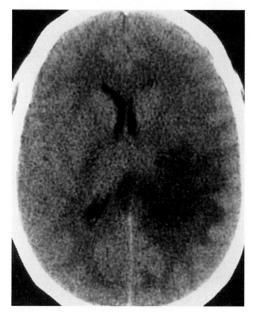 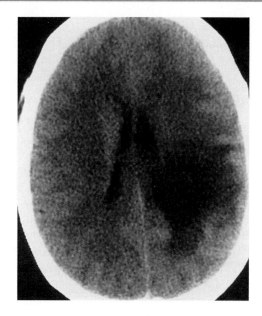

1. What is the differential diagnosis in this case?
2. What clinical and imaging factors might help differentiate demyelinating disease from a glioma?
3. What percentage of patients with multiple sclerosis present after 50 years of age?
4. What findings may be present in the CSF in patients with multiple sclerosis?

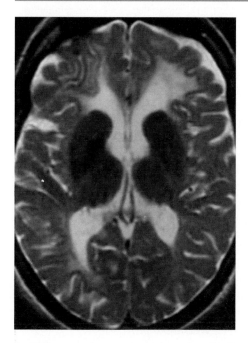

1. What are the pertinent imaging findings?
2. Positive Perls' staining indicates the presence of what type of products?
3. What deep gray matter nucleus is associated with increasing amounts of iron deposition with age?
4. Regardless of age, what deep gray matter structures typically do not have hypointensity on T2W images in normal patients?

Tumefactive Multiple Sclerosis

1. Glioma, demyelinating disease, and encephalitis.

2. Young age, the presence of additional lesions separate from the mass, and neurologic symptoms spaced over time and location favor demyelinating disease.

3. Approximately 10%.

4. Elevated oligoclonal bands (≥ 90% of cases) and elevated IgG (approximately 75% of patients).

Reference

Dagher AP, Smirniotopoulos J: Tumefactive demyelinating lesions, *Neuroradiology* 38:560-565, 1996.

Cross-Reference

Neuroradiology: THE REQUISITES, pp 202-209.

Comment

Although the etiology of multiple sclerosis is unknown, several causative factors have been implicated. These include autoimmune disease, infection (viral agent), and genetic factors. The prevalence of multiple sclerosis varies with geographic location.

Variants of multiple sclerosis may be present on a clinical and/or imaging basis. The majority of patients with multiple sclerosis present in the third or fourth decade of life; however, a virulent form of acute multiple sclerosis (Marburg type) infrequently occurs and is usually seen in younger patients. It may be preceded by fevers and is typically rapidly progressive, often resulting in death. In such cases there is extensive demyelination. A variety of multiple sclerosis that may involve the optic nerves and spinal cord (either simultaneously or, less commonly, separately) is Devic's disease or neuromyelitis optica. Concentric sclerosis or Balo type sclerosis is characterized by alternating rings of demyelination and myelination (normal brain or areas of remyelination) and has a characteristic MRI appearance.

Multiple sclerosis and other demyelinating diseases, such as acute disseminated encephalomyelitis and progressive multifocal leukoencephalopathy, may present as a mass lesion with or without enhancement. "Tumefactive" multiple sclerosis on imaging may be mistaken for a neoplasm or occasionally an abscess, particularly in the absence of a clinical history. The age of the patient may be helpful (multiple sclerosis typically occurs in younger patients). In addition, there are often additional clinical and/or imaging findings to suggest the diagnosis of multiple sclerosis. On close questioning, patients often have neurologic symptoms that are spaced both in time and in location. Furthermore, MRI evaluation may demonstrate white matter lesions separate from the mass that are suggestive of multiple sclerosis. Unlike neoplasms, tumefactive multiple sclerosis often has relatively little mass effect for the amount of signal abnormality present. Multiple sclerosis less commonly involves the gray matter.

Notes

Accelerated Iron Deposition in the Deep Gray Matter

1. Diffuse T2W hypointensity in the deep gray matter of the basal ganglia and thalami.

2. Iron (ferric)-containing compounds.

3. The lentiform nucleus, especially the globus pallidus.

4. The caudate nucleus and thalamus.

Reference

Milton WJ, Atlas SW, Lexa FJ, Mozley PD, Gur RE: Deep gray matter hypointensity patterns with aging in healthy adults: MR imaging at 1.5 T, *Radiology* 181:715-719, 1991.

Cross-Reference

Neuroradiology: THE REQUISITES, p 206.

Comment

Detection of iron deposition within the deep gray matter of the brain (globus pallidus, putamen, caudate nucleus, thalamus), as well as the dentate nuclei, substantia nigra, and red nuclei, manifests as hypointensity on T2W images and may serve as an indirect marker of cerebral neurodegenerative processes. Although there is a spectrum of normal iron deposition within the basal ganglia and brain stem nuclei noted at pathology and to some extent confirmed on MRI, certain trends are clear. Specifically, in healthy subjects hypointensity on T2W images within the substantia nigra, red nucleus, and dentate nucleus is present in young adults. Both evaluation of pathologic specimens and MRI suggests that the volume of iron products in these structures does not significantly increase with age. Although hypointensity in the globus pallidus is often present in young adults, the amount of hypointensity (reflective of iron deposition) increases with age. In addition, whereas hypointensity may be seen in the putamen, in normal subjects this typically is not seen before the sixth decade of life. Of note, hypointensity in the thalamus or caudate nucleus is generally not present in normal subjects regardless of age, and hypointensity in these locations is indicative of CNS disease.

The presence of a variety of CNS disorders may be suggested by the detection of hypointensity within the deep gray matter and nuclei that is different than the expected normal patterns. Increased brain iron may be seen in a variety of pathologic states, including demyelinating disease (multiple sclerosis), the leukodystrophies, brain anoxia and infarction, movement disorders (Wilson's disease, Hallervorden-Spatz disease), metabolic disorders, and significant closed head trauma. The patient in this case has an underlying leukodystrophy.

Notes

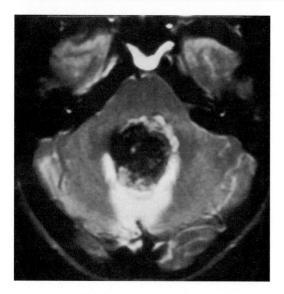

1. How would this mass appear on unenhanced CT?
2. What primitive neuroectodermal tumor occurs in the pineal gland?
3. In adults, where in the posterior fossa do medulloblastomas characteristically present?
4. Approximately what percentage of patients with medulloblastomas present with subarachnoid seeding of tumor?

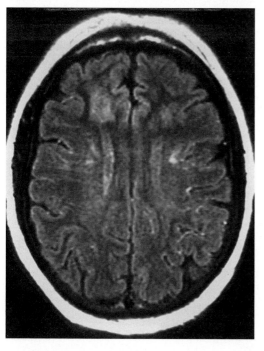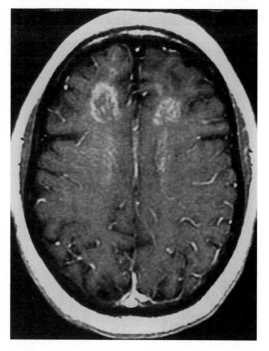

1. What disease is caused by a deficiency of β-galactosidase?
2. What dysmyelinating disorder is associated with an advancing edge of enhancing active demyelination as well as relative sparing of the subcortical U fibers?
3. Papovavirus is associated with what acquired demyelinating disorder?
4. What is the name of the fulminant form of ADEM associated with diffuse demyelination and white matter hemorrhage?

Medulloblastoma

1. Hyperdense.

2. Pineoblastoma.

3. The lateral cerebellar hemisphere.

4. Approximately 30%.

Reference

Mueller DP, Moore SA, Sato Y, Yuh WTC: MR spectrum of medulloblastoma, *Clin Imaging* 16:250-255, 1992.

Cross-Reference

Neuroradiology: THE REQUISITES, pp 82-85.

Comment

Medulloblastomas comprise up to one third of all pediatric posterior fossa tumors. They occur more commonly in boys than in girls (approximately 3:1) and arise from the superior medullary velum of the fourth ventricle from primitive neuroectoderm. In children they are typically midline masses associated with the inferior vermis. Importantly, subarachnoid seeding of the leptomeninges is very common at presentation (reported in up to 30% of cases in some series); therefore patients should have a screening contrast enhanced spine MRI study to exclude this type of spread. On unenhanced CT medulloblastomas are typically hyperdense relative to brain parenchyma because of their dense cellularity. They are demarcated masses and calcification, cystic change, and/or hemorrhage may be present in up to 10% to 20% of lesions. On MRI most medulloblastomas are mildly hypointense to brain parenchyma on T1W imaging. However, their signal characteristics on T2W imaging may vary considerably depending on the presence of hemorrhage and the degree of cellularity. Following the administration of intravenous contrast, most medulloblastomas demonstrate avid but heterogeneous enhancement. Typically they efface the fourth ventricle and present with hydrocephalus. The major differential diagnostic consideration of a midline posterior fossa mass in children is a fourth ventricular ependymoma. These typically arise in the fourth ventricle and expand rather than compress it. Unlike medulloblastomas, ependymomas characteristically grow through the foramina of Magendie and Luschka. Less commonly, cerebellar astrocytomas may occur in the midline; however, they usually are hemispheric lesions.

Notes

Enhancing Demyelinating Disease

1. Krabbe's disease (an obscure disorder that presents in the first 6 months of life with psychomotor retardation, seizures, and spasticity).

2. Adrenoleukodystrophy.

3. Progressive multifocal leukoencephalopathy.

4. Acute hemorrhagic encephalomyelitis.

Reference

Stewart WA, Alvord EC Jr, Hruby S, Hall LD, Paty DW: Magnetic resonance imaging of experimental allergic encephalomyelitis in primates, *Brain* 114:1069-1096, 1991.

Cross-Reference

Neuroradiology: THE REQUISITES, pp 212-213.

Comment

Acute disseminated encephalomyelitis does not have pathognomonic clinical or imaging findings; however, the diagnosis may be made with a high index of suspicion in the appropriate clinical setting (antecedent viral illness, vaccination). It is a monophasic demyelinating process that is immune-mediated and/or allergic in nature. Pathologic findings of ADEM include a variable perivascular inflammatory reaction (depending on whether tissue sampling was done during the acute or subacute phase), edema, varying degrees of perivenous demyelination, and the presence of macrophages containing myelin particles. Deposition of circulating immune complexes, complement activation, and localization of viral antigens in the walls of cerebral arteries may result in vascular damage. During active demyelination, there may be breakdown of the blood-brain barrier leading to enhancement of such lesions on MRI. In ADEM the development of new lesions should not occur after approximately 6 months following the initial onset of disease. Lesions most commonly involve the cerebrum; however, they also occur in the spinal cord and brain stem. Treatment is usually with high-dose steroids. Although results of therapy are often excellent, ADEM may be associated with significant morbidity and neurologic deficits. Death has been reported in up to one third of cases; a fulminant form of ADEM, acute hemorrhagic leukoencephalomyelitis, is associated with disseminated white matter demyelination and hemorrhage, as well as a high incidence of death.

Notes

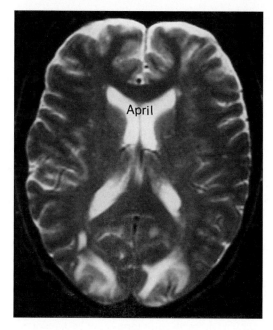 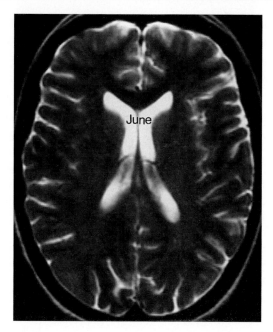

1. What intravenous drugs have been associated with transient white matter abnormalities?

2. What common immunosuppressive agent used following organ transplantation may be associated with white matter disease?

3. What is the most common location for cyclosporine toxicity in the CNS?

4. How is neurotoxicity secondary to cyclosporine managed?

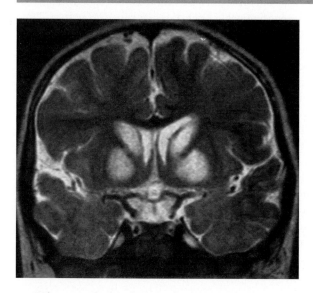

1. What metabolic abnormality does this patient have?

2. In Leigh disease, enzyme deficiencies result in a failure to properly metabolize what compound?

3. What are the characteristic signs and symptoms of Kearns-Sayre syndrome?

4. What mitochondrial disorder may be associated with bilateral subdural hematomas and cerebral atrophy?

Cyclosporine Neurotoxicity

1. Cocaine, methamphetamine, and heroin.

2. Cyclosporine; FK506 (tacrolimus) and OKT3 may also be associated with neurotoxicity.

3. The occipital lobes.

4. By aggressive management of hypertension, as well as temporary reduction or discontinuation of cyclosporine.

References

Schwartz RB, Bravo SM, Klufas RA, et al: Cyclosporine neurotoxicity and its relationship to hypertensive encephalopathy: CT and MR findings in 16 cases, *AJR Am J Roentgenol* 165:627-631, 1995.

de Groen PC, Aksamit AJ, Rakela J, Forbes GS, Krom RA: Central nervous system toxicity after liver transplantation. The role of cyclosporine and cholesterol, *N Engl J Med* 317:861-866, 1987.

Cross-Reference

Neuroradiology: THE REQUISITES, pp 216-217.

Comment

This case illustrates typical MRI findings in cyclosporine toxicity. Increased T2W signal intensity is most commonly seen in the deep and subcortical white matter of the occipital lobes; however, the remainder of the cerebrum may be involved. Imaging findings are similar in pattern to those of hypertensive encephalopathy. Management of hypertension and/or a reduction in the dose or temporary discontinuation of cyclosporine may result in reversibility of the clinical and imaging findings. In some cases, patients may be switched to FK506.

Cyclosporine has been an extremely successful immunosuppressant in adults following bone marrow transplantation, following whole organ transplantation, and following transplantation in children to reduce the effects of steroids on growth and the development of Cushing's syndrome. The use of cyclosporine must be closely monitored because of the significant side effects associated with it including toxicity to the liver, CNS, and kidney, as well as hypertension. Neurotoxicity is seen in 25% of patients and may manifest as visual disturbance including cortical blindness, seizures, change in mental status, cerebellar ataxia, paresthesias, and headache. A proposed mechanism for neurotoxicity has been suggested in which the neuropeptide endothelin results in focal vasoconstriction. Reported risk factors for the development of neurotoxicity in patients on cyclosporine in addition to hypertension include hypomagnesemia, hypoalbuminemia, and low total serum cholesterol levels following transplantation. Other conditions that may produce similar, potentially reversible white matter changes include intravenous drugs such as cocaine, chemotherapeutic agents (cytosine arabinoside, methotrexate, cisplatin), radiation therapy, hypertensive encephalopathy, and eclampsia.

Notes

Leigh Disease (Subacute Necrotizing Encephalomyelopathy)

1. Lactic acidosis.

2. Pyruvate.

3. Ophthalmoplegia, retinitis pigmentosa, ataxia, and cardiac abnormalities (heart block).

4. Menkes "kinky hair" disease.

Reference

Barkovich AJ, Good WV, Koch TK, Berg BO: Mitochondrial disorders: analysis of their clinical and imaging characteristics, *AJNR Am J Neuroradiol* 14:1119-1137, 1993.

Cross-Reference

Neuroradiology: THE REQUISITES, pp 245-246.

Comment

Infants and children with Leigh disease typically present in the first few years of life (although adult forms have been reported) with typical clinical manifestations, including hypotonia, ophthalmoplegia, nystagmus, ataxia, delayed psychomotor development, and metabolic lactic acidosis. Most cases are sporadic. Leigh disease has been associated with enzyme deficiencies, particularly enzymes related to metabolism of pyruvate. There may be a deficiency of pyruvate dehydrogenase, pyruvate carboxylase, or cytochrome C oxidase. Other biochemical and genetic abnormalities have also been recognized in patients with clinical symptoms consistent with those of Leigh disease.

Imaging findings in Leigh disease may be detected on CT and MRI and include hypoattenuation and T2W hyperintensity, respectively, within the deep gray matter (including the globus pallidus, putamen, and the caudate nuclei). Bilateral putamenal hyperintensity is classic. Abnormalities have also been identified within the periaqueductal gray matter, the cerebral peduncles, and, less commonly, the cortical gray matter. A spectrum of findings may be present on pathology, including vascular proliferation, neuronal loss, demyelination, and cystic cavitation in involved structures (most notably the basal ganglia, brain stem, cerebellar dentate nuclei, and, less common, the cerebral white matter). MR spectroscopy has identified reduced levels of *N*-acetyl-aspartate and elevated lactic acid levels. In general, the degree of elevation of lactate corresponds to the severity of imaging findings, being most pronounced in those regions of the brain shown on imaging to be most severely affected.

Notes

Challenge Cases

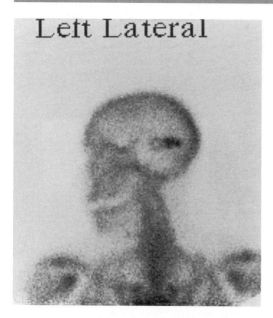

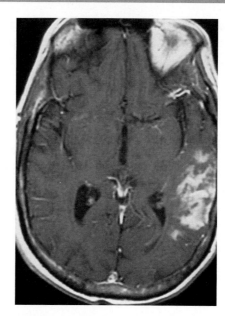

1. Using only the bone scan, what are the diagnostic considerations?
2. What radiopharmaceuticals are most commonly used for bone scanning?
3. What factors affect the accumulation of technetium-labeled radiopharmaceuticals in bone?
4. Using the bone scan and enhanced MRI, what is your best diagnosis?

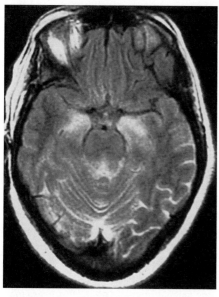

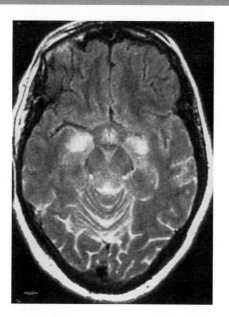

1. What is the differential diagnosis?
2. In limbic encephalitis, what structures are most commonly involved?
3. In CNS paraneoplastic syndromes, what are the two most common sites of involvement?
4. What malignancy is most commonly associated with this entity?

Subacute Middle Cerebral Artery Territory Stroke Simulating a Bone Metastasis

1. Metastatic disease, primary bone neoplasm, bone dysplasia (e.g., Paget's disease).

2. Technetium-labeled phosphate analogues.

3. Blood supply, the amount of mineralized bone, bone turnover, and systemic factors (medications such as hormones/vitamins).

4. A subacute-chronic stroke in the left middle cerebral artery territory simulating a bone lesion.

Reference

Rappaport AH, Hoffer PB, Genant HK: Unifocal bone findings by scintigraphy: clinical significance in patients with known primary cancer, *West J Med* 129:188-192, 1978.

Cross-Reference

Neuroradiology: THE REQUISITES, pp 106-114.

Comment

The left lateral projection from the patient's delayed bone scan demonstrates increased radiotracer activity projecting over the temporal bone region (it is important to remember that an anteroposterior view is necessary to accurately localize the abnormality). This was the only abnormality on the patient's bone scan. Corresponding enhanced MRI demonstrates mild local mass effect in the superficial portion of the posterior left temporal lobe with cortical enhancement; the imaging findings are consistent with a stroke. In this patient with renal cell carcinoma, the bone scan was initially interpreted as metastatic disease. It is important to remember that any process that stimulates deposition of calcium within soft tissues, the solid organs, or areas of infarction may result in increased uptake of technetium-labeled radiopharmaceuticals. Similarly, in circumstances in which there is increased blood flow or luxury perfusion, there will also be increased radiotracer uptake. Infarctions in the brain may take up radionuclides as can brain metastases from systemic cancers, which have a predilection for calcification (mucinous adenocarcinomas including breast and gastrointestinal carcinomas; sarcomas; and in children neuroblastomas). In a patient with a known systemic malignancy, an isolated region of increased radiotracer uptake in the cranium should be further assessed with additional imaging (plain films, CT, and/or MRI as needed) before it is assumed to represent metastatic disease. MRI in this patient was obtained 1 week following the bone scan because of new-onset left upper extremity weakness. Images showed an acute infarct in the distal right middle cerebral artery territory (not shown) and at the same time confirmed a subacute to chronic infarct in the left middle cerebral artery territory. In addition, no calvarial lesion was identified on MRI.

Notes

Paraneoplastic Syndrome—Limbic Encephalitis (Ovarian Carcinoma)

1. Limbic encephalitis, viral encephalitis (herpes), carbon monoxide intoxication (when globus pallidus is also involved).

2. The hippocampal formations, the amygdala, and the insula. The gyri may also be involved.

3. The medial temporal lobes (limbic encephalitis) and the cerebellum.

4. Small cell carcinoma of the lung.

Reference

Kodama T, Numaguchi Y, Gellad FE, Dwyer BA, Kristt DA: Magnetic resonance imaging of limbic encephalitis, *Neuroradiology* 33:520-523, 1991.

Cross-Reference

Neuroradiology: THE REQUISITES, p 229.

Comment

Neurologic paraneoplastic syndromes represent a spectrum of neurologic manifestations that are associated with extracranial cancers but are not the result of direct invasion of the CNS by tumor. They occur in less than 1% of patients with cancer; however, one third to one half of patients with a paraneoplastic syndrome develop it before the diagnosis of systemic neoplasm. Such syndromes include limbic encephalopathy, cerebellar degeneration, opsoclonus/myoclonus, retinal degeneration, Lambert-Eaton myasthenic syndrome, and myelopathy. Lung cancer, particularly small cell carcinoma, is the most common malignancy associated with neurologic paraneoplastic syndromes. However, these syndromes may be seen in gynecologic malignancies (ovarian carcinoma), gastrointestinal cancer, Hodgkin's disease, breast cancer, and neuroblastoma in children. The cause of paraneoplastic syndromes is unknown; however, the most widely accepted theory is that they occur as a result of an autoimmune disorder. Circulating autoantibodies have been identified in several paraneoplastic syndromes. Anti-Yo is specific in paraneoplastic cerebellar degeneration associated with breast and ovarian cancer, and One anti-Hu is associated with lung cancer.

The clinical presentation of limbic encephalitis is a change in mental status, including personality changes and memory impairment. Imaging findings are nonspecific. CT may be unremarkable. On MRI, high signal intensity on T2W images may be identified in the medial temporal lobes. Mild enhancement may occur. Involvement of the hypothalamus may also be noted. On pathologic evaluation, nonspecific inflammatory changes/cellular infiltrates are identified without the presence of tumor or viral inclusions. Treatment of the primary malignancy may result in improvement of the neurologic symptoms.

Notes

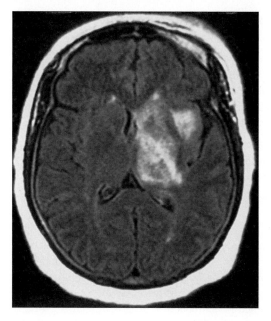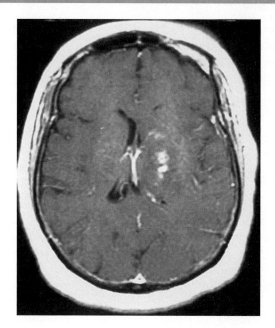

1. Where are the regions of abnormal T2W signal intensity and enhancement in this case?
2. How often is there gray matter involvement in patients with multiple sclerosis?
3. What is the characteristic clinical presentation in Behçet's syndrome?
4. Persons of what ethnic backgrounds have a predilection for this condition?

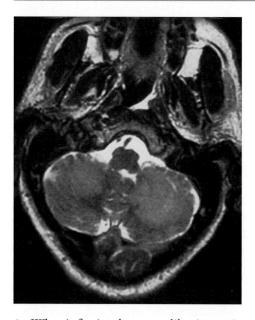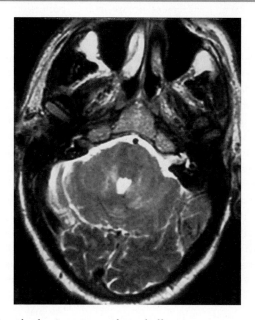

1. What infection has a predilection to involve the brain stem and cerebellum?
2. Who is at risk for CNS infection with *Listeria*?
3. What is the most common cause (infectious agent) of encephalitis?
4. What are the common viral encephalitides in the immunocompromised host?

Behçet's Syndrome

1. The deep gray matter of the basal ganglia including the caudate and lentiform nuclei, the associated white matter tracts of the corpus striatum, and the left thalamus.

2. In 5% to 7% of cases. However, there is usually still a predominance of white matter disease in these cases.

3. Recurrent oral cavity and genital ulcerations as well as uveitis.

4. Mediterranean and Japanese.

Reference

Morrissey SP, Miller DH, Hermaszewski R, et al: MRI of the CNS in Behçet's disease, *Eur Neurol* 33:287-293, 1993.

Cross-Reference

Neuroradiology: THE REQUISITES, p 197.

Comment

Behçet's syndrome is a systemic disorder that is believed to be secondary to an immune-related necrotizing vasculitis. Most patients present with mucosal ulcerations in the oral cavity, ulcers along the genitalia, and relapsing orbital inflammation, including uveitis and iridocyclitis. Depending on which reported series is being cited, Behçet's syndrome may affect the CNS in up to 40% of cases. Other organ systems may be involved, including the gastrointestinal tract, the skin (macules and papules), and the lungs. Lung involvement occurs in approximately 5% of patients and is characterized by lymphocytic vasculitis.

The MRI appearance of CNS involvement in Behçet's syndrome is nonspecific. Lesions may involve the gray and white matter (believed to be secondary to vasculitis). On T2W imaging, hyperintense lesions may be seen within the brain parenchyma. Although the radiologic appearance is nonspecific, there is a predilection for lesions to occur in the basal ganglia, brain stem, and the cerebral white matter. Abnormalities may also occur in the cerebellum and spinal cord and along the optic nerves. The enhancement pattern is variable. Some lesions may not enhance, whereas others may demonstrate either ring or solid enhancement. Because of the spectrum of imaging findings, in the absence of clinical history it may difficult to distinguish Behçet's disease from other CNS arteritides, inflammatory disorders such as sarcoid, or demyelinating disease (multiple sclerosis).

Notes

Rhombencephalitis—*Listeria monocytogenes**

1. *Listeria monocytogenes.*

2. Immunocompromised patients (particularly those with impaired cellular immunity), individuals working with farm animals, and individuals who eat unpasteurized cheese. Patients with no predisposing factors may occasionally be infected.

3. Most cases are related to viral infections, with herpes simplex being the most common viral agent in the United States.

4. HIV, CMV, and papovaviruses.

References

Salgado MJ, Damani NN, Llewellyn CG, et al: Magnetic resonance imaging of abscesses of the brain stem and cerebellum complicating *Listeria monocytogenes* rhombencephalitis, *Can Assoc Radiol J* 47:431-433, 1996.

Aladro Y, Ponce P, Santullano V, Angel-Moreno A, Santana MA: Cerebritis due to *Listeria monocytogenes*: CT and MR findings, *Eur Radiol* 6:188-191, 1996.

Cross-Reference

Neuroradiology: THE REQUISITES, p 189.

Comment

Listeria monocytogenes is most commonly seen in immunocompromised patients; however, it may also be seen in patients with certain occupational exposures and even in patients without risk factors. Listerial infection may cause meningitis, meningoencephalitis, and, less frequently, brain abscesses. It may infect any portion of the CNS, although it has a predilection for involvement of the intracranial contents, particularly the brain stem. *Listeria* occasionally affects the spinal cord.

Listeria is a gram-positive rod that is hard to isolate from the CSF when there is CNS infection. It is commonly mistaken for a diphtheroid in the CSF and disregarded as a contaminant. It may be isolated from blood cultures in infected patients. The key to diagnosing listerial encephalitis is in remembering to consider it in the differential diagnosis of patients with suspected bacterial meningitis. There are no characteristic radiologic findings; however, like other encephalitides *Listeria* causes increased T2W signal intensity in involved areas with mild local mass effect. Enhancement may or may not be present. Again, the pattern of rhombencephalitis should raise a red flag and should be considered *Listeria*. Less frequently, listerial rhombencephalitis may present with brainstem and cerebellar abscesses. Other infectious processes that may involve the brain stem and cerebellum include tuberculosis and syphilis; noninfectious inflammatory conditions to consider include sarcoid, multiple sclerosis, and acute disseminated encephalomyelitis.

Notes

---

*Figures for Case 154 courtesy Robert A. Zimmerman, MD.

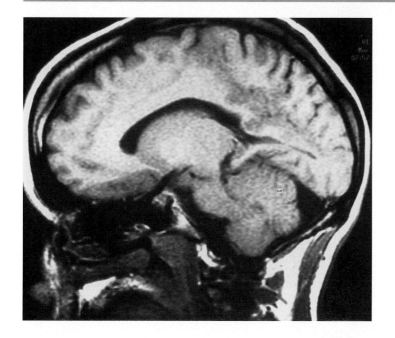
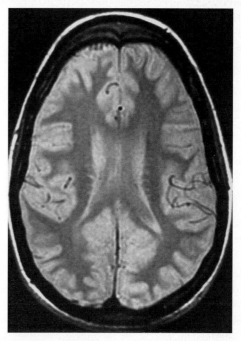
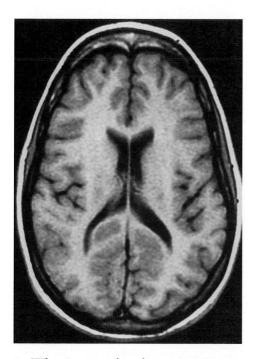
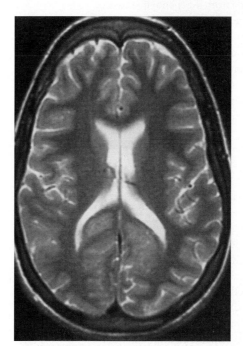

1. What is meant by a hamartoma?
2. What was this patient's clinical presentation?
3. What finding is characteristic of focal heterotopias?
4. From what embryologic structure is the cerebral cortex derived?

Focal Heterotopia—Subcortical

1. Proliferation of normal brain tissue in an abnormal location.

2. Seizures.

3. The presence of gray matter in the deep and subcortical white matter.

4. The germinal matrix.

Reference
Barkovich AJ: Subcortical heterotopia: a distinct clinicoradiologic entity, *Am J Neuroradiol* 17:1315-1322, 1996.

Cross-Reference
Neuroradiology: THE REQUISITES, pp 255-258.

Comment
The germinal matrix resides in the subependymal layer of the lateral ventricles and is the origin of the cells destined to become the cerebral cortex. As early as 7 to 8 weeks' gestational age, cells in the germinal matrix begin to undergo proliferation and migration. Radial glial fibers extend from the ependymal layer of the lateral ventricles to the surface of the brain, and it is along these fibers that neurons migrate to the cerebral cortex. Neuronal migration from the germinal matrix to the cortical layers follows a specific pattern. Migration occurs from the inside out, with gray matter cells destined to reside within the deepest cortical layer migrating first. Following migration, the neurons are arranged in laminae and ultimately form the six-layered cortex.

Migration anomalies result from insults that either prevent or interrupt normal migration such as in utero infections (CMV), ischemia, and metabolic abnormalities. Heterotopias represent the presence of normal gray matter in abnormal locations. There are several types of heterotopia, including subependymal, focal, and diffuse. A common clinical presentation of migrational abnormalities is seizures. Some patients may also have developmental delay and mental retardation.

In this case there is gray matter abnormally located within the subcortical white matter of the medial occipital lobes bilaterally, as well as within the splenium. On MRI heterotopias have a characteristic appearance and follow the signal characteristics of gray matter on all pulse sequences. Enhancement should not be present.

Notes

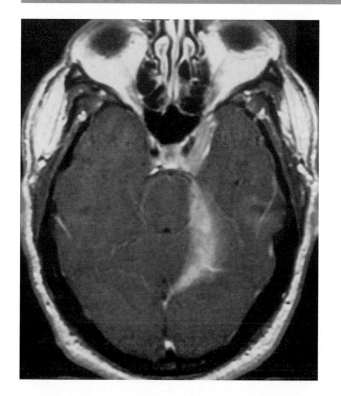
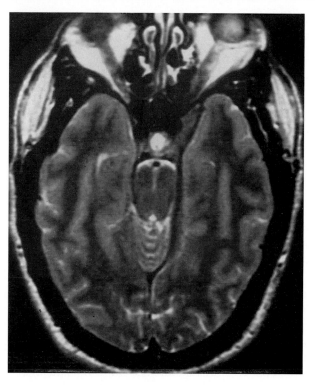
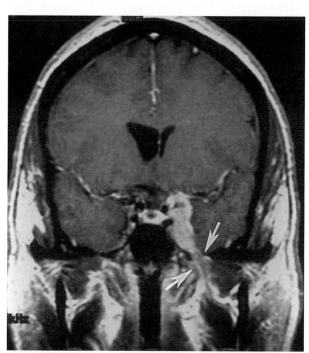

1. From what structure does the mass arise?
2. What skull base foramen is marked by the arrows?
3. What is the most common dural-based neoplasm?
4. What are the histologic findings of a plasma cell granuloma?

Intracranial Plasmacytoma

1. The dura.

2. The foramen ovale.

3. Meningioma.

4. Benign polyclonal plasma cells, lymphocytes, and histiocytes.

Reference

Provenzale JM, Schaefer P, Traweek ST, et al: Craniocerebral plasmacytoma: MR features, *Am J Neuroradiol* 18: 389-392, 1997.

Cross-Reference

Neuroradiology: THE REQUISITES, pp 297, 308-309, 326-330.

Comment

Craniocerebral plasmacytomas are plasma cell neoplasms that involve the cranium or the intracranial contents in the absence of other systemic manifestations (no laboratory or radiologic evidence of a plasma cell dyscrasia). Isolated craniocerebral plasmacytoma is a clinically distinct entity from multiple myeloma. These tumors may arise from the cranium or from the contents within the cranium (the dura and, rarely, the brain). Isolated craniocerebral plasmacytoma has a much better prognosis than does multiple myeloma.

In this case there is a broad-based mass along the tentorium cerebelli with extension into the left cavernous sinus. The mass is hypointense to brain on T2W images and enhances homogeneously. The most common neoplasm with this imaging appearance is a meningioma. However, invasion of the cavernous sinus in the absence of encasement and/or narrowing of the internal carotid artery, which is so typical of meningioma, should at least raise suspicion of other disease processes. The differential diagnosis includes lymphoma and sarcoid. Although craniocerebral plasmacytomas are uncommon, they too may mimic a meningioma on imaging. Biopsy should be performed when possible because craniocerebral plasmacytomas may sometimes be treated with radiation therapy alone rather than surgical resection. Once the histologic diagnosis of plasmacytoma is established, a full workup must be performed to exclude multiple myeloma. Some craniocerebral plasmacytomas may produce monoclonal immunoglobulin that may be detected in the urine or blood. When present, this is a convenient way to follow the patient's response to therapy.

Notes

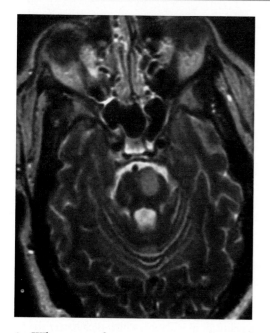
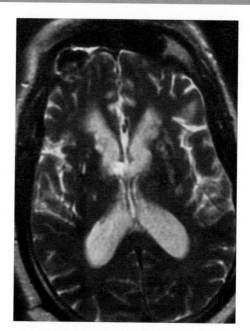

1. What type of treatment was used several years previously to treat this middle-aged adult's craniopharyngioma?
2. What are the major findings on the MRI?
3. What types of injury can occur when radiation is used with adjuvant chemotherapy?
4. At what time interval following radiation therapy are hemorrhagic parenchymal abnormalities typically seen?

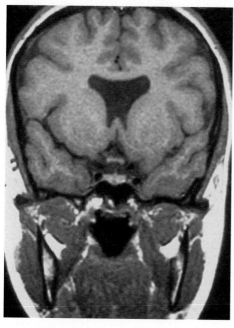
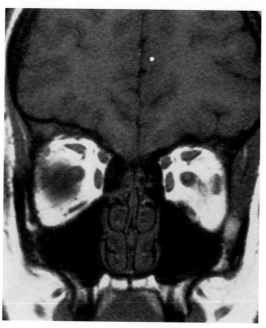

1. What midline structures are absent on these images?
2. What congenital syndromes are associated with this finding?
3. In addition to the olfactory nerves, what other cranial nerve is typically hypoplastic in midline ventral induction anomalies?
4. Seizures in holoprosencephaly and septo-optic dysplasia usually are due to what associated anomaly?

CASE 157

Radiation Vasculitis With Small Vessel Infarctions

1. Radiation therapy.

2. Multiple regions of abnormal T2W signal intensity within the pons and basal ganglia. The lesion in the left pons is the largest, is rounded in configuration, and is associated with mild mass effect, suggesting that it is more acute (clinically the patient had right hemiparesis).

3. Disseminated necrotizing leukoencephalopathy, mineralizing microangiopathy, atrophy, and occult cerebral vascular malformations.

4. Months to years following therapy. In early injury (weeks to months) when symptoms and imaging findings may be reversible, hemorrhage is infrequent. Occult cerebrovascular malformations occur late.

Reference

Hecht-Leavitt C, Grossman RI, Curran WJ Jr, et al: MR of brain radiation injury: experimental studies in cats, *Am J Neuroradiol* 8:427-430, 1987.

Cross-Reference

Neuroradiology: THE REQUISITES, pp 100-102, 118.

Comment

Arteritis resulting in ischemic changes of the brain may result from radiation therapy. In addition, these effects may be accelerated with adjuvant chemotherapy (intravenous or intrathecal). Symptoms of radiation arteritis are dependent on the regions of the brain affected and may include change in mental status, focal neurologic deficits, and occasionally seizures (which may simulate a mass lesion). MRI is frequently of value in differentiating radiation vasculitis from recurrent tumor. The location of the lesions in relation to the location of the patient's primary tumor and radiation port may be helpful in distinguishing radiation change from primary lesion recurrence. Ischemic lesions related to radiation vasculitis often occur in the distribution of the perforating vessels (the basal ganglia, white matter tracts of the corpus striatum, and brain stem), as well as within the deep white matter. Although the white matter T2W hyperintensity seen in early radiation arteritis may be transient, the changes related to chronic arteritis may be quite marked.

Mineralizing microangiopathy occurs most commonly in children being treated with both brain radiation and chemotherapy for acute leukemia or lymphoma. Radiologic findings typically include calcification within the basal ganglia and at the gray-white matter junction. The underlying pathophysiology of radiation- and/or chemotherapy-induced neurologic toxicity is believed to be related to a vasculitis. Vessel injury results in endothelial thickening with fibrinoid necrosis of small arteries and arterioles.

Notes

CASE 158

Septo-optic Dysplasia (deMorsier's Syndrome)

1. The septum pellucidum and the olfactory bulbs.

2. Holoprosencephaly and septo-optic dysplasia.

3. The optic nerves and chiasm.

4. Migrational abnormalities.

Reference

Barkovich AJ, Fram EK, Norman D: Septo-optic dysplasia: MR imaging, *Radiology* 171:189-192, 1989.

Cross-Reference

Neuroradiology: THE REQUISITES, p 253.

Comment

This case demonstrates absence of the olfactory bulbs (as well as a dysmorphic right inferior olfactory sulcus). Abnormalities of the olfactory bulbs and tracts are common in Kallmann's syndrome, holoprosencephaly, and septo-optic dysplasia. In this case the septum pellucidum is absent, which is characteristic of ventral induction congenital defects (although it is not part of Kallmann's syndrome).

Septo-optic dysplasia (first described by deMorsier) is characterized radiologically by complete (two thirds of patients) or partial (one third of patients) absence of the septum pellucidum, hypoplasia of the optic nerves and chiasm (when severe, the optic canals may be hypoplastic), and dysgenesis of the olfactory bulbs and tracts. On imaging, evidence of optic hypoplasia is noted in approximately one half of cases. Visual symptoms may be absent, or patients may have decreased visual acuity and/or nystagmus. In addition, as many as 50% to 60% of these patients have abnormalities of the hypothalamic-pituitary axis resulting in deficiency of growth hormone in particular (but also thyroid stimulating hormone). As a result, patients with septo-optic dysplasia may present with short stature. The posterior pituitary "bright spot" may be ectopic. Seizures are common and are usually related to migrational abnormalities. The most common of these is schizencephaly, which is present in 50% of cases of septo-optic dysplasia; however, focal heterotopias may also occur. White matter hypoplasia and ex vacuo enlargement of the ventricles may be present in some patients.

Notes

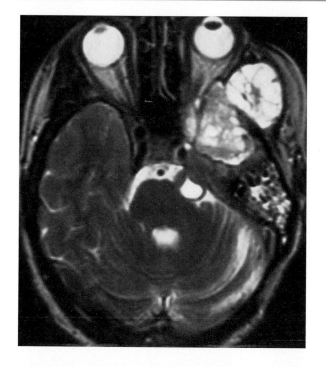 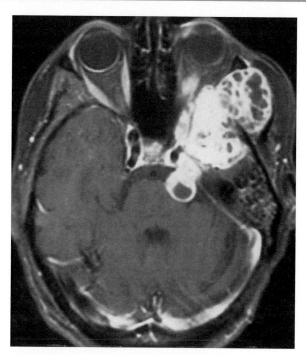

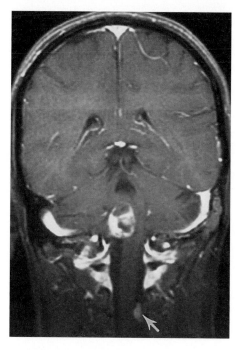 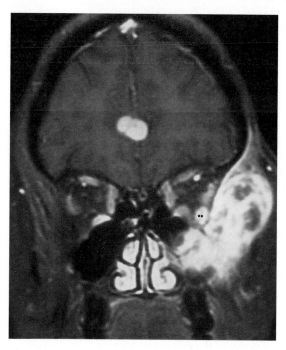

1. Which cranial nerve is this (**)?

2. What neurocutaneous syndrome does this patient have?

3. What glial neoplasm is this disorder associated with?

4. From what type of nerves do schwannomas typically arise?

Neurofibromatosis Type 2

1. V2, which is the maxillary division of the trigeminal nerve.

2. Neurofibromatosis type 2.

3. Ependymoma.

4. Sensory nerves. Uncommonly, they may be associated with motor nerves.

Reference

Aoki S, Barkovich AJ, Nishimura K, et al: Neurofibromatosis types 1 and 2: cranial MR findings, *Radiology* 172:527-534, 1989.

Cross-Reference

Neuroradiology: THE REQUISITES, pp 267-268.

Comment

This case illustrates a patient with radiologic findings consistent with neurofibromatosis type 2. A large, circumscribed, solid and cystic mass involves cranial nerve V (trigeminal) on the left, extending from its cisternal portion and growing along the course of the nerve to extend extracranially to the superficial zygomatic masticator space. Tumor along the second division of the trigeminal nerve (*) is also noted. There are also schwannomas involving cranial nerve IX on the right and the upper left cervical spine (*arrow*), as well as an anterior falcine meningioma.

Neurofibromatosis type 2 is an autosomal dominant disorder transmitted on chromosome 22. It typically presents in adolescence or young adulthood, and the most common clinical presentation is bilateral sensorineural hearing loss. The radiologic hallmark of neurofibromatosis type 2 is the presence of bilateral acoustic schwannomas. Otherwise, the diagnosis of neurofibromatosis type 2 can be made if a patient has a unilateral vestibular schwannoma and a first-degree relative with neurofibromatosis type 2, or a if patient has a first-degree relative with neurofibromatosis type 2 and at least two schwannomas, meningiomas, and/or ependymomas. Unlike neurofibromatosis type 1, cutaneous manifestations in neurofibromatosis type 2 are rare. CNS lesions are present in virtually 100% of patients with neurofibromatosis type 2. Schwannomas most commonly involve cranial nerve VIII. The trigeminal nerve is the next most common site of schwannomas. Although most of these tumors are sporadic, those arising from more than one cranial nerve or from the cranial nerves III through VI should prompt a search for NF-2. Other imaging findings that may be present in neurofibromatosis type 2 include prominent calcifications along the choroid plexus or occasionally along the cerebral or cerebellar cortex. Lesions within the spinal canal are common and include schwannomas and meningiomas. Intramedullary tumors are typically ependymomas.

Notes

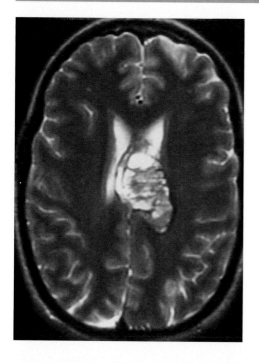
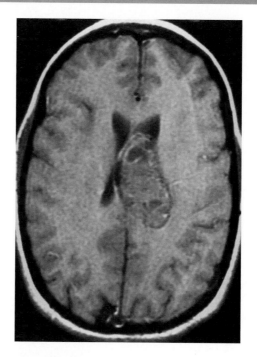
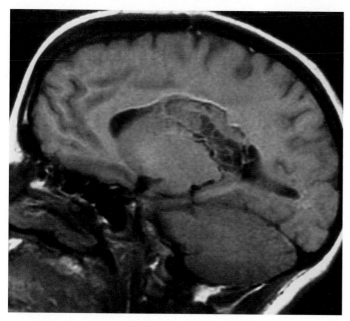

1. Where is this mass arising?

2. What neoplasms arise in the body of the lateral ventricle along the foramen of Monro or septum pellucidum?

3. What is the characteristic location of choroid plexus papillomas?

4. Both on imaging and on histologic evaluation, the tumor in this case is frequently indistinguishable from what other neoplasm?

Central Neurocytoma

1. The lateral ventricle/septum pellucidum.

2. Oligodendroglioma, central neurocytoma, fibrillary astrocytoma, pilocytic astrocytoma, ependymoma, hemangioma, and subependymal giant cell astrocytoma. The patient's age and the imaging appearance of the mass may be useful in limiting the differential considerations.

3. In children, the atria of the lateral ventricles. In adults, the fourth ventricle.

4. Oligodendroglioma. Electron microscopy and immuno-histochemistry reveal neurosecretory granules and the neuronal marker synaptophysin, respectively, which are characteristic of central neurocytoma.

References

Yasargil M, von Ammon K, von Deimling A, Valavanis A, Wichmann W, Wiestler OD: Central neurocytoma: histopathological variants and therapeutic approaches, *J Neurosurg* 76:32-37, 1992.

Goldstein JH, Haas RA, Tung GA: General case of the day: intraventricular neurocytoma, *RadioGraphics* 16:971-973, 1996.

Cross-Reference

Neuroradiology: THE REQUISITES, pp 93-94.

Comment

Central neurocytomas typically have a homogeneous cell population with neuronal differentiation. These neoplasms occur in young and middle-aged adults. Patients may be asymptomatic or may present with headache and signs of increased intracranial pressure. Central neurocytomas arise most commonly within the lateral ventricle (and, less frequently, the third ventricle) adjacent to the septum pellucidum and the foramen of Monro. The vast majority of cases are confined to the ventricles.

On CT neurocytomas typically are heterogeneous lesions that contain multiple cysts resulting in regions of hypodensity. In addition, there are frequently regions of isodensity or hyperdensity within the mass when compared with the adjacent brain parenchyma. In most neurocytomas calcifications are present. On MRI, neurocytomas frequently demonstrate regions of cyst formation. The more solid component of these masses tend to follow the signal characteristics of gray matter on T1W and T2W imaging (as in this patient). Signal voids may be related to calcification or tumor vascularity. Contrast enhancement is variable, ranging from none to moderate. On imaging and conventional pathology (light microscopy), these tumors are frequently indistinguishable from oligodendrogliomas. The distinctions between these two neoplasms are important because central neurocytomas have a more benign course and treatment may differ. Although neurocytomas have a favorable prognosis, anaplastic malignant variants and recurrences have been reported.

Notes

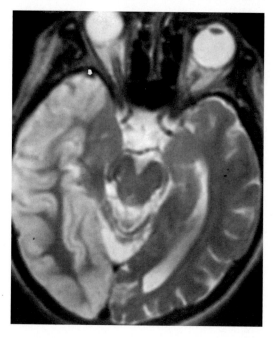

1. Abnormal signal intensity in the right cerebral hemisphere predominantly involves what structure?

2. Many of the mitochondrial encephalomyopathies, particularly Leigh disease and MELAS (mitochondrial encephalomyopathy, lactic acidosis, and stroke) syndrome, are characterized by what biochemical abnormality?

3. Which MRI sequence is useful in establishing elevated levels of lactic acid?

4. In Leigh disease, what structures are characteristically involved on MRI?

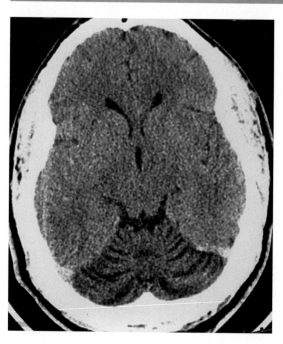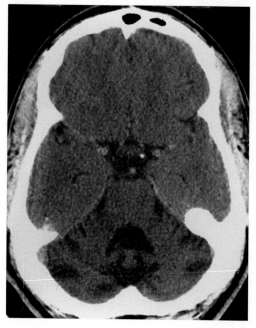

1. What is the most common clinical presentation of patients with cerebellar degenerative processes?

2. In olivopontocerebellar degeneration (OPCD), myelin loss and gliosis usually begins in what structure?

3. What are common causes of acquired cerebellar degeneration?

4. What feature is useful in distinguishing cerebellar cortical degeneration from OPCD?

MELAS Syndrome (Mitochondrial Encephalomyopathy, Lactic Acidosis, and Stroke)

1. The gray matter.

2. Lactic acidosis.

3. Spectroscopy.

4. The putamen typically have abnormal T2W signal intensity that is frequently bilaterally symmetric.

References

Allard JC, Tilak S, Carter AP: CT and MR of MELAS syndrome, *Am J Neuroradiol* 9:1234-1238, 1988.

Castillo M, Kwock L, Green C: MELAS syndrome: imaging and proton MR spectroscopic findings, *Am J Neuroradiol* 16:233-239, 1995.

Cross-Reference

Neuroradiology: THE REQUISITES, pp 245-246.

Comment

The mitochondrial encephalomyopathies represent a group of disorders that tend to be characterized by enzymatic defects within the mitochondria. These disorders are systemic, resulting in a spectrum of abnormalities related to involvement of both the CNS and peripheral nervous system, skeletal muscle, bone marrow, and gastrointestinal tract. Prominent overlap of the clinical, biochemical, and imaging findings make differentiation among the mitochondrial defects difficult in many cases. Most mitochondrial disorders present in childhood; however, a few, such as MERRF (myoclonus, epilepsy, and ragged red fibers) syndrome, present in adults.

In general, CNS imaging findings in the mitochondrial disorders are varied and include signal alterations within the basal ganglia, cortical strokes, cortical atrophy, white matter disease (demyelination), and spinal cord atrophy. In many instances, MELAS syndrome can be differentiated from other mitochondrial disorders by the clinical presentation of cortical blindness and hemiparesis. On imaging, ischemic injury especially involving the cerebral cortex is usually present. These regions of cortical signal abnormality may be bilaterally symmetric or asymmetric and often are not confined by a single vascular territory. Follow-up imaging of the cortical abnormalities frequently shows evolution of the stroke(s) with associated cortical atrophy; however, it is not uncommon for some of the regions of cortical signal abnormality to resolve. Serologic studies and MR spectroscopy demonstrate elevated lactic acid levels.

Notes

Olivopontocerebellar Degeneration

1. Ataxia.

2. The pons. Degeneration begins in the pontine nuclei and progresses along pontocerebellar tracts, which course through the middle cerebellar peduncles and into the cerebellum.

3. Substance abuse (alcohol), medications (particularly anticonvulsants such as phenytoin), paraneoplastic syndromes, and certain chemotherapeutic agents.

4. OPCD typically involves the pontocerebellar tracts with cerebellar atrophy (the hemispheres are more involved than the vermis). In contrast, in cerebellar cortical degeneration there is relative sparing of the pontocerebellar tracts and cerebellar atrophy typically affects the vermis.

Reference

Savoiardo M, Strada L, Girotti F, et al: Olivopontocerebellar atrophy: MR diagnosis and relationship to multisystem atrophy, *Radiology* 174:693-696, 1990.

Cross-Reference

Neuroradiology: THE REQUISITES, pp 227-229.

Comment

Olivopontocerebellar degeneration may be transmitted through autosomal dominant inheritance or may occur sporadically. Although the onset of symptoms in OPCD may span several decades, it most commonly presents in young adults. The main clinical presentation is truncal ataxia first involving the legs and then the arms. Patients may also have nystagmus, dysarthria, and tremors.

Pathologically, in OPCD there is loss of myelin and gliosis of the pontocerebellar pathways beginning in the pontine nuclei and progressing into the cerebellum (hemispheres and, to a lesser degree, the vermis) with neuronal loss of the cerebellar cortex. The development of MRI has greatly enhanced our ability to evaluate the degenerative processes of the cerebellum, brain stem, and spinal cord. On MRI, atrophy of the involved structures (pons, middle cerebellar peduncle, and cerebellum) is evident. In addition, there may be mild hyperintensity on T2W images in the involved structures in OPCD.

Notes

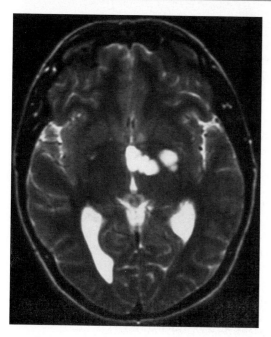
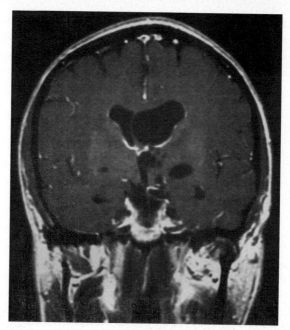

1. What are the MRI criteria for an uncomplicated cyst?
2. What cystlike lesions may occur in the ventricles?
3. What type of cystlike lesions may be seen in the region of the basal ganglia?
4. What is the characteristic anatomic location of an intracranial colloid cyst?

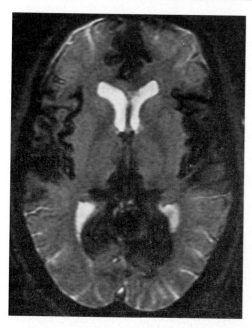
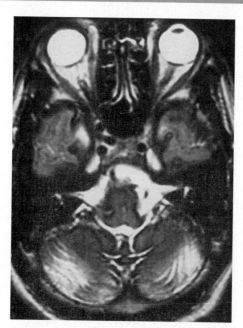

1. What is the clinical presentation of these patients?
2. In CNS siderosis, what are common locations for hemosiderin deposition?
3. What are causes of diffuse hemosiderosis?
4. How would one proceed in the workup of this patient?

Parasitic Infection

1. Circumscribed lesion that follows the signal characteristics of CSF on all pulse sequences. Following contrast, the cysts do not enhance.

2. Arachnoid cysts, colloid cysts, cysts related to a neoplasm, epidermoid cysts, parasitic infection (cysticercosis, echinococcus), ependymal cysts, and a cyst of the cavum septum pellucidum.

3. Perivascular (Virchow-Robin) space, infections (especially parasitic), and cysts related to tumors.

4. Foramen of Monro/superior aspect of the third ventricle at the columns of the fornices.

Reference

Van Tassel P, Cure JK: Non-neoplastic intracranial cysts and cystic lesions, *Ultrasound CT MRI* 16:186-211, 1995.

Cross-Reference

Neuroradiology: THE REQUISITES, pp 193-196.

Comment

These images demonstrate multiple cystlike lesions in the regions of the anterior third ventricle, cavum septum pellucidum, and basal ganglia that are isointense to CSF on T1W and T2W images (uncomplicated cysts must also be isointense to CSF on intermediate and FLAIR imaging). Following contrast, there is no enhancement of these lesions. Due to its multiplanar capabilities and its superior tissue resolution, MRI allows excellent characterization of cystlike lesions, as well as anatomic localization (intraparenchymal versus intraventricular), and in many instances allows differentiation of intratumoral cysts from nonneoplastic intracranial cysts.

Nonneoplastic cystic lesions can have a variety of causes. Cysts may be developmental (cavum septum pellucidum/vergae, arachnoid cyst, perivascular space, neuroepithelial cyst) or related to infection (particularly parasitic disease), or they may occur in a region of previous injury (e.g., prior ischemia, hemorrhage, and/or surgery). History may be useful in some instances in differentiating among the various types of cysts. In particular, the location of the cyst(s) (supratentorial or infratentorial; within the brain, ventricles, and/or subarachnoid space) may be extremely useful in helping to limit the differential considerations of nonneoplastic intracranial cystlike lesions.

Notes

Diffuse Hemosiderosis of the Central Nervous System

1. Gait disturbance, cranial neuropathies (especially cranial nerve VIII), and cognitive impairment.

2. The cerebellum, brain stem, and cranial nerves.

3. Chronic subarachnoid hemorrhage from a brain or spinal cord tumor, amyloid angiopathy, and vascular malformations.

4. Clinical correlation regarding the patient's history is first advised. Then, in the absence of an intracranial abnormality (aneurysm, tumor), further evaluation should include MRI of the spine to look for a spinal cord tumor. If no source is found, it may be necessary to perform catheter angiography to exclude a dural AVM (DAVM).

References

Castelli ML, Husband A: Superficial siderosis of the central nervous system: an underestimated cause of hearing loss, *J Laryngol Oto* 3:60-62, 1997.

Fearnley JM, Stevens JM, Rudge P: Superficial siderosis of the central nervous system, *Brain* 118:1051-1066, 1995.

Cross-Reference

Neuroradiology: THE REQUISITES, pp 135, 346-347.

Comment

This case shows marked hypointensity along the surface of the brain stem, the cerebellum, and throughout the subarachnoid spaces (most notably in the Sylvian cisterns). Diffuse hemosiderosis (deposition of hemosiderin along the pial, subpial, and ependymal surfaces in proximity to CSF) may be seen in a spectrum of disease processes that result in recurrent subarachnoid hemorrhage. Chronic or recurrent subarachnoid hemorrhage from a primary brain tumor, DAVM, or ependymoma of the conus medullaris are potential causes of superficial hemosiderosis. A source of bleeding is identified in approximately 55% of cases. Deposition of hemosiderin is associated with neuronal loss, demyelination, and gliosis. Patients may be asymptomatic for months to years. Clinical presentation typically includes cerebellar ataxia in over 80% of cases, cranial neuropathies in over 90% of cases (most commonly hearing loss), pyramidal signs, anosmia, progressive cognitive decline, bladder dysfunction, and sensory symptoms. Men are affected more often than are women (approximately 3:1). Treatment is surgical or endovascular ablation of the source of bleeding.

On T2W and gradient echo susceptibility MRI hemosiderosis is manifested by hypointensity along the parenchymal surfaces of the brain, cranial nerves, and spinal cord. In particular, the cerebellum is a common location for hemosiderin deposition, and there is often associated atrophy. On histologic evaluation hemosiderin-laden macrophages may be identified within the leptomeninges and subpial regions.

Notes

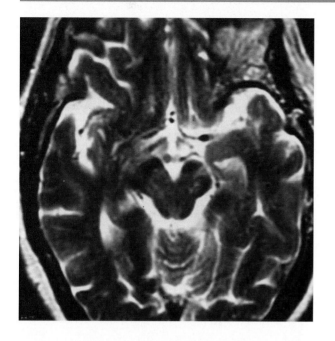

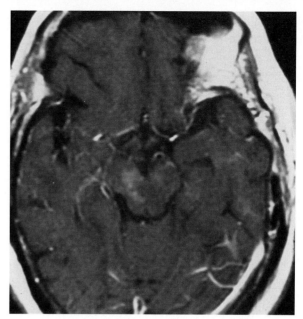

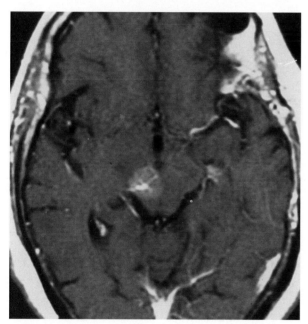

1. What is the most common location of these lesions?

2. What is the most common clinical presentation of these abnormalities?

3. On MRI what is the most useful finding in distinguishing capillary telangiectasias from other pathologic lesions (such as inflammatory disease or lymphoma)?

4. What other occult vascular malformations can capillary telangiectasias be associated with?

Capillary Telangiectasia and Venous Angioma of the Brain Stem

1. The brain stem/pons.

2. Typically, capillary telangiectasias and venous angiomas are clinically silent, incidental lesions detected on MRI performed for other indications.

3. The absence of signal abnormality on unenhanced images, particularly T2W images.

4. Venous angiomas and cavernomas.

References

Barr RM, Dillon WP, Wilson CB: Slow-flow vascular malformations of the pons: capillary telangiectasias? *Am J Neuroradiol* 17:71-78, 1996.

Lee C, Pennington MA, Kenney CM: MR evaluation of developmental venous anomalies: medullary venous anatomy of venous angiomas, *Am J Neuroradiol* 17:61-70, 1996.

Cross-Reference

Neuroradiology: THE REQUISITES, pp 141-142.

Comment

Capillary telangiectasias represent a cluster of abnormally dilated capillaries with intervening normal brain tissue. They usually represent clinically silent lesions that are detected on imaging studies acquired for unrelated reasons. Angiographically, they are most often occult. On MRI a capillary telangiectasia is typically recognized as a poorly demarcated region of contrast enhancement. Importantly, on the unenhanced images no significant associated signal abnormality should be identified. Gradient echo susceptibility images may demonstrate hypointensity associated with these lesions, and it has been postulated that this T2W shortening may be related to intravascular deoxyhemoglobin from stagnant blood flow. Capillary telangiectasias may coexist with other vascular malformations, including cavernomas and venous angiomas.

Venous angiomas are typically incidental vascular malformations representing a developmental anomaly of venous drainage. Within the venous network is intervening normal brain tissue, and no arterial elements are associated with these lesions. The angiomas are comprised of a tuft of enlarged venous channels that drain into a common venous trunk, which then subsequently drains into the deep or superficial venous system. Typically they are clinically silent lesions, although they may be associated with intracranial hemorrhage. These lesions have a characteristic MRI appearance representing a cluster of veins oriented in a "radial" pattern that drain into a large central vein. There is usually no signal abnormality in the adjacent brain parenchyma. Angiographically the arterial and capillary phases are normal, and there may be opacification of the venous angioma during the venous phase.

Notes

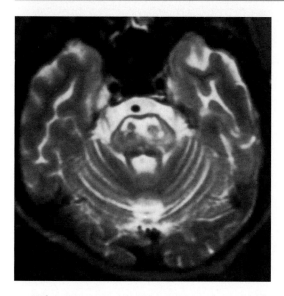

1. What anatomic structures are represented by the two central, symmetric regions of isointensity within the pons that are surrounded by abnormal T2W hyperintensity?

2. This condition is frequently associated with overzealous correction of what electrolyte abnormality?

3. What extrapontine structures may be involved in this case?

4. What type of patients typically present with this disorder?

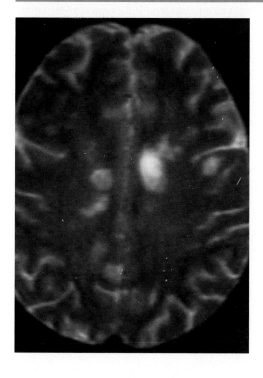
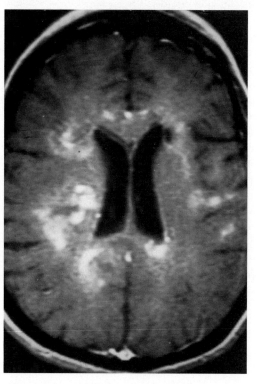

1. What should be included in the differential diagnosis?

2. What is the most common MRI finding in patients with Lyme disease?

3. In addition to multiple bilateral periventricular and subcortical hyperintense lesions on T2W images, what other MRI findings may be present in patients with Lyme disease?

4. What is the other spirochetal infection that may involve the CNS?

Osmotic Demyelination (Central Pontine Myelinolysis)

1. Descending corticospinal tracts.

2. Hyponatremia.

3. The deep gray matter (thalami, lentiform nuclei); the deep white matter, including the tracts around the corpus striatum (external and internal capsules); and the cerebellum.

4. Alcoholics and the malnourished.

Reference

Sterns RH, Riggs JE, Schochette SS Jr: Osmotic demyelination syndrome following correction of hyponatremia, *N Engl J Med* 314:1535-1542, 1986.

Cross-Reference

Neuroradiology: THE REQUISITES, pp 215-216.

Comment

Osmotic demyelination is a demyelinating disorder that may be seen in a variety of underlying systemic processes that have a predilection for electrolyte abnormalities. It is most commonly seen in alcoholics or chronically debilitated and malnourished patients following rapid correction of hyponatremia. It is not the low serum level but rather the rapidity with which it is corrected that is felt to be responsible for this disorder. Overzealous correction of serum sodium levels may be followed by an acute or subacute clinical deterioration, including a change in mental status, coma, quadriparesis, extrapyramidal signs, and, if unrecognized, death. This process not uncommonly involves extrapontine structures. Pathologically, demyelination is noted without a significant inflammatory response with relative sparing of axons. There is an associated reactive astrocytosis. When osmotic demyelination is localized only in the pons, it is characterized by high signal intensity on T2W images in the central pons in the region of demyelination. There typically is sparing of the peripheral pons. Commonly the descending corticospinal tracts are spared (as in this patient). Usually central pontine myelinolysis is not associated with enhancement or significant mass effect. When osmotic demyelination is localized only to the pons, the radiologic diagnosis is usually easy. However, if there is pontine and extrapontine involvement or involvement only in extrapontine structures, the differential diagnosis is somewhat broad, including other demyelinating disorders, encephalitis, and ischemia.

Notes

Lyme Disease

1. Demyelinating disease, vasculitis, infectious disease (Lyme disease), and other inflammatory processes such as neurosarcoid.

2. A normal examination.

3. Enhancement of the meninges and/or cranial nerves, focal lesions in the deep gray matter (basal ganglia, thalami) and brain stem, and hydrocephalus.

4. Syphilis (*Treponema pallidum*). Symptomatic neurosyphilis may be on the basis of parenchymal or meningovascular disease.

Reference

Pachner AR, Duray P, Steere AC: Central nervous system manifestations of Lyme disease, *Arch Neurol* 46:790-795, 1989.

Cross-Reference

Neuroradiology: THE REQUISITES, pp 190, 209.

Comment

Lyme disease is a multisystem disorder caused by a spirochetal (*Borrelia burgdorferi*) infection that is transmitted most commonly by the deer tick (*Ixodes dammini*). The characteristic initial bull's-eye skin lesion (erythema chronicum migrans) is pathognomonic of this infection and is the typical presentation of the first of the three recorded clinical stages. In this clinical stage, the rash is usually accompanied by constitutional symptoms, including myalgia, headache, and low grade fevers. Stage II disease is characterized by disseminated infection and is normally manifest by neurologic and cardiac abnormalities. Stage II typically occurs weeks to months following the initial infection. In stage III (persistent infection), patients usually present with neurologic (meningitic) and/or rheumatologic symptoms. Neurologic manifestations typically develop in up to 15% of patients with Lyme disease and include cranial neuropathies (especially Bell's palsy), meningitis, cerebellar findings, ophthalmic involvement (conjunctivitis, keratitis, and ocular inflammation), and/or encephalitis. The diagnosis of Lyme disease is made based on clinical presentation and serology. Treatment is with antibiotics.

Notes

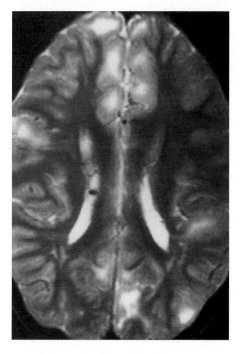
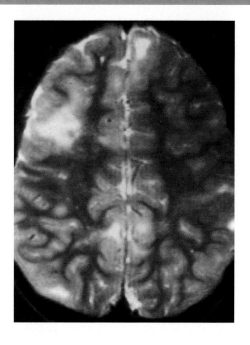

1. How might this pediatric patient have presented clinically?
2. What neoplasm is associated with this syndrome?
3. What is the CNS imaging hallmark seen in 98% of patients with this disorder?
4. What organ systems in addition to the CNS are affected in patients with tuberous sclerosis?

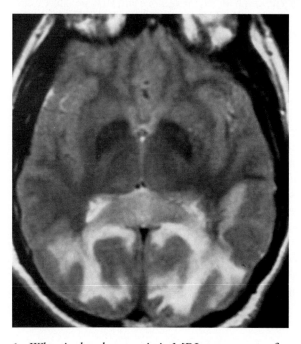
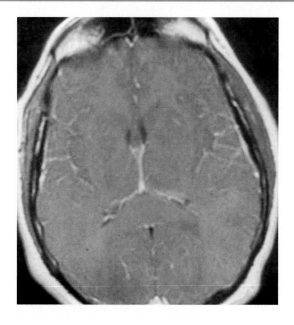

1. What is the characteristic MRI appearance of metachromatic leukodystrophy?
2. What do the areas of enhancement represent in this case?
3. How is adrenoleukodystrophy transmitted?
4. What is the most common pattern of white matter disease on MRI in adrenoleukodystrophy?

CASE 168

Tuberous Sclerosis (Bourneville's Disease)

1. With seizures, mental retardation, and/or adenoma sebaceum. Other clinical signs and symptoms include skin lesions (ash-leaf spots, shagreen patches, and subungual fibromas).

2. Subependymal giant cell astrocytoma.

3. Subependymal nodules (tubers).

4. Hamartomas may occur in the retina or kidneys (angiomyolipomas), rhabdomyomas may occur along the ventricular septum in the heart, the lungs may be affected by angiomyomatosis, and the liver and pancreas may have adenomas. A variety of skeletal lesions and occasionally vascular lesions (aneurysms and stenoses) may be present.

Reference

Takanashi J-I, Sugita K, Fujii K, Niimi H: MR evaluation of tuberous sclerosis: increased sensitivity with fluid-attenuated inversion recovery and relation to severity of seizures and mental retardation, *Am J Neuroradiol* 16:1923-1928, 1995.

Cross-Reference

Neuroradiology: THE REQUISITES, pp 268-270.

Comment

Tuberous sclerosis most commonly occurs as a sporadic mutation (chromosome 11); it also may be an autosomal dominant disorder transmitted by a mutation in chromosome 9. There are a spectrum of clinical signs and symptoms in these patients; however, the imaging manifestations should be sufficient to make the diagnosis in the majority of cases. Seizures, mental retardation, and/or adenoma sebaceum is the classic clinical triad described in tuberous sclerosis; however, the three together are seen in less than 50% of patients with this diagnosis.

The CNS manifestations of tuberous sclerosis are numerous and include subependymal nodules, cortical tubers, white matter lesions (believed to represent dysplastic white matter and/or foci of hypomyelination), subependymal giant cell astrocytomas, and ventriculomegaly. Subependymal tubers are seen in essentially all patients with tuberous sclerosis, and over 75% are calcified. Cortical tubers are present in approximately 50% of these patients, and about half are calcified. Cortical tubers are hyperintense on long TR images and are frequently bilateral and symmetric (as in this case). They affect the frontal, parietal, occipital, and temporal lobes in descending order of frequency. Up to one third of subependymal nodules and 5% of cortical tubers may enhance. Because of their high incidence of calcification, subependymal nodules are easily detected on CT, but they can be difficult to detect on MRI. Gradient echo and unenhanced T1W imaging may enhance detection of these lesions, which are hypointense and often mildly hyperintense to brain, respectively.

Notes

CASE 169

Adrenoleukodystrophy

1. Confluent, symmetric white matter abnormalities that usually begin in the frontal lobes and progress posteriorly. There is usually relative sparing of the subcortical U fibers and the white matter within the basal ganglia.

2. Active demyelination and inflammation.

3. X-linked recessive.

4. Bilaterally symmetric T2W hyperintensity in the deep periventricular white matter of the parietal and occipital lobes that extends across the splenium and posterior body of the corpus callosum.

Reference

Demaerel P, Faubert C, Wilms G, Casaer P, Piepgras U, Baert AL: MR findings in leukodystrophy, *Neuroradiology* 33:368-371, 1991.

Cross-Reference

Neuroradiology: THE REQUISITES, pp 219-220.

Comment

Adrenoleukodystrophy is an X-linked recessive disorder that is related to a single enzyme deficiency (acyl coenzyme A synthetase) within intracellular peroxisomes. This enzyme is necessary for β oxidation in the breakdown of very long-chain fatty acids that accumulate in erythrocytes, plasma, and fibroblasts, as well as the CNS white matter and adrenal cortex. Male patients typically present between the ages of 4 and 10 years. The clinical presentation may be that of behavioral disturbance, visual symptoms, hearing loss, seizures, and eventually spastic quadriparesis. Patients often present with adrenal insufficiency (Addison's disease), which may occur before or after the development of neurologic symptoms.

As in other demyelinating and dysmyelinating disorders, MRI is the imaging modality of choice for the detection of white matter disease, being far superior to CT. In adrenoleukodystrophy, the most common pattern of white matter disease is bilaterally symmetric abnormalities within the parietal and occipital white matter, extending across the splenium of the corpus callosum. From here, the disease may continue to progress anteriorly to involve the frontal and temporal lobes. The region of active demyelination usually along the anterior margin of the disorder may demonstrate contrast enhancement. Less typical presentations include predominantly frontal lobe involvement or holohemispheric involvement. Adrenoleukodystrophy also involves the cerebellum, spinal cord, and the peripheral nervous system.

Notes

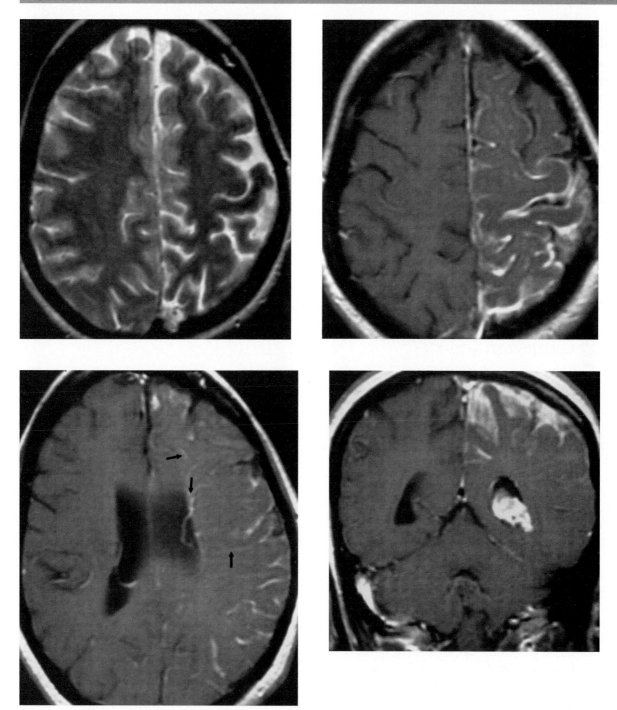

1. What is the inheritance pattern of this neurocutaneous disorder?

2. What is the classic cutaneous manifestation of this phakomatosis, and in what distribution does it typically occur?

3. What is the cause of the intracranial lesion associated with this syndrome?

4. In this syndrome, calcification is frequently present in what area of the brain?

Sturge-Weber Syndrome
(Encephalotrigeminal Angiomatosis)

1. Unlike most phakomatoses, Sturge-Weber syndrome occurs sporadically and has a relatively equal predilection in both men and women.

2. Port wine stain (nevus flammeus), which typically occurs in the trigeminal nerve distribution; the ophthalmic division (V1) is most common.

3. Leptomeningeal venous angiomatosis develops as a result of failure of development of normal cortical venous drainage in involved areas of the brain.

4. The cortex.

Reference

Griffiths PD, Blaser S, Boodram MB, Armstrong D, Harwood-Nash D: Choroid plexus size in young children with Sturge-Weber syndrome, *Am J Neuroradiol* 17:175-180, 1996.

Cross-Reference

Neuroradiology: THE REQUISITES, pp 270-271.

Comment

The precise cause of Sturge-Weber syndrome is uncertain; however, it is believed to result from persistence of the primitive vascular plexus as a result of failure of development of the normal cortical venous drainage in affected areas of the brain. A pial vascular malformation develops that is characterized pathologically by thin-walled, dilated capillaries and venules. The pial angiomatous malformation is usually ipsilateral to the port-wine nevus on the face and most commonly affects the posterior cerebral hemisphere (the occipital lobe most frequently followed by the parietal and temporal lobes).

There are several characteristic imaging manifestations. In patients older than 2 years of age, plain film radiography or CT may show "tram-track" calcifications representing calcification in opposing gyri. Enhanced MRI is particularly useful in demonstrating the extent of the angiomatous malformation because there is enhancement of the pia in regions of the vascular abnormality. Collateral venous drainage is manifest by an increase in both the size and number of medullary and subependymal veins. There is also enhancement of the ipsilateral choroid plexus, which is secondarily hypertrophied, and often enlargement of the internal cerebral veins. The involved brain may have abnormal T2W signal intensity within the white matter related to gliosis and demyelination, cortical enhancement related to anoxic injury, and atrophy. Secondary calvarial changes include compensatory hypertrophy of the diploic space, and enlargement of the ipsilateral paranasal sinuses and mastoid air cells. This case shows many of these abnormalities including the extent of the pial vascular malformation, cortical enhancement, dilated medullary and subependymal veins (*arrows*), and ipsilateral enlargement of the choroid plexus.

Notes

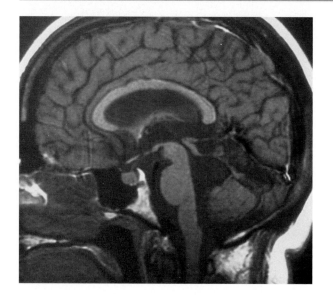

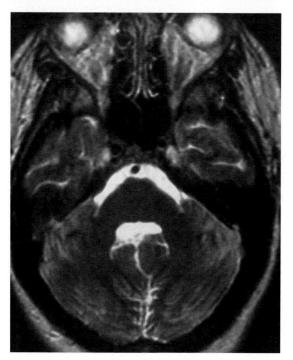

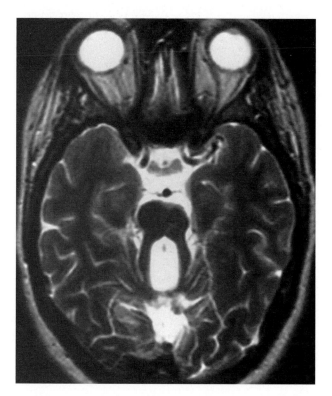

1. How can a Dandy-Walker malformation be distinguised from cerebellar hypoplasia/dysplasia?

2. What are common causes of acquired cerebellar volume loss/atrophy?

3. Which type of Chiari malformation is associated with a lumbosacral myelomeningocele?

4. In Joubert's syndrome, what part of the cerebellum is predominantly affected?

Joubert's Syndrome

1. Dandy-Walker malformations are typified by a retrocerebellar cyst that communicates with the fourth ventricle. In true Dandy-Walker malformations the posterior fossa is usually enlarged. In addition, up to 75% of patients with these malformations have associated hydrocephalus and/or supratentorial anomalies that are not typical of most cerebellar hypoplasias.

2. Alcohol, phenytoin, malnutrition.

3. Chiari II malformation.

4. The superior vermis.

Reference

Friede RL, Boltshauser E: Uncommon syndromes of cerebellar vermis aplasia. I: Joubert syndrome, *Dev Med Child Neurol* 20:758-763, 1978.

Cross-Reference

Neuroradiology: THE REQUISITES, pp 227-229, 259-262.

Comment

A spectrum of cerebellar developmental anomalies have been loosely categorized into complete or incomplete cerebellar agenesis, median aplasia/hypoplasia, and lateral aplasia/hypoplasia. These aberrations in cerebellar development may result in prominent CSF spaces or CSF collections/cystic dilation of the fourth ventricle (giant cisterna magna, Dandy-Walker malformations) in the posterior fossa. Other rarer entities are associated with enlargement and/or an abnormal configuration of the fourth ventricle. Such entities include aplasia or a spectrum of hypoplasias involving the cerebellar hemispheres, vermis, and/or brain stem. Unlike Dandy-Walker malformations, these cerebellar hypoplasias are not associated with posterior fossa cysts and less commonly have associated hydrocephalus or other supratentorial anomalies.

The predominant abnormality in Joubert's syndrome is aplasia or hypoplasia of the vermis, particularly the superior portion. In addition, these patients have dysplastic cerebellar tissue, including heterotopic and dysplastic cerebellar nuclei; abnormal development of the inferior olivary nuclei; and incomplete formation of the pyramidal decussation. It is an autosomal recessive disorder.

Magnetic resonance images in these patients show a somewhat characteristic appearance. Specifically, sagittal T1W images demonstrate a diminutive vermis. Axial images in particular show an enlarged fourth ventricle that is "bat-wing shaped" in configuration. The superior cerebellar peduncles are vertically oriented and elongated in the anteroposterior direction. Because of the dysgenesis of the vermis, the hallmark of Joubert's syndrome is separation or disconnection of the cerebellar hemispheres, which are apposed but not fused in the midline.

Notes

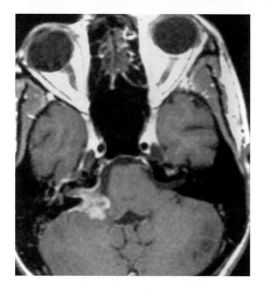
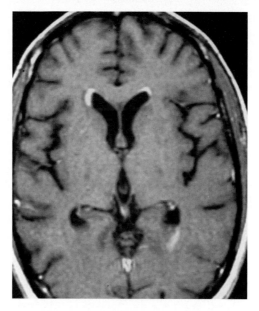

1. What major disease categories should be considered when there is ependymal enhancement?
2. What is the differential diagnosis of an enhancing cerebellopontine angle mass?
3. In immunocompromised patients, what CNS manifestations may occur in the reactivation of CMV?
4. What imaging findings are common in infants infected in utero by transplacental transmission of maternal CMV infection?

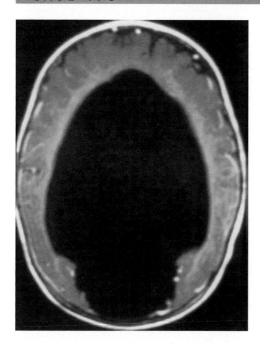
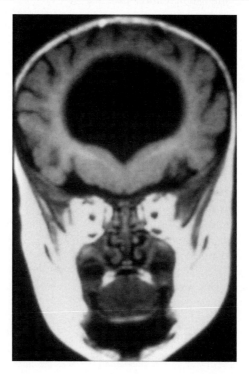

1. How can maximal pressure hydrocephalus be distinguished from alobar holoprosencephaly?
2. The hallmark of all holoprosencephalies (alobar, semilobar, and lobar) is the absence of what structure?
3. What is the triad of lesions seen in septo-optic dysplasia (deMorsier's syndrome)?
4. What is the presumed cause of hydranencephaly?

Cytomegalovirus Meningitis and Ependymitis in a Patient with Human Immunodeficiency Virus Infection

1. Infection (ventriculitis, ependymitis) and neoplasm (lymphoma, or seeding from other systemic and primary brain neoplasms).

2. Schwannoma, meningioma, metastasis, and inflammatory processes (e.g., infection, sarcoid).

3. Meningoencephalitis and ependymitis.

4. Bilateral ventricular subependymal calcification, ventricular enlargement, periventricular hypodensity on CT or hyperintensity on T2W MRI, atrophy, and migrational anomalies (pachygyria/polymicrogyria).

Reference

Post MJ, Hensley GT, Moskowitz LB, Fischl M: Cytomegalic inclusion virus encephalitis in patients with AIDS: CT, clinical and pathologic correlation, *Am J Neuroradiol* 146: 1229-1234, 1986.

Cross-Reference

Neuroradiology: THE REQUISITES, pp 180, 187, 264-265.

Comment

Cytomegalovirus is present in the latent form in the majority of the U.S. population. Reactivation usually results in a subclinical or mild flulike syndrome. In immunocompromised patients, however, reactivation not infrequently results in disseminated infection. CMV infection more often involves the respiratory and gastrointestinal tract; however, it may also result in infection of the nervous system. In the CNS, CMV may cause meningoencephalitis and ependymitis. Symptomatology in patients with CNS CMV may be acute or chronic, developing over months. Patients may have fever, change in mental status, and cognitive decline. Patients may also present with cranial neuropathies (as in this case).

Magnetic resonance imaging is clearly the diagnostic study of choice in assessing immunocompromised patients suspected of having CNS infection. Imaging may demonstrate atrophy; high signal intensity, which is poorly demarcated in the periventricular white matter and typically not associated with significant mass effect; and retinitis (frequently seen in the AIDS population) in patients with CMV infection. Although patients with CNS infection may also have subependymal involvement, associated imaging findings often are not present. However, the presence of T2W signal abnormalities and enhancement along the subependyma are valuable in establishing this diagnosis when present. At present, the most common cause of subependymal enhancement in the setting of AIDS is lymphoma.

Notes

Alobar Holoprosencephaly

1. In the latter there is absence of the interhemispheric fissure and midline structures, resulting in a monoventricle with failure of separation of the right and left cerebral hemispheres. In maximal-pressure hydrocephalus the midline structures are present (although chronic ventricular enlargement may result in failure to visualize the septum pellucidum).

2. The septum pellucidum.

3. (1) Complete or partial absence of the septum pellucidum; (2) optic nerve hypoplasia; and (3) hypothalamic-pituitary dysfunction, which typically manifests as growth retardation and short stature (this may be accompanied by an ectopic posterior pituitary gland).

4. Ischemia in the anterior and middle cerebral artery territories.

Reference

Fitz CR: Holoprosencephaly and related entities, *Neuroradiology* 25:225-238, 1983.

Cross-Reference

Neuroradiology: THE REQUISITES, pp 251-253.

Comment

The holoprosencephalies represent a spectrum of disorders characterized by hypoplasia of both the rostral end of the neural tube and the premaxillary segment of the face (lack of forebrain induction). With this comes failure of separation of the telencephalon and diencephalon into the right and left cerebral hemispheres and basal ganglia/thalami, respectively. Because the optic vesicles and olfactory bulbs evaginate from the prosencephalon, visual disturbances and incomplete formation of the olfactory system are frequently present. Hypoplasia of the premaxillary segment results in facial anomalies, including cleft lip and palate; abnormalities of the orbit (cyclopia, hypotelorism); and forehead proboscis.

Holoprosencephaly may be divided into three subtypes: alobar (the most severe form and usually incompatible with life), semilobar, and lobar (the mildest form). There is no clear distinction between subtypes. This case presents the characteristic appearance of alobar holoprosencephaly. There is absence of the interhemispheric fissure, the falx, and the septum pellucidum. There is resultant failure of separation of the cerebrum and the ventricular system into right and left halves. There is a monoventricle that is contiguous with a dorsal cyst. In semilobar holoprosencephaly the interhemispheric fissure and falx cerebri are usually formed posteriorly and absent anteriorly. In lobar holoprosencephaly, the interhemispheric fissure and falx anteriorly are hypoplastic. In semilobar and lobar holoprosencephaly, the ventricular system shows variable degrees of development.

Notes

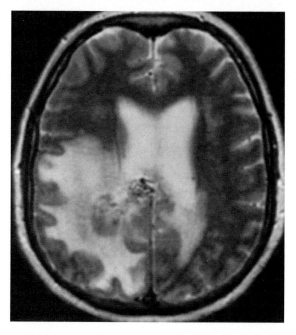
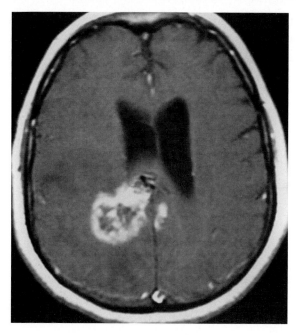

1. What are treatment options for AVMs and what factors are important in determining treatment?

2. What is the accepted size of an AVM nidus that is considered suitable for radiosurgery or stereotactic external beam radiation?

3. What is the incidence of radiation necrosis following radiosurgery for an AVM?

4. What factors contribute to the development of radiation necrosis?

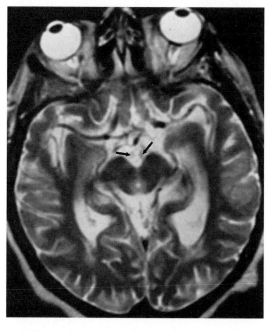
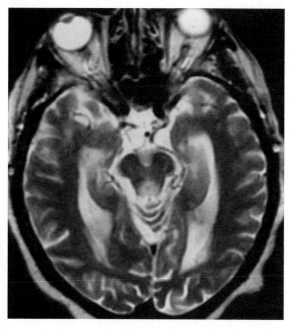

1. What is the cause of Wernicke's encephalopathy?

2. What structures are typically affected in Wernicke-Korsakoff syndrome?

3. What vascular abnormalities can result in bithalamic signal alterations?

4. What are the typical clinical manifestations of Wernicke's encephalopathy?

Radiation Necrosis After Radiosurgery of a Pericallosal Arteriovenous Malformation

1. Intravascular embolization, surgery, radiotherapy, or a combination of these modalities. Treatment depends on the size of the AVM as well as its location in the brain.

2. The nidus should be less than 3.5 cm.

3. Approximately 3% to 10%. Symptomatic radiation necrosis is reported in less than 5% of patients.

4. Total radiation dose and the time interval over which it is given, number and size of fractions per irradiation, and patient age.

Reference

Rabin BM, Meyer JR, Berlin JW, Marymount MH, Palka PS, Russell EJ: Radiation-induced changes in the central nervous system and head and neck, *RadioGraphics* 16:1055-1072, 1996.

Cross-Reference

Neuroradiology: THE REQUISITES, pp 100-102.

Comment

This case shows a pericallosal AVM with extensive signal abnormality in the adjacent parietal and occipital lobes (right greater than left) associated with enhancement and necrosis. In the management of AVMs, intravascular embolization and/or surgery for cure are favored when possible. Radiation therapy is particularly useful in treating AVMs in inoperable locations; however, the AVM should meet criteria for radiation. In some instances endovascular embolization is performed to reduce the size of the nidus and is followed with radiation therapy.

Brain changes due to radiation may be divided into those occurring early (during therapy) and those that are delayed. Delayed radiation changes may be further divided into early (within 3 to 4 months of therapy) and late (months to years following therapy). In early radiation injury, as well as early delayed injury, MRI typically demonstrates T2W-hyperintensity (edema) in the white matter that is frequently reversible. Late delayed injury is usually related to vascular injury and demyelination and appears as focal or diffuse abnormal T2W signal intensity with mass effect and enhancement.

In AVMs managed with radiation therapy, the diagnosis of radiation necrosis is not difficult to make. However, in patients treated with radiation for brain tumors, the distinction between recurrent tumor and radiation necrosis may be difficult because both present as enhancing necrotic masses. Recurrent tumor often has increased activity relative to normal brain tissue on positron emission tomography, whereas radiation necrosis typically shows reduced activity. Radiation necrosis sometimes can only be distinguished from recurrent tumor by surgical biopsy. When the mass is remote from the primary tumor site, the diagnosis of radiation necrosis may be easier to establish.

Notes

Wernicke's Syndrome

1. Thiamine deficiency.

2. The mamillary bodies (essentially in all patients), hypothalamus, periaqueductal gray matter, and thalami.

3. Venous ischemia/infarction (due to deep vein thrombosis such as with the internal cerebral veins) and artery of Persheron (a single vascular pedicle that supplies the paramedian thalamic arteries) infarction.

4. Ocular symptoms (nystagmus and gaze paralysis), change in mental status, and ataxia.

Reference

Gallucci M, Bozzao A, Splendiani A, et al: Wernicke encephalopathy: MR findings in five patients, *Am J Neuroradiol* 11:887-892, 1990.

Cross-Reference

Neuroradiology: THE REQUISITES, pp 222, 227-228.

Comment

This case demonstrates many of the radiologic findings seen in Wernicke's encephalopathy. Specifically, best appreciated is abnormal signal intensity in the periaqueductal gray matter and in the mamillary bodies (*arrows*) in this patient with a long history of alcoholism. On MRI, which is much more sensitive than is CT in evaluating the small structures affected in this syndrome, one typically sees abnormalities involving the mammillary bodies. Also commonly involved is the periaqueductal gray matter, hypothalamus, floor of the fourth ventricle, and medial portions of the thalami. Imaging findings are often bilaterally symmetric. Typically there is increased T2W signal intensity in these structures. In the acute setting there may be mild swelling associated with the signal alterations, and enhancement has also been reported. In the late stages, atrophy (particularly of the mammillary bodies) may be the main finding. Resolution of the signal alterations following treatment with thiamine has been reported.

Wernicke's encephalopathy is related to thiamine deficiency and is found most commonly in alcoholics; however, this vitamin deficiency may also be present in other circumstances resulting in chronic malnutrition, as well as long-term parenteral therapy. Whereas Wernicke's encephalopathy clinically manifests with ocular abnormalities and confusion, Korsakoff psychosis is manifested by retrograde amnesia and difficulty acquiring new information. The two not uncommonly occur together.

Notes

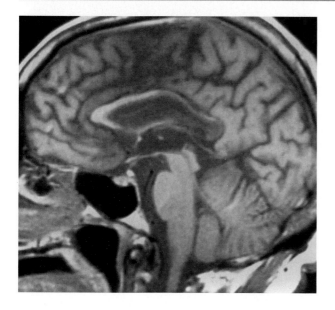

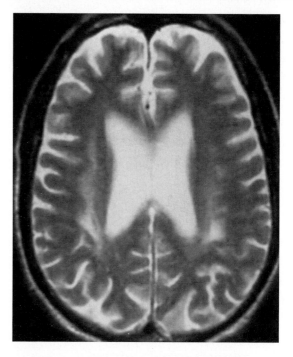

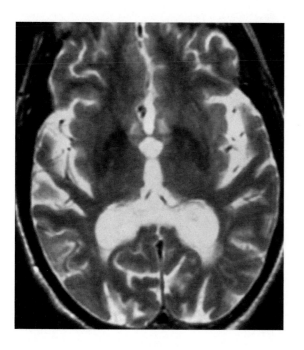

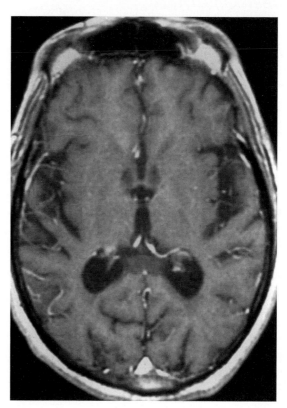

1. What are the major MRI findings?

2. What is the most likely underlying causes of these abnormalities?

3. Marchiafava-Bignami disease can be considered in what category of demyelinating disease?

4. What is the characteristic location for osmotic demyelination?

Marchiafava-Bignami Disease

1. Abnormal signal intensity in the splenium of the corpus callosum, which is hypointense on unenhanced T1W images and is atrophied. In addition, there is global atrophy of the cerebrum and multiple additional foci of increased T2W signal intensity in the periventricular white matter.

2. Demyelinating disease.

3. Extrapontine osmotic demyelination.

4. The pons.

References

Chang KH, Cha SH, Hahn MH, et al: Marchiafava-Bignami disease: serial changes in the corpus callosum on MRI, *Neuroradiology* 34:480-482, 1992.

Caparros-Lefebvre D, Pruvo JP, Josien E, Pertuzon B, Clarisse J, Petit H: Marchiafava-Bignami disease: use of contrast media in CT and MRI, *Neuroradiology* 36:509-511, 1994.

Cross-Reference
Neuroradiology: THE REQUISITES, pp 215-216.

Comment

Marchiafava-Bignami disease is a demyelinating disorder that was initially described in patients who consumed large quantities of red wine in Italy (it is also associated with poor nutrition). However, it has been described in other populations and with other alcoholic delights. The disease may present acutely with rapid deterioration or may exist in a chronic form over a period of years. On pathologic evaluation, Marchiafava-Bignami disease is typified by demyelination and occurs most commonly in the corpus callosum; however, there may be extensive demyelination involving multiple areas of the brain, including the deep and periventricular white matter (as in this case), as well as other commissural fibers. Sagittal T1W images are valuable in assessing these patients because these images show the extensive callosal atrophy and the associated focal necrosis as demarcated regions of signal abnormality that are hypointense on T1W imaging and hyperintense on T2W imaging. This case nicely demonstrates all of these findings. In the absence of history, it would be difficult to distinguish this diagnosis from the other demyelinating processes that are more common, such as multiple sclerosis. However, Marchiafava-Bignami disease should be considered in patients with encephalopathy with a history of chronic alcoholism.

Notes

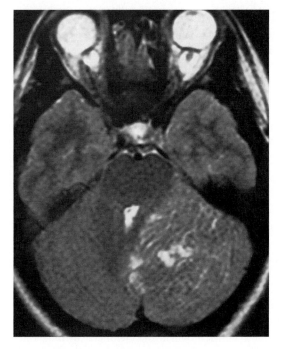 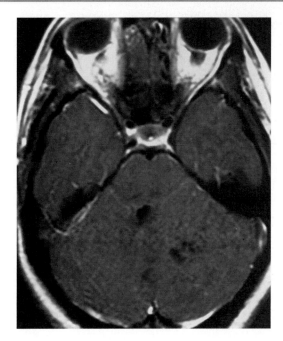

1. In children and young adults, what are the most common cerebellar hemispheric neoplasms?
2. What are the typical MRI findings seen with dysplastic gangliocytomas?
3. In general, are dysplastic gangliocytomas considered true neoplasms?
4. With what uncommon neurocutaneous syndrome are dysplastic gangliocytomas associated?

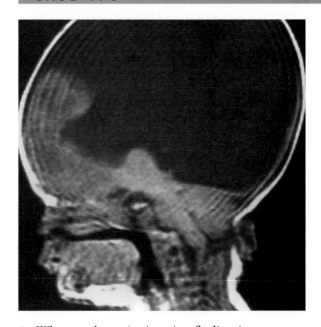

1. What are the major imaging findings?
2. The combination of imaging findings is consistent with what congenital abnormality?
3. What is the most common location for congenital meningoencephaloceles?
4. What syndrome is characterized by the presence of an encephalocele, microcephaly, polydactyly, and cystic kidneys?

Lhermitte-Duclos Disease (Dysplastic Gangliocytoma of the Cerebellum)

1. Astrocytoma (frequently pilocytic), hemangioblastoma, and (uncommonly) metastases.

2. Typically there is T2W hyperintensity and thickening of involved cerebellar folia giving a laminated appearance. These lesions typically do not demonstrate avid enhancement, but they often exert mass effect.

3. Although controversial, dysplastic gangliocytomas are considered complex hamartomatous malformations rather than true neoplasms.

4. Cowden disease.

References

Vieco PT, del Carpio-O'Donovan R, Melanson D, et al: Dysplastic gangliocytoma (Lhermitte-Duclos disease): CT and MR imaging, *Pediatr Radiol* 22:366-369, 1992.

Meltzer CC, Smirniotopoulos JG, Jones RV: The striated cerebellum: an MR imaging sign in Lhermitte-Duclos disease (dysplastic gangliocytoma), *Radiology* 194:699-703, 1995.

Cross-Reference

Neuroradiology: THE REQUISITES, p 99.

Comment

When symptomatic, Lhermitte-Duclos disease or dysplastic gangliocytoma of the cerebellum typically presents with symptoms related to mass effect in the second and third decades of life. Lhermitte-Duclos disease has been associated with Cowden disease (multiple hamartoma syndrome), an autosomal dominant disorder associated with an increased incidence of neoplasms in the pelvis, breast, colon, and thyroid. Intracranial meningiomas have also been noted with this syndrome.

Although controversial, Lhermitte-Duclos disease is considered to represent a complex hamartomatous malformation, not a true neoplasm. Dysplastic gangliocytomas often occur in the cerebellar hemispheres. Unlike neoplasms, which tend to be circumscribed, these lesions tend to be poorly demarcated, presenting on CT as a mildly hypodense mass. Calcification has been reported. On MRI these lesions have a more characteristic appearance in which the gray and white matter of the cerebellar hemisphere are both involved and are thickened and hyperintense on T2W imaging, showing a somewhat characteristic laminated or "corduroy" appearance. They typically are poorly demarcated, and may exert mass effect. Hydrocephalus may be present. Following contrast administration, these lesions do not demonstrate significant enhancement. On pathologic evaluation they usually appear as dysplasia with cellular disorganization of the normal laminar structure of the cerebellum and hypertrophied granular cell neurons. Histologically there is hypermyelination of axons, and pleomorphic ganglion cells replace the granular and Purkinje cell layers.

Notes

Chiari III Malformation

1. Herniation of the cerebellum and caudal displacement of the brain stem into the foramen magnum/upper cervical canal, high cervical/low occipital encephalocele, and agenesis of the corpus callosum.

2. Chiari III malformation.

3. Meningoencephaloceles are usually midline lesions, most commonly occurring in the occipital region.

4. Meckel-Gruber syndrome.

Reference

Castillo M, Quencer RM, Dominguez R: Chiari-III malformation: imaging features, *Am J Neuroradiol* 13:107-113, 1992.

Cross-Reference

Neuroradiology: THE REQUISITES, pp 249-250, 261-262.

Comment

Meningoceles and meningoencephaloceles may be congenital or acquired abnormalities in which the meninges (meningocele) and/or brain tissue (encephalocele) protrudes through an osseous defect in the calvaria. Encephaloceles almost always contain meninges in addition to brain tissue, hence the term *meningoencephalocele*. Congenital meningoencephaloceles are more common than are meningoceles. They are typically midline lesions that most commonly occur in the occipital region (65% to 75%), followed by the parietal and frontal regions (each has about a 10% incidence). The presence of an off-midline encephalocele (a lateral encephalocele, such as in the temporal region) should raise suspicion of amniotic bands or limb-body complex syndrome. In the Asian population there is an increased incidence of meningoencephaloceles in the sphenoethmoid and nasofrontal regions that may be clinically occult. Alternatively, they may present with CSF leaks and/or recurrent infection/meningitis.

The most sensitive imaging modality to confirm the presence of a meningocephalocele is MRI. The diagnosis can be clinched by establishing continuity of the tissue protruding through the calvarial defect with that in the intracranial compartment. Brain tissue within an encephalocele may be normal in signal intensity or may be hyperintense on T2W images due to gliosis.

In the Chiari III malformation, patients typically have all of the imaging findings of a Chiari II malformation in addition to a high cervical/low occipital meningoencephalocele (which usually contains the cerebellum but may also contain the brain stem). In Chiari III malformations, a lumbosacral myelomeningocele is not present. Chiari III malformations are often associated with agenesis or dysgenesis of the corpus callosum (as in this case), migrational abnormalities, and anomalies of the upper cervical spine.

Notes

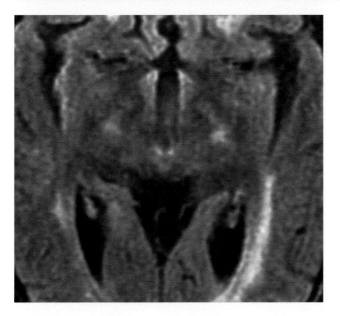
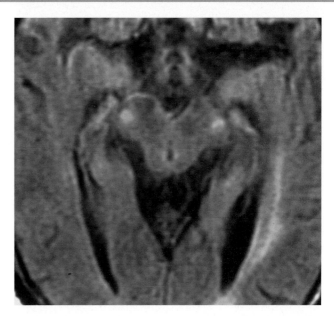

1. What are the findings on the MRI?

2. In what part of the brain stem is the pyramidal decussation located?

3. Abnormality extending from the precentral gyrus to the level of the ventral and lateral spinal cord is characteristic of what neurodegenerative disorder?

4. What cranial nerve is most commonly involved in amyotrophic lateral sclerosis?

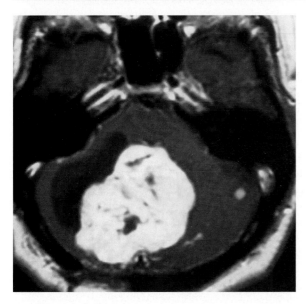
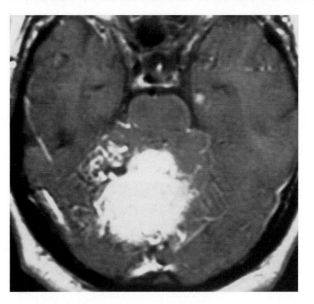

1. What is the most common cause of multiple cerebellar masses in adults?

2. What neoplasms may present as a cystic mass with an enhancing mural nodule?

3. What finding makes the diagnosis of pilocytic astrocytoma highly unlikely?

4. What neurocutaneous syndrome is associated with multiple hemangioblastomas?

Amyotrophic Lateral Sclerosis

1. Bilaterally symmetric high signal intensity within the pyramidal tracts in the posterior part of the posterior limb of the internal capsule, and extending into the cerebral peduncles.

2. The medulla.

3. Amyotrophic lateral sclerosis (Lou Gehrig's disease).

4. The hypoglossal nerve, resulting in denervation atrophy of the tongue.

Reference

Udaka F, Sawada H, Seriu N, Shindou K, Nishitani N, Kameyama M: MRI and SPECT findings in amyotrophic lateral sclerosis: demonstration of upper motor neuron involvement by clinical neuroimaging, *Neuroradiology* 34: 389-393, 1992.

Cross-Reference

Neuroradiology: THE REQUISITES, p 236.

Comment

Amyotrophic lateral sclerosis (Lou Gehrig's disease) is the most common of the neurodegenerative disorders involving the motor neurons. It occurs in approximately 1 in every 100,000 people annually. Most cases are sporadic, although autosomal dominant transmission may occur. Amyotrophic lateral sclerosis typically presents in the sixth decade of life; clinical manifestations include hyperreflexia, weakness of the hands and forearms, spasticity, and cranial neuropathies. The hypoglossal nerve is most commonly affected, and its involvement may be detected on imaging as denervation atrophy with fatty replacement of the tongue. Amyotrophic lateral sclerosis typically involves the corticospinal tracts and lower motor neurons. Progression is usually relentless, with death frequently occurring within 3 to 6 years from disease onset. The cause is unknown. In extreme cases abnormal T2W signal intensity may extend from the cortex along the precentral gyrus of the motor strip (the pyramidal Betz's cells/upper motor neurons), through the corona radiata, the posterior part of the posterior limb of the internal capsule, the cerebral peduncles, and brain stem, and down to the ventral and lateral portions of the spinal cord. Abnormal hypointensity may be present along the cerebral cortex in the motor strip and is believed to be related to deposition of iron and/or other minerals. SPECT with *N*-isopropyl-p-I123 iodoamphetamine may reveal decreased uptake in the cerebral cortex, including the motor cortex. MRI evaluation of the spinal cord may demonstrate atrophy along the corticospinal tracts.

Notes

von Hippel-Lindau Disease

1. Metastases.

2. Pilocytic astrocytoma, hemangioblastoma, and metastases.

3. The multiplicity of lesions (pilocytic astrocytomas are usually isolated neoplasms in children).

4. von Hippel-Lindau disease.

Reference

Neumann HP, Eggert HR, Scheremet R, et al: Central nervous system lesions in von Hippel-Lindau syndrome, *J Neurol Neurosurg Psychiatry* 55:898-901, 1995.

Cross-Reference

Neuroradiology: THE REQUISITES, pp 81-82, 271, 289.

Comment

This case shows multiple enhancing cerebellar lesions. The largest lesion is a cystic mass with an enhancing mural nodule. Because this patient is an adult and the lesions are multiple, juvenile pilocytic astrocytoma is not a consideration. The differential diagnosis includes metastases or multiple hemangioblastomas seen in von Hippel-Lindau disease.

Von Hippel-Lindau disease is a neurocutaneous syndrome (neurocutaneous is a misnomer in that there are no cutaneous manifestations in this disorder). The hallmark lesion is the hemangioblastoma. Approximately 20% of patients with hemangioblastomas have von Hippel-Lindau disease. Conversely, up to 45% of patients with von Hippel-Lindau disease have CNS hemangioblastomas. In von Hippel-Lindau disease, these neoplasms are multiple in at least 40% of cases. Hemangioblastomas occur most commonly in the cerebellum and retina, although they may also arise in the brain stem (especially the medulla), the spinal cord, and (rarely) the cerebrum and viscera outside of the CNS. In addition to CNS lesions, patients with von Hippel-Lindau disease also have a spectrum of findings in other organs. Cysts in the pancreas occur in the majority of patients but may also be seen in the kidneys, liver, and epididymis in men and ovaries in women. Renal cell carcinomas are common and are different from the garden variety renal cell adenocarcinoma in that in von Hippel-Lindau disease they are frequently bilateral, small, and less malignant. There is an approximately tenfold increase in the incidence of pheochromocytomas in these patients. Polycythemia related to production of erythropoietin by the hemangioblastoma(s) is not uncommon. Diagnostic criteria for von Hippel-Lindau disease include more than one CNS and/or retinal hemangioblastoma; a CNS hemangioblastoma and at least one visceral abnormality; or a family history of von Hippel-Lindau disease and at least one of the visceral manifestations.

Notes

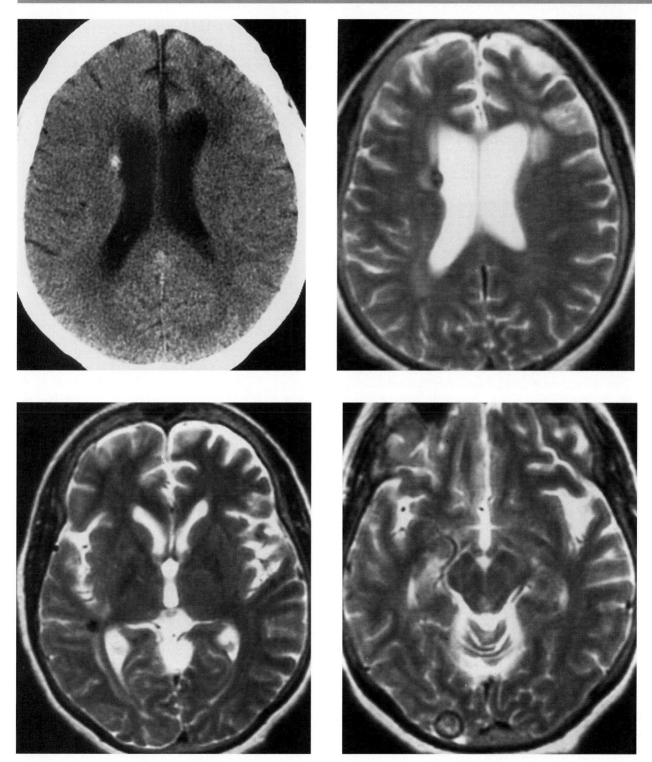

1. What disease processes should be considered in the presence of both calcified and "ring" lesions?
2. What infectious agents are commonly associated with calcified parenchymal lesions?
3. In immunocompromised patients, how do fungal infections such as aspergillus and mucormycosis infect the CNS?
4. What type of metastases are associated with calcification?

Aspergillus Emboli

1. Infection (especially cysticercos, is as well as granulomatous and fungal agents) and metastatic disease. The presence of the two together suggests an infectious process.

2. Tuberculosis, cysticercosis, toxoplasmosis, fungal infections, and in utero infection with CMV.

3. By direct extension from sinonasal infection or by hematogenous dissemination.

4. Mucinous adenocarcinomas, as well as sarcomatous lesions (osteogenic sarcoma).

Reference

Cox J, Murtagh FR, Wilfong A, Brenner J: Cerebral aspergillosis: MR imaging and histopathologic correlation, *Am J Neuroradiol* 13:1489-1492, 1992.

Cross-Reference

Neuroradiology: THE REQUISITES, pp 192-193.

Comment

These images show multiple lesions that are characterized by small, punctate regions of calcification in the periventricular region on the right, as well as a "ring" lesion in the right occipital lobe. Prior imaging studies showed hemorrhage in the regions of calcification seen as high density on an unenhanced CT. The lesions are surrounded by a small amount of edema seen as T2W hyperintensity. Differential considerations include an infectious process and metastatic disease. The presence both of calcified lesions (with relatively little surrounding edema) and ring lesions favors an infectious etiology. On biopsy, the patient was found to have CNS aspergillosis.

The CNS is affected with aspergillus either by direct extension from a sinonasal cavity infection or hematogenous dissemination (emboli), most commonly from a pulmonary source (as in this case). Unlike most patients infected with *Aspergillus* who are immunocompromised, this patient had a normal immune system. When *Aspergillus* infects the CNS by direct extension from the sinonasal cavity, there is frequently vascular invasion of the cavernous sinus and/or the vessels in the basal cisterns that may result in thrombosis and infarction due to direct invasion of the vessel wall. Similarly, in embolic transmission of infection the organism directly invades the walls of distal vessels and may result in regions of hemorrhage (as in this case, in which the areas of calcification on the images presented were preceded by small areas of hemorrhage).

Notes

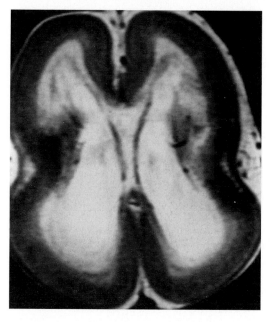

1. What is the major imaging finding?
2. What is the name of this disorder when it involves only a focal area of the brain?
3. What in utero infection has been implicated in this entity?
4. What is the cause of high signal intensity in the peripheral cortex of this lesion?

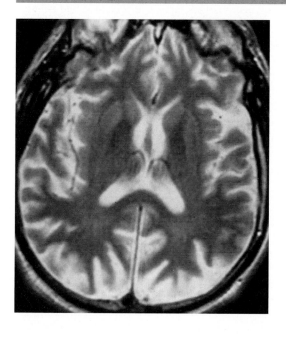 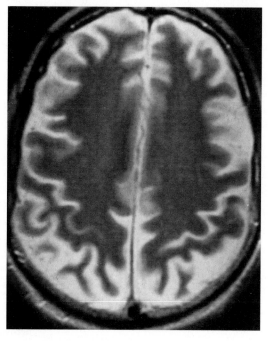

1. In this 44-year-old patient, what is the most striking abnormality?
2. What other finding is present?
3. What is the typical clinical presentation of Creutzfeldt-Jakob disease?
4. In addition to eating bad meat (beef, sheep), what other modes of transmission have been associated with this infection?

CASE 182

Lissencephaly

1. Global broad, thickened cortex with lack of sulcation and gyral formation.

2. Pachygyria.

3. CMV.

4. Laminar necrosis in the cell sparse zone.

Reference

Barkovich AJ, Gressens P, Evrard P: Formation, maturation, and disorders of brain neocortex, *Am J Neuroradiol* 13: 423-446, 1992.

Cross-Reference

Neuroradiology: THE REQUISITES, p 258.

Comment

Complete lissencephaly, or "agyria," is the most severe of the gray matter migrational abnormalities. It is the result of abnormal neuronal migration during the second half of the first trimester and first weeks of the second trimester of pregnancy. There is absence of sulcation and gyration of the cerebral cortex with failure in the development of the normal six cortical layers. Pachygyria or incomplete lissencephaly refers to a focal abnormality in sulcation/gyration. Lissencephaly has been linked to genetic causes (chromosome 17), muscular dystrophy, and in utero CMV infection. Global involvement of the entire brain results in its smooth hourglass appearance. This hourglass appearance is due to lack of opercularization of the sylvian cisterns, which are vertically or obliquely oriented. Lissencephaly can be divided into several subtypes categorized on the basis of cortex morphology and associated brain anomalies.

Imaging findings include a diffuse broad, thickened cortex with a smooth outer surface, as well as a smooth transition at the gray-white matter interface. The gray matter abnormality is associated with underdevelopment or hypoplasia of the underlying white matter. High signal intensity may be seen within the cortical layer and is believed to be related to laminar necrosis. In addition, signal abnormality may be seen in the underlying white matter as a result of delayed myelination and/or gliosis.

Notes

CASE 183

Creutzfeldt-Jakob Disease

1. Diffuse cortical atrophy.

2. Mild increased signal intensity in the anterior putamen and the heads of the caudate nuclei bilaterally.

3. Rapidly progressive dementia.

4. Corneal transplantation, cerebral electrode implantation, and cannibalism.

References

Finkenstaedt M, Szudra A, Zerr I, et al: MR imaging of Creutzfeldt-Jakob disease, *Radiology* 199:793-798, 1996.

Falcone S, Quencer RM, Bowen B, Bruce JH, Naidich TP: Creutzfeldt-Jakob disease: focal symmetrical cortical involvement demonstrated by MR imaging, *Am J Neuroradiol* 13:403-406, 1992.

Cross-Reference

Neuroradiology: THE REQUISITES, pp 231-232.

Comment

Creutzfeldt-Jakob, or "prion," disease is a rare degenerative disorder that affects the CNS. Approximately 1 in every 1 million persons worldwide is infected. It is believed to be caused by a slow virus, an organism devoid of active nucleic acid. The most common clinical presentation is that of rapidly progressive dementia. Other neurologic symptoms may occur and include upper motor neuron signs, ataxia, myoclonus, and sensory deficits. The prognosis is poor, with death usually occurring within a year from the onset of symptoms. Histologic evaluation demonstrates neuronal degeneration and gliosis in the gray matter, especially the cortex, but also in the deep gray matter of the corpus striatum and thalami. Spongiform changes are characteristic. Inflammatory changes are usually not present. The disease is best known in association with mad cow disease (bovine spongiform encephalopathy) in the United Kingdom; however, there have been scattered sporadic cases described with corneal transplantation, as well as with implantation of cerebral electrodes.

Computed tomography usually demonstrates no abnormality; however, atrophy (most commonly cortical) represents the next most common presentation. With the advent of MRI additional lesions have been detected. In addition to atrophy, T2W signal alterations have been described, especially in the caudate and putamen nuclei but also in the thalami. Lesions typically are bilateral and not associated with enhancement or significant mass effect. In addition, abnormalities involving the gray and white matter have been noted within the cerebral hemispheres.

Notes

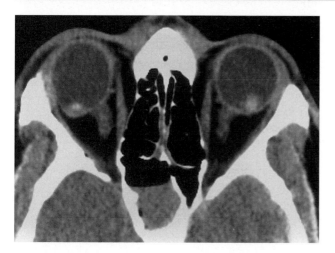 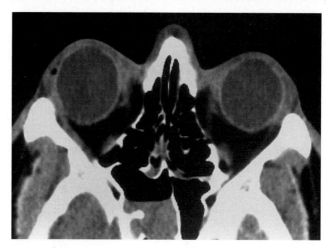

1. Regarding ocular foreign bodies, what is the CT and MRI appearance of wood?

2. What is the salient finding in this case?

3. What is the best initial imaging modality in assessing orbital trauma?

4. What connective tissue disorders (mesodermal abnormalities) are associated with dislocation and/or subluxation of the lens?

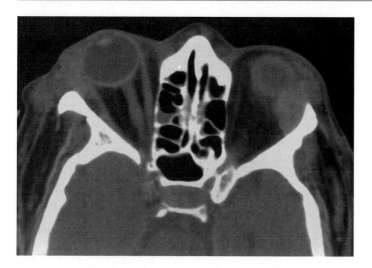 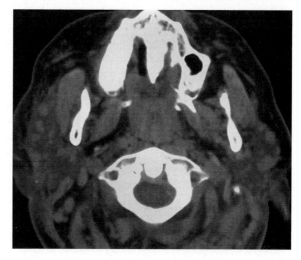

1. What are the salient imaging findings?

2. What is the most common benign epithelial tumor of the lacrimal gland?

3. Mikulicz's syndrome is associated with what other conditions?

4. With what systemic condition is Sjögren's syndrome frequently associated?

CASE 184

Bilateral Lens Dislocations—Marfan Syndrome

1. Wood is hypodense and hypointense, respectively. On CT the orbits should be viewed on wide (bone) windows in order to distinguish wood from orbital emphysema, because wood can look like air on soft tissue windows.

2. Bilateral lens dislocations.

3. CT.

4. Marfan syndrome, Ehler-Danlos syndrome, and homocystinuria.

References

Maguire AM, Enger C, Eliott D, Zinreich SJ: Computerized tomography in the evaluation of penetrating ocular injuries, *Retina* 11:405-411, 1991.

Weissman JL, Beatty RL, Hirsch WL, Curtin HD: Enlarged anterior chamber: CT finding of a ruptured globe, *Am J Neuroradiol* 16(Suppl):936-938, 1995.

Cross-Reference

Neuroradiology: THE REQUISITES, p 289.

Comment

This case illustrates bilateral lens dislocations. On imaging, lens dislocation may be differentiated from other intraocular foreign bodies by identifying that the intraocular density has the configuration of a lens and, importantly, in observing that the lens in that eye is not located in its normal position. Lens dislocation may be confirmed on physical examination. In this case, intraocular foreign bodies would be unusual given that the disease is bilateral and there are no other imaging findings of orbital trauma. CT is the imaging modality of choice in the initial assessment of patients with orbital trauma due to its availability, as well as the ease and rapidity in which the examination can be performed. In addition, CT readily establishes the presence of orbital foreign bodies, delineates orbital fractures, and assesses for retrobulbar complications of trauma.

Subluxation and/or dislocation of the lens may be seen in settings that are unrelated to trauma. Subluxations or dislocations may occur spontaneously or may be related to infection. In addition, there are hereditary disorders that may be associated with this condition. Most inherited disorders associated with lens subluxation/dislocation result from abnormalities of the connective (mesodermal) tissues and include Marfan syndrome (as in this case), Ehlers-Danlos syndrome, and homocystinuria. In Marfan syndrome the lenses are usually subluxed superiorly and at the periphery of the globe, whereas in homocystinuria the subluxations are inferior ("down and out"). Marfan syndrome is typically associated with skeletal anomalies, cardiovascular disease (dissections), and arachnodactyly. Lens subluxation or dislocation is present in most patients with Marfan syndrome and is usually bilateral.

Notes

CASE 185

Sjögren's Syndrome

1. Bilaterally symmetric enlargement of the lacrimal glands.

2. Pleomorphic adenoma.

3. Tuberculosis, sarcoid, leukemia, and lymphoma.

4. Connective tissue disorders.

Reference

Stewart WB, Krohel GB, Wright JE: Lacrimal gland and fossa lesions: an approach to diagnosis and management, *Ophthalmology* 86:886-895, 1979.

Cross-Reference

Neuroradiology: THE REQUISITES, pp 300, 418.

Comment

The lacrimal glands are histologically similar to the salivary glands and therefore are involved by similar disease processes. Involvement of both lacrimal glands is frequently due to chronic systemic disorders usually related to lymphocytic infiltration or inflammatory lesions. Inflammation of the lacrimal glands may be an isolated process, may be part of diffuse orbital inflammation, or may be associated with a spectrum of systemic disorders. Acute inflammation of the lacrimal gland is usually seen in younger patients, is frequently unilateral, and is most commonly related to a postviral syndrome. Chronic dacryoadenitis may occur with Sjögren's syndrome, Mikulicz's syndrome, sarcoid, and Wegener's granulomatosis. Mikulicz's syndrome represents a nonspecific inflammation and enlargement of the lacrimal and salivary glands and is associated with sarcoidosis, hematologic malignancies (leukemia and lymphoma), and tuberculosis. In Sjögren's syndrome there is lymphocytic infiltration of the lacrimal and salivary glands that results in dry eyes (keratoconjunctivitis sicca) and xerostomia, respectively (note in this case the involvement of the parotid glands with hyperplastic lymph nodes and lymphoepithelial cysts). Sjögren's syndrome is usually associated with connective tissue disorders, especially rheumatoid arthritis but also systemic lupus erythematosus, polymyositis, and scleroderma.

In Sjögren's syndrome on cross-sectional imaging there is usually enlargement of both lacrimal glands (without a demarcated mass) that is not distinguishable from other inflammatory conditions and lymphoproliferative disorders. In the late stages of disease, atrophy of the glands may be present.

Notes

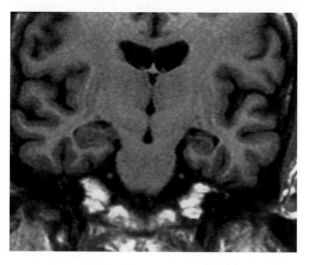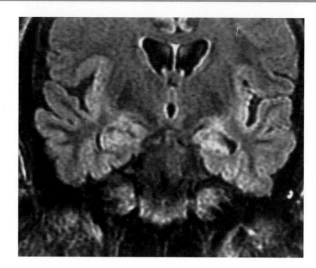

1. What are the pertinent imaging findings?
2. What is the patient's clinical history?
3. What benign neoplasm has a predilection for the temporal lobe?
4. What imaging features help differentiate mesial temporal sclerosis from a neoplasm?

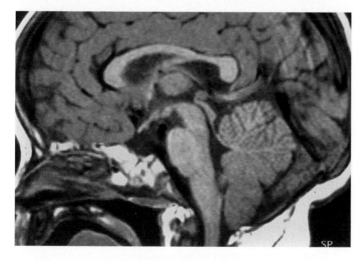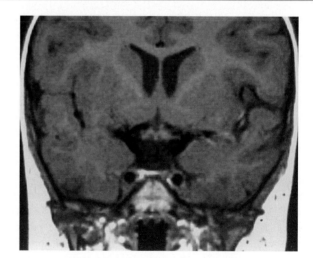

1. What is the normal T1W signal intensity of the posterior lobe of the pituitary gland?
2. In what circumstances is the anterior lobe of the pituitary gland normally hyperintense on T1W imaging?
3. What is the pertinent finding in this case?
4. What are common locations for a Rathke's cleft cyst?

CASE 186

Hippocampal (Mesial Temporal) Sclerosis

1. The hippocampus is atrophic and focally hyperintense on T2W imaging compared with the contralateral normal side, and there is ipsilateral enlargement of the adjacent temporal horn.

2. Seizure disorder.

3. Ganglioglioma.

4. Hippocampal sclerosis is manifest by hyperintensity on T2W images associated with volume loss, whereas neoplasms involving the hippocampus are typically associated with hippocampal enlargement and mass effect.

References

Jack CR Jr, Rydberg CH, Krecke KN, et al: Mesial temporal sclerosis: diagnosis with fluid-attenuated inversion-recovery versus spin-echo MR imaging, *Radiology* 199:367-373, 1996.

Bronen RA, Fulbright RK, Spencer DD, et al: Refractory epilepsy: comparison of MR imaging, CT, and histopathologic findings in 117 patients, *Radiology* 201:97-105, 1996.

Cross-Reference

Neuroradiology: THE REQUISITES, pp 45-47.

Comment

Magnetic resonance imaging has emerged as the imaging modality of choice for evaluating patients with seizure disorders because of its multiplanar capabilities and superior tissue resolution and contrast. This case illustrates the MRI appearance of hippocampal sclerosis in which there is abnormal T2W hyperintensity within the hippocampus, which is also atrophied. There is mild asymmetry of the temporal horns of the lateral ventricles, with mild ipsilateral dilation compared with the normal side. The hippocampal formations are best visualized on coronal MRI using thin sections. In my experience, 1-mm T1W spoiled gradient echo images are especially useful, as are 3-mm thick fast spin echo T2W and FLAIR images. In addition, coronal T1W gradient volumetric images provide extremely thin sections and are useful for detecting anatomic abnormalities (such as migrational anomalies). Thin section imaging in the coronal plane is also important because thick section images may result in misinterpretation of partial volume averaging of CSF in the temporal horn for abnormal signal intensity within the hippocampus. The major differential considerations for hippocampal sclerosis are cortical dysplasias or a primary brain neoplasm. Although hippocampal sclerosis may be hyperintense on T2W imaging and, importantly, is associated with volume loss, neoplasms involving the hippocampus are usually associated with focal mass effect. In addition, extension of mass effect and/or signal alteration outside of the hippocampus into other structures in the medial temporal lobe should also raise suspicion for a neoplasm.

Notes

CASE 187

Panhypopituitarism With Absence of the Infundibulum*

1. Hyperintense to white matter.

2. During pregnancy and the first 3 months of life.

3. Absence of the pituitary stalk and the anterior lobe of the gland.

4. The anterior sella and/or suprasellar cistern.

Reference

Colombo N, Berry I, Kucharczyk J, et al: Posterior pituitary gland: appearance on MRI in normal and pathologic states, *Radiology* 165:481-485, 1987.

Cross-Reference

Neuroradiology: THE REQUISITES, pp 311-312, 318.

Comment

This case shows an absent/diminutive anterior pituitary lobe, absence of the pituitary stalk, and absence of the normal posterior pituitary "bright" spot in the sella. High signal intensity at the apex-median eminence of the pituitary stalk is characteristic of an ectopic posterior pituitary gland. The differential diagnosis of high signal intensity along the apex of the stalk at the floor of the third ventricle includes a tuber cinereum lipoma or fat in the marrow of the tip of the dorsum sella. In the latter two conditions, the normal posterior pituitary "bright" spot in the sella is present. Absence of the normal posterior pituitary high signal intensity may be seen in Langerhans cell histiocytosis and hemosiderosis.

The neurohypophysis is ectopic in a subset of patients with pituitary dwarfism. Specifically, low growth hormone levels associated with other pituitary hormonal deficiencies may be accompanied on MRI by an ectopic posterior pituitary gland and absence of the infundibulum. Failure of development of the infundibulum and posterior pituitary gland may be an isolated condition or may be part of a larger brain anomaly. It is believed that an ectopic posterior pituitary gland is related to an insult to the pituitary infundibulum, which, through a rich venous plexus normally transmits hormonal mediators from the hypothalamus to the neurohypophysis. An ectopic posterior pituitary gland has also been associated with traumatic transection of the pituitary stalk. The normal neurohypophysis is of high signal intensity on unenhanced T1W images; however, the exact etiology of this is debated, with explanations including vasopressin, phospholipid, and neurophysin stored in neurosecretory granules of the posterior pituitary gland.

Notes

---

*Figures for Case 187 courtesy Robert A. Zimmerman, MD.

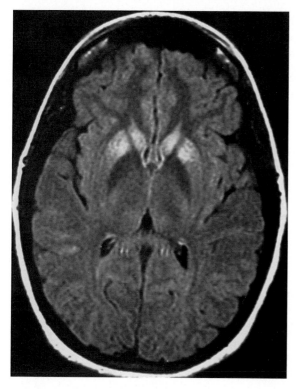
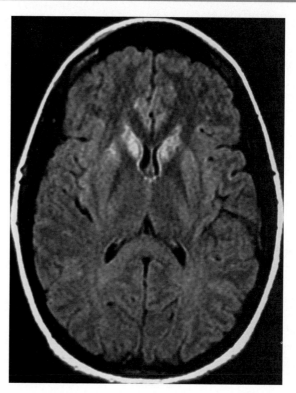

1. Wilson's disease is caused by abnormal metabolism of what mineral?
2. Abnormal metabolism of this mineral is due to deficiency of what carrier protein?
3. How is this disorder transmitted?
4. What is the characteristic finding in the eye that is diagnostic of this condition?

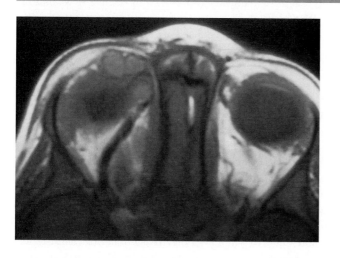
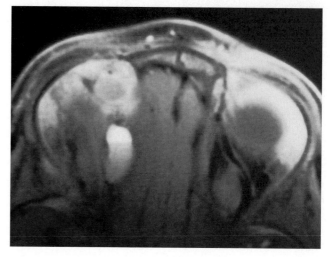

1. What are the three most common orbital vascular tumors?
2. What is the most common intraconal mass in adults?
3. Which vascular neoplasm is seen almost exclusively in infancy?
4. Are lymphangiomas more commonly intraconal or extraconal in location?

CASE 188

Wilson's Disease

1. Copper.

2. Ceruloplasmin.

3. In an autosomal recessive pattern.

4. Kayser-Fleischer rings (copper deposition in the cornea).

Reference

van Wassenaer-van Hall HN, van den Heuvel AG, Algra A, Hoogenrad TU, Mali WP: Wilson's disease: findings at MR imaging and CT of the brain with clinical correlation, *Radiology* 198:531-536, 1996.

Cross-Reference

Neuroradiology: THE REQUISITES, pp 235-236.

Comment

Wilson's disease (hepatolenticular degeneration) results from abnormal metabolism of copper caused by deficiency of its carrier protein, ceruloplasmin. As a result, there is extensive abnormal deposition of copper in multiple organ systems (most pronounced in the liver and brain). Although neurologic symptoms may be directly related to copper deposition within the brain parenchyma, they may also be a manifestation of hepatic encephalopathy due to liver failure. Neurologic signs and symptoms may include a pseudoparkinsonian-like syndrome with rigidity, gait disturbance, and difficulty with fine motor skills. Dysarthria and cognitive and psychiatric disturbances may also be present. The condition is fatal unless treated with D-penicillamine (chelation therapy).

On MRI, the most common finding may be atrophy. Regions of abnormal T2W signal intensity in particular are noted to involve the deep gray matter of the basal ganglia and thalami, as well as the white matter. In particular, the putamen of the lentiform nucleus and caudate are involved. In addition to signal abnormality, atrophy of the caudate nuclei may be present. Regions of T2W hypointensity have also been noted in the basal ganglia and have been attributed either to the paramagnetic effects of copper or possibly associated iron deposition. Signal alteration involving the globus pallidus has been strongly associated with the presence of a portosystemic shunt and total parenteral nutrition with a high manganese content. MRI abnormalities may also be present in the brain stem and in the white matter tracts of the cerebellum. The diagnosis is made by laboratory analysis in which there is elevated copper within the urine and low serum ceruloplasmin levels.

Notes

CASE 189

Orbital Lymphangioma

1. Cavernous hemangioma, capillary hemangioma, and lymphangioma.

2. Cavernous hemangioma.

3. Capillary hemangioma.

4. Extraconal.

Reference

Kazim M, Kennerdell JS, Rothfus W, Marguardt M: Orbital lymphangioma: correlation of magnetic resonance images and intraoperative findings, *Ophthalmology* 99:1588-1594, 1992.

Cross-Reference

Neuroradiology: THE REQUISITES, p 301.

Comment

The most common vascular neoplasms in the orbit include cavernous hemangioma, capillary hemangioma, and lymphangioma. They are usually distinguishable based on their location in the orbit, their imaging appearance, and the age of the patient. Capillary hemangiomas are seen almost exclusively in children and usually present clinically within the first months of life. Although they may undergo rapid expansion, they usually peak in size within the first 18 months of life and then often undergo spontaneous regression. They are typically infiltrative lesions that may secondarily extend into the periorbita, eyelid, and conjunctiva. Because of their vascularity, they may increase in size during crying or coughing (Valsalva maneuvers). On imaging, capillary hemangiomas may involve any portion of the orbit and are frequently associated with vascular flow voids on MRI. Cavernous hemangiomas are the most common retrobulbar mass lesion in adults. Their imaging appearance is distinctly different from that of capillary hemangiomas. Typically these are demarcated lesions that are hyperdense on unenhanced CT, hypointense on T1W imaging, and markedly hyperintense on T2W imaging. Following contrast, they enhance avidly. Although calcified phleboliths may be present, this is not as common as with hemangiomas found in other parts of the body.

Lymphangiomas are poorly demarcated, infiltrating lesions that are less common than hemangiomas. They are usually extraconal and may extend to involve the adjacent extraocular muscles as well as the soft tissues in the periorbita and conjunctiva. Small lesions may be asymptomatic; however, patients may become acutely symptomatic due to hemorrhage within the lesion. On MRI lymphangiomas have a somewhat characteristic appearance: They are usually multilobular, and regions of cystic change with peripheral enhancement are often present. Hemorrhage within cystic regions of the neoplasm is quite common and usually appears hyperintense on T1W imaging. A key to the diagnosis is identifying fluid hemorrhage levels within the lesion. Because lymphangiomas are not encapsulated, surgical resection is difficult and recurrence common.

Notes

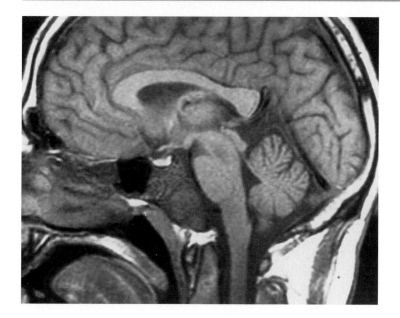
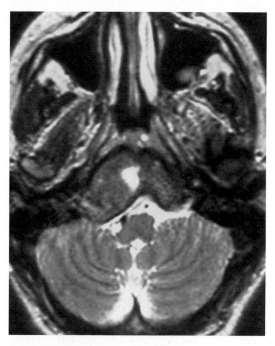
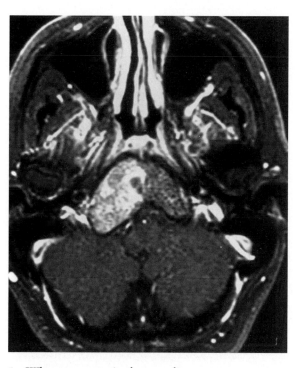
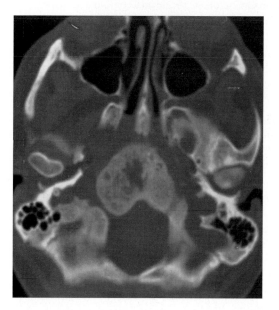

1. What structure is abnormal?
2. What is the differential diagnosis of a clival mass?
3. Cortical thickening is characteristic of what bone dysplasia?
4. How often does fibrous dysplasia undergo malignant degeneration?

Fibrous Dysplasia of the Clivus/Skull Base

1. The clivus.

2. Chordoma, chondrosarcoma, plasmacytoma (multiple myeloma), metastatic disease, lymphoma, fibrous dysplasia, and occasionallly nonossifying fibromas.

3. Paget's disease.

4. General less than 1%, although the incidence is slightly higher in the facial bones and skull base.

Reference

Gee WH, Choi KH, Choe BY, Park JM, Shinn KS: Fibrous dysplasia: MR imaging characteristics with radiopathologic correlation, *Am J Neuroradiol* 167:1523-1527, 1996.

Cross-Reference

Neuroradiology: THE REQUISITES, pp 352, 390, 425.

Comment

This case shows diffuse decreased signal intensity of the clival marrow on T1W and T2W imaging. The clivus is expanded; however, the enlargement follows the normal contour and shape of the clivus. Conditions that may cause diffuse marrow signal abnormality include hematopoietic marrow seen in chronic anemia, infiltrative processes such as hematologic malignancies (leukemia, lymphoma) or granulomatous disease (sarcoid, tuberculosis), and bone dysplasias. A spectrum of neoplasms may also arise from the clivus, including chordoma, chondrosarcoma, plasmacytoma, and metastatic disease. However, these tend to be more focal and destructive in appearance.

On MRI, the signal characteristics of fibrous dysplasia are variable. Typically, on T1W imaging it is hypointense. On T2W imaging it may be hypointense (approximately 33%) or hyperintense (over 60% of cases). Cystic changes, internal septations, and blood products may be present. The majority of cases demonstrate enhancement, frequently homogeneous. In clival and skull base lesions, CT is complimentary to MR in providing information about the underlying bony architecture. Calcified matrix may be seen in chondroid lesions, whereas calcification (bone destruction) may be seen in chordomas and other malignant lesions. In this case, CT demonstrates expansion of the clivus with preservation of the cortical margins. In fibrous dysplasia, involved bones are typically enlarged; the enlargement often follows the normal contour of the bone. The cortex is preserved. The medullary space may have a variety of appearances including sclerotic and ground glass, and at the skull base there may be areas of cystic change. In Paget's disease, which is also typically associated with expansion of bone, there is characteristic thickening of the cortex (unlike fibrous dysplasia). The age of the patient frequently allows differentiation of these conditions. Paget's disease is seen in older patients, whereas fibrous dysplasia tends to be seen in young patients.

Notes

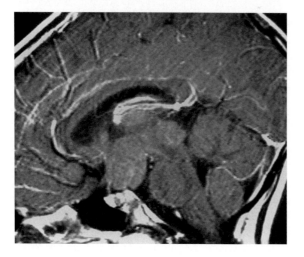
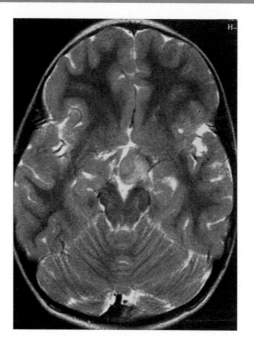

1. Where anatomically is the lesion located?
2. What is the typical clinical presentation of this lesion?
3. What is the typical imaging appearance of this entity?
4. What is the differential diagnosis?

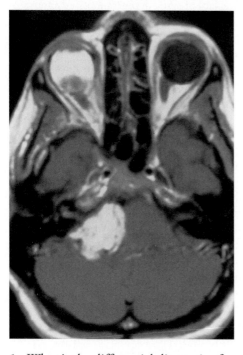
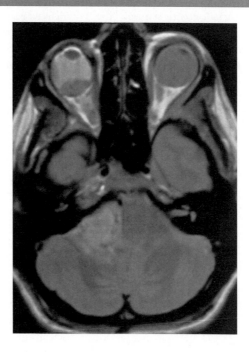

1. What is the differential diagnosis of an enhancing mass in the cerebellopontine angle?
2. Which tumor is most likely to involve the IAC?
3. What are the T1W and T2W signal characteristics of melanotic melanoma?
4. What is the most common primary intraocular malignancy in adults?

Hypothalamic Hamartoma*

1. At the tuber cinereum (floor of the third ventricle), anterior to the mammillary bodies.

2. Precocious puberty and gelastic seizures.

3. These lesions usually follow the signal characteristics of gray matter on T1W imaging but may be isointense or hyperintense on intermediate and T2W imaging. They do not enhance.

4. Hypothalamic glioma; however, the anatomic location of a tuber cinereum hamartoma, its imaging appearance, and the clinical history usually allow correct diagnosis.

Reference

Boyko OB, Curnes JT, Oakes WJ, Burger PC: Hamartomas of the tuber cinereum: CT, MR, and pathologic findings, *Am J Neuroradiol* 12:309-314, 1991.

Cross-Reference

Neuroradiology: THE REQUISITES, pp 324-325.

Comment

This case illustrates the characteristic appearance of a hamartoma of the tuber cinereum. The mass is isointense to gray matter on T1W imaging and sits just anterior to the mammary bodies at the level of the floor of the third ventricle. Hamartomas are benign nonneoplastic lesions that are likely congenital in nature. Many are asymptomatic, but symptoms may be more common in children and typically include gelastic seizures, "fits of laughter," and precocious puberty. Knowledge of this lesion and its radiologic and clinical presentations usually allows the diagnosis to be established in most cases. Occasionally, atypical imaging findings (marked hyperintensity on T2W imaging or a lesion larger than 1.5 cm) raise the possibility of a hypothalamic glioma. In this case follow-up imaging at several-month intervals can be obtained (hamartomas should not grow).

Notes

---

*Figures for Case 191 courtesy Robert A. Zimmerman, MD.

Metastasis to the Cerebellopontine Angle—Ocular Melanoma

1. Schwannoma, meningioma, metastatic disease (hematogenous dissemination or subarachnoid seeding), ependymoma, lymphoma, and inflammatory disorders.

2. Schwannoma.

3. Hyperintense on T1W imaging and hypointense on T2W imaging.

4. Melanoma.

Reference

Bedikian AY, Legha SS, Maviigit G, Carrasco CH, Khorana S, Plager C, Papadopoulos N, Benjamin RS: Treatment of uveal melanoma metastatic to the liver: a review of the M.D. Anderson Cancer Center experience and prognostic factors, *Cancer* 76:1665-1670, 1995.

Cross-Reference

Neuroradiology: THE REQUISITES, pp 70, 287.

Comment

This case shows a poorly demarcating enhancing mass in the right cerebellopontine angle with extension into the IAC. The differential diagnosis includes schwannoma, meningioma, metastatic disease, and an inflammatory mass. The appearance is atypical for a meningioma, given the extension into the IAC and the poorly demarcated margins of the mass. Similarly, poorly defined boundaries, lack of cystic degeneration, and absence of expansion of the IAC in conjunction with abnormality within it is atypical for schwannoma.

Malignant melanoma of the uveal tract represents the most common intraocular malignancy of adults. It is usually unilateral and commonly presents in the fifth and sixth decades of life. On CT ocular melanomas are typically hyperdense relative to the vitreous and enhance following contrast. On MRI, melanotic melanomas are characteristically hyperintense on T1W and hypointense on T2W images. The signal characteristics are related to paramagnetic affects of melanin. In the absence of intravenous contrast, melanoma could be mistaken for hemorrhage such as that seen with retinal detachment. However, enhanced images typically demonstrate solid enhancing tissue with melanomas. The most common site of orbital metastases is also along the uveal tract, and this may be confused with melanoma. Metastatic mucinous-secreting adenocarcinomas to the uveal tract have been noted to have signal characteristics similar to those of ocular melanoma. The most important role of MRI is in detecting extraocular extension of melanoma. Episcleral involvement, retrobulbar extension, and occasional perineural and intracranial subarachnoid spread may be observed. Systemic metastases may occur with primary ocular melanoma; these are most commonly noted in the liver and lungs but may also be seen in the bone and brain. Therefore a careful metastatic workup is required to prevent unnecessary enucleation.

Notes

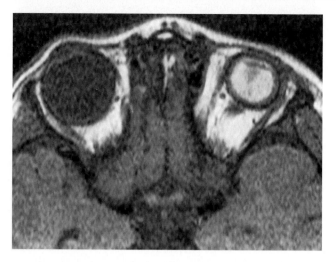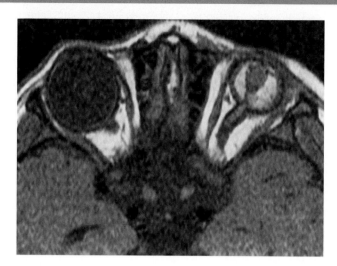

1. What conditions are associated with microphthalmia?

2. What is the most common cause of leukokoria in infancy?

3. Use of high concentrations of oxygen in premature infants is associated with what ocular abnormality?

4. How can persistent hyperplastic primary vitreous be distinguised from retinoblastoma in infancy?

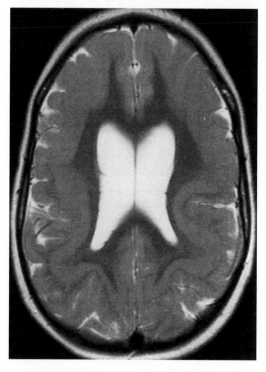

1. What are the types of heterotopia?

2. What other gray matter abnormality is often associated with band heterotopia?

3. What is the pathologic substrate of hemimegalencephaly?

4. In hemimegalencephaly is the ipsilateral ventricle typically enlarged or decreased in size?

Persistent Hyperplastic Primary Vitreous

1. Congenital rubella, retinopathy of prematurity (retrolental fibroplasia), persistent hyperplastic primary vitreous, Aicardi's syndrome (seen in female patients and includes agenesis of the corpus callosum, seizures due to heterotopia, choroidal abnormalities, and vertebral anomalies), and oculocerebral renal disease (Lowe syndrome; how's that for trivia)?

2. Retinoblastoma.

3. Retinopathy of prematurity (retrolental fibroplasia).

4. The presence of microphthalmia and the absence of ocular calcification are features of persistent hyperplastic primary vitreous but not of retinoblastoma.

Reference
Mafee MF, Goldberg MS: CT and MR imaging for diagnosis of persistent hyperplastic primary vitreous (PHPV), *Radiol Clin North Am* 25:683-692, 1987.

Cross-Reference
Neuroradiology: THE REQUISITES, p 286.

Comment
Persistent hyperplastic primary vitreous (PHPV) is a congenital disorder caused by failure of regression of portions of the primary vascular vitreous. Patients may have associated microphthalmia, cataract formation, shallow anterior chambers, and leukokoria on physical examination. The entity occurs much more frequently in boys.

On CT the density of the vitreous is prominently increased. The presence of microphthalmia and the absence of intraocular calcification distinguish PHPV from retinoblastoma. Fibrovascular tissue may be seen extending in a somewhat S-shaped configuration along Cloquet's canal. When present, this persistent hyaloid canal is recognized as tissue that extends through the vitreous toward the optic nerve head insertion at the back of the globe. Blood may be present within the vitreous as a result of retrohyaloid hemorrhage and may outline the hyaloid canal. The MRI appearance of PHPV is variable; however, the vitreous chamber is often markedly hyperintense on T1W, proton-density, and T2W images. Retinal detachments may be present and vitreous blood levels may occur. Retrolental fibroplasia may have a strikingly similar MRI appearance to PHPV, but is usually readily differentiated by the clinical history of prematurity and management with high concentrations of oxygen. Retrolental fibroplasia may also have calcifications that are difficult to identify on MRI but may be readily detected on CT imaging.

Coats' disease, a degenerative process affecting the retina, is associated with subretinal hemorrhage and retinal detachment. The globe is usually normal in size, and there are no calcifications present.

Notes

Band Heterotopia—Pachygyria

1. Subependymal, focal, and diffuse (band, laminar).

2. Cortical dysplasia.

3. Hamartomatous overgrowth of a cerebral hemisphere.

4. Enlarged.

Reference
Barkovich AJ, Jackson DE Jr, Boyer RS: Band heterotopias: a newly recognized neuronal migration anomaly, *Radiology* 171:455-458, 1989.

Cross-Reference
Neuroradiology: THE REQUISITES, pp 256-257.

Comment
Focal, subependymal, and diffuse (laminar, band) are the three well-recognized types of heterotopia. Heterotopias are migrational abnormalities in which normal neurons occur in abnormal locations. The cortical dysplasias are different from the heterotopias in that they do not represent a failure of normal migration, but rather a failure in development of a normal six-layered cortex following migration to the cortical region. Diffuse or band heterotopia refers to a layer of gray matter whose migration has arrested such that it is localized between the subcortical white matter laterally and the deep white matter medially. Therefore the band of gray matter is separated from the overlying cortex by a mantle of subcortical white matter. Band heterotopias are frequently associated with overlying cortical dysplasias. The severity of the cortical dysplasia is directly related to the severity of the band heterotopia: The thicker the band, the more severe the overlying dysplasia (pachygyria, polymicrogyria) will be. Similarly, patients with band heterotopia tend to have more pronounced clinical symptomatology. In addition to seizures, many patients have moderate to severe developmental delay.

Hemimegalencephaly refers to hamartomatous overgrowth of a cerebral hemisphere. Migrational abnormalities are usually present within the affected hemisphere, but they may also be present on the contralateral side. On imaging, there is usually enlargement of the affected cerebral hemisphere and the ipsilateral lateral ventricle, as well as associated cortical dysplasias.

Notes

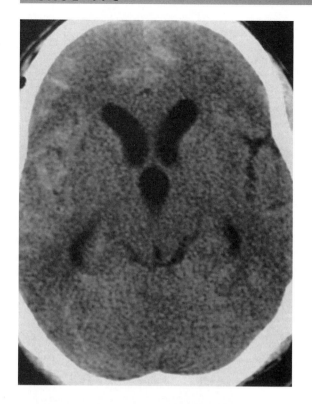
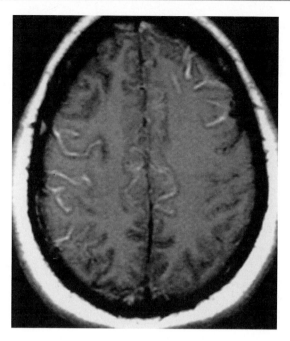

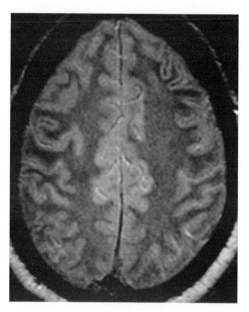

1. What is the differential diagnosis of hyperdensity within the subarachnoid spaces on unenhanced CT?

2. Define neurocutaneous melanosis.

3. What criteria must be met to establish a diagnosis of primary leptomeningeal melanoma?

4. What imaging findings are characteristic of malignant degeneration of leptomeningeal melanosis?

Primary Leptomeningeal Melanosis*

1. Acute hemorrhage, iodinated contrast material (such as is seen following myelography), and a proteinaceous exudate such as is seen in meningitis.

2. A phakomatosis characterized by cutaneous nevi and proliferation of melanocytes within the leptomeninges.

3. Demonstration of proliferation of melanocytes within the meninges, absence of cutaneous or ocular melanoma and absence of systemic metastases.

4. Parenchymal invasion of the brain or spinal cord.

Reference

Byrd SE, Reyes-Mugica M, Darling CF, Chou P, Tomita T: MR of leptomeningeal melanosis in children, *Eur J Radiol* 20:93-99, 1995.

Cross-Reference

Neuroradiology: THE REQUISITES, p 272.

Comment

Leptomeningeal melanosis refers to an increase in the number of melanocytes in the leptomeninges. Melanoblasts (precursors to melanocytes) are derived from the neural crest. Proliferation of melanocytes along the leptomeninges may be seen in a variety of forms, including primary leptomeningeal melanosis, primary leptomeningeal melanoma, and metastatic melanoma. Metastatic melanoma is the most common cause of such proliferation.

The diagnosis of primary leptomeningeal melanosis can be made when the following criteria are met: (1) there is a proliferation of melanocytes within the meninges and/or melanocytosis (high melanocyte count in the CSF); (2) there is no cutaneous or ocular melanoma; and (3) an extensive workup, including a bone scan as well as CT of the chest, abdomen, and pelvis, reveals no metastatic lesions. Primary CNS melanocytic proliferation carries a poor prognosis, with patients living only months following diagnosis. Patients may present with signs of increased intracranial pressure (nausea, vomiting, headaches), seizures, and cranial neuropathies. Leptomeningeal melanosis may be benign or malignant. When malignant, there is characteristically invasion of the adjacent brain (cerebral cortex and subcortical region) or the spinal cord.

Leptomeningeal melanosis associated with cutaneous nevi is referred to as neurocutaneous melanosis and is classified as a phakomatosis. These patients typically have multiple congenital hyperpigmented and/or giant hairy pigmented cutaneous nevi.

Malignant transformation of meningeal melanosis may occur in as many as 50% of patients and often presents with seizures when the intracranial compartment is involved due to direct brain invasion. Leptomeningeal melanosis responds poorly to radiation and chemotherapy. Reported cases suggest that intrathecal recombinant interleukin-2 may provide a more promising response.

Because melanocytosis in the CSF may be associated with a high protein content, unenhanced CT may show a hyperdense exudate in the subarachnoid spaces that may be mistaken for acute hemorrhage. On MRI, unenhanced T1W images may demonstrate en plaque and nodular hyperintense lesions along the leptomeninges within the subarachnoid space or within the cortex/subcortical white matter (when there is malignancy with brain invasion). Involved leptomeninges and brain may show regions of T2W hypointensity due to the paramagnetic effects of melanin. Involved leptomeninges demonstrate prominent enhancement.

Notes

---

*Figures for Case 195 courtesy David M. Yousem, MD.

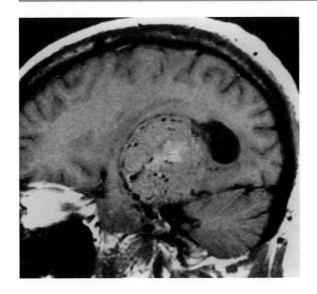
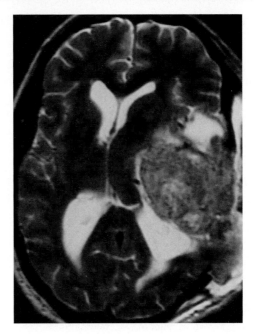

1. What is the most likely diagnosis in this case?
2. How would this mass most likely appear on unenhanced CT?
3. Which tumor is more commonly associated with calcification, meningioma or hemangiopericytoma?
4. With hemangiopericytomas, what type of bony reaction may be present?

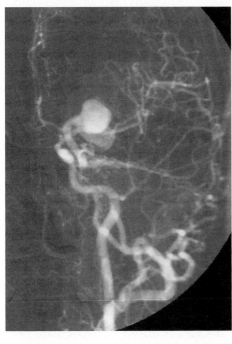
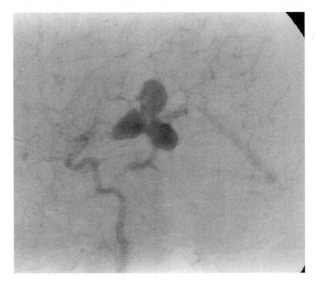

1. What are proposed mechanisms for development of these lesions?
2. What types of intracranial hemorrhage may be associated with these lesions?
3. Which type of dural arteriovenous malformation (DAVM) is associated with hemorrhage, those whose drainage is isolated to the dural venous sinuses or those with leptomeningeal/cortical venous drainage?
4. DAVMs most commonly involve what dural venous sinuses?

Hemangiopericytoma

1. Meningioma.

2. Hyperdense.

3. Meningioma. On pathology, hemangiopericytomas do not calcify.

4. Erosion. In contrast, meningiomas are much more commonly associated with hyperostosis.

Reference

Chiechi MV, Smirniotopoulos JG, Mena H: Intracranial hemangiopericytomas: MR and CT features, *Am J Neuroradiol* 17:1365-1371, 1996.

Cross-Reference

Neuroradiology: THE REQUISITES, pp 68-73, 289.

Comment

Hemangiopericytomas were first reported in 1928; however, at that time they were referred to as angioblastic meningiomas. Several reported cases of identical tumors occurred over subsequent years, sometimes referred to as angioblastic meningiomas and other times as hemangiopericytomas. According to the WHO, the term *angioblastic meningioma* has fallen out of favor and these tumors are now referred to as *hemangiopericytomas*. Hemangiopericytomas represent less than 1% of all intracranial neoplasms. They arise from pericytes in the meninges, presenting most commonly in the fifth decade of life. Headaches are the most common symptom.

Like meningiomas (the main diagnostic consideration) hemangiopericytomas are extraaxial masses that are attached to the dura. Over 50% of hemangiopericytomas have a broad-based attachment to the dura; the remaining have narrow dural attachments. They are usually large tumors (the majority are over 2 cm in size). When large enough, they frequently erode the adjacent calvaria. Unlike meningiomas, hyperostosis is unusual with hemangiopericytomas and calcifications do not occur. These neoplasms are usually hyperdense on unenhanced CT and may be associated with edema (hypodensity) in the adjacent brain. On MRI, hemangiopericytomas tend to be heterogeneous masses that are usually isointense on T1W and T2W images. The presence of vascular flow voids is characteristic. Following contrast, enhancement may be heterogeneous but is usually avid. Approximately 50% of hemangiopericytomas are associated with a "dural tail."

Hemangiopericytomas are aggressive tumors that have a high rate of local recurrence even after total resection. Hemangiopericytomas frequently invade adjacent dural venous sinuses and bone or cranial nerves when they occur at the skull base. Treatment usually includes surgical resection with adjuvant radiation and/or chemotherapy. Extracranial metastases have been reported in the liver, lung, bone, pancreas, and adrenal glands.

Notes

Dural Arteriovenous Malformation/Fistula

1. Venous thrombosis is the most widely accepted etiology; however, these lesions may also be seen as a consequence of trauma, surgery, or venous hypertension without venous thrombosis.

2. Intraparenchymal or subarachnoid hemorrhage.

3. Leptomeningeal/cortical venous drainage.

4. The sigmoid and transverse sinuses.

References

Guo W-Y, Pan DHC, Wu H-M, et al: Radiosurgery as a treatment alternative for dural arteriovenous fistulas of the cavernous sinus, *Am J Neuroradiol* 19:1081-1087, 1998.

Willinski R, Terbrugge K, Montanera W, et al: Venous congestion: an MR finding in dural arteriovenous malformations with cortical venous drainage, *Am J Neuroradiol* 15:1501-1507, 1994.

Cross-Reference

Neuroradiology: THE REQUISITES, pp 144-145.

Comment

DAVMs comprise approximately 12% of all intracranial vascular malformations. Over half occur in the posterior fossa. DAVMs may be categorized based on the dural venous sinus involved by the vascular malformation. These lesions most commonly involve the sigmoid and/or transverse sinuses, representing as many as 70% of all DAVMs. The cavernous sinus region is the next most common site for DAVMs, representing approximately 10% to 15% of these lesions.

Most DAVMs present clinically in older adults. They are believed to be acquired lesions. At present it is believed that these lesions arise as a consequence of dural venous sinus thrombosis. As a result, there is development of a collateral network of vessels, including enlargement of normally present microscopic arteriovenous shunts within the dura. In addition, as arteriovenous shunting increases, venous hypertension develops. In certain DAVMs the venous hypertension may result in retrograde filling of leptomeningeal and/or cortical veins that communicate with the involved sinus. In such cases, rupture of the enlarged venous collaterals may occur. Approximately 10% to 15% of DAVMs are associated with intracranial hemorrhage, which is usually intraparenchymal and/or subarachnoid in nature. Hemorrhage is associated with lesions in which there is development of dilated leptomeningeal veins. DAVMs in which drainage is strictly to the dural venous sinuses are not associated with hemorrhage.

Notes

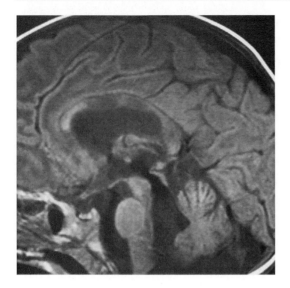

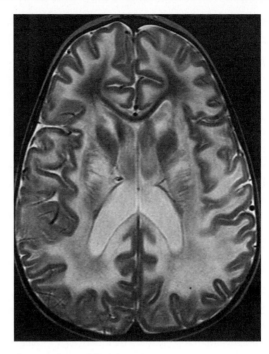

1. What leukodystrophies are typically associated with an enlarged head?

2. What is the typical clinical presentation of the leukodystrophies?

3. What leukodystrophy is unusual in that it begins in the subcortical white matter rather than the deep white matter?

4. Canavan's disease is usually seen in what ethnic group?

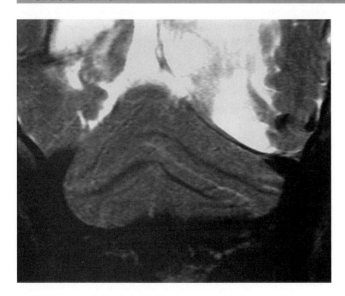

1. What structure is absent?

2. In this condition what other posterior fossa abnormalities are present?

3. What other posterior fossa anomalies are associated with vermian dysgenesis or agenesis?

4. Among Dandy-Walker malformations, Joubert's syndrome, and rhombencephalosynapsis, which is associated with agenesis of the corpus callosum?

Canavan's Disease*

1. Alexander's and Canavan's diseases.

2. Progressive deterioration of motor function, cognitive decline, hypotonia, and/or spasticity.

3. Canavan's disease.

4. Ashkenazi Jews.

Reference

Brismar J, Brismar G, Gascon G, Oznan P: Canavan disease: CT and MR imaging of the brain, *Am J Neuroradiol* 11: 805-810, 1990.

Cross-Reference

Neuroradiology: THE REQUISITES, pp 220-221.

Comment

The leukodystrophies, or dysmyelinating disorders, represent a spectrum of inherited diseases that usually result in both abnormal formation and abnormal maintenance of myelin. Many of the more common of these rare disorders are inherited in an autosomal recessive pattern. In many of these diseases, enzyme deficiencies have been identified as the cause.

Canavan's disease is transmitted as an autosomal recessive disorder usually identified in infants of Ashkenazi Jewish descent. It is the result of a deficiency of *N*-acetylaspartase. Infants may have macrocephaly due to enlargement of the brain. On histologic evaluation there is diffuse demyelination and the white matter is replaced by cystic spaces, giving it a "spongy" appearance. In contrast to most of the other dysmyelinating syndromes, Canavan's disease preferentially begins in the subcortical white matter and later spreads to diffusely involve the deep white matter. There may be sparing of the internal capsules. Usually the ventricles remain normal or slightly small in size; however, in the late stages of disease when cerebral atrophy occurs there may be proportionate dilation of the ventricles and sulci.

Alexander's disease is different from many of the leukodystrophies in that no familial pattern has been recognized. Like Canavan's disease, it presents with macrocephaly in addition to developmental delay and spasticity. The deep white matter is usually involved early, and the internal capsules are typically involved (in contrast to Canavan's disease, where they are often relatively spared).

Notes

Rhombencephalosynapsis

1. The cerebellar vermis.

2. Fusion anomalies of the cerebellar hemispheres, the colliculi, the middle cerebellar peduncles, and the dentate nuclei.

3. Dandy-Walker malformation and Joubert's syndrome.

4. Dandy-Walker malformation.

Reference

Truwit CL, Barkovich AJ, Shanahan R, Maroldo TV: MR imaging of rhombencephalosynapsis: report of three cases, *Am J Neuroradiol* 12:957-965, 1991.

Cross-Reference

Neuroradiology: THE REQUISITES, pp 227-229, 259-262.

Comment

Rhombencephalosynapsis is an anomaly of the cerebellar vermis, which is agenetic or hypoplastic. There is fusion of the cerebellar hemispheres with variable fusion of other posterior fossa structures, including the middle cerebellar peduncles, the cerebellar dentate nuclei, and the superior and inferior colliculi. In the cerebellar hemispheres the orientation of the folia is disorganized. They are usually transverse in configuration, extending across the midline without intervening vermis. MRI imaging typically shows an absent or severely hypoplastic vermis with fusion of the cerebellar hemispheres. There is usually posterior pointing of the fourth ventricle. Associated supratentorial anomalies include partial or complete absence of the septum pellucidum, a hypoplastic anterior commissure, ex vacuo enlargement of the ventricular system related to surrounding volume loss of the brain parenchyma, and fusion of the thalami. Hypertelorism, as well as migrational anomalies, have also been reported with this condition. The clinical presentation is more commonly related to the associated supratentorial anomalies.

Joubert's syndrome, another dysplasia of the posterior fossa contents, is characterized by severe hypoplasia or aplasia of the cerebellar vermis. It has a characteristic imaging appearance, including a "bat-wing" configuration of the fourth ventricle, as well as a horizontal orientation of the superior cerebellar peduncles. Unlike rhombencephalosynapsis, the cerebellar hemispheres are apposed in the midline but are not fused. Associated supratentorial anomalies are uncommon.

Notes

---

*Figures for Case 198 courtesy Jill Hunter, MD.

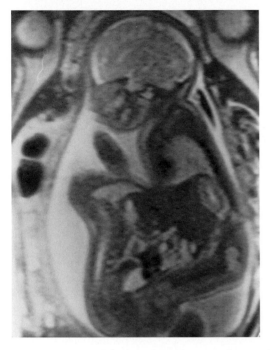
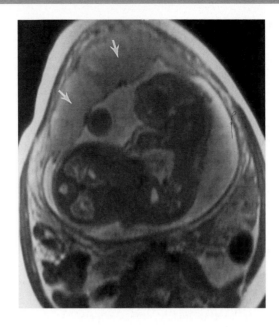

1. Evaluation of potential CNS anomalies in the fetus is typically done with what imaging modality?
2. What structure is labeled by the *arrows*?
3. What type of imaging study is presented in this case?
4. On obstetric ultrasound, what is the upper limit of normal for the transverse diameter of the ventricular atrium?

Fetal Magnetic Resonance Imaging—
Siamese Twins

1. Ultrasonography.

2. The placenta.

3. Prenatal fetal MRI.

4. 10 mm. Mild ventriculomegaly is defined by a maximal transverse atrial diameter of 10 to 15 mm.

References

Sonigo PC, Rypens FF, Carteret M, Delezoide A-L, Brunelle FO: MR imaging of fetal cerebral anomalies, *Pediatr Radiol* 28:212-222, 1998.

Levine D, Barnes PD, Madsen JR, Li W, Edelman RR: Fetal central nervous system anomalies: MR imaging augments sonographic diagnosis, *Radiology* 204:635-642, 1997.

Comment

Anomalies of the CNS occur in approximately 6000 newborns in the United States each year. Many of these anomalies can be detected by maternal serum AFP and obstetric ultrasonography. However, sonography in many cases is not specific. Studies comparing sonographic findings with those of fetal MRI have shown several anomalies that are better detected with MRI. In particular, MRI was more sensitive in detecting migrational abnormalities, anomalies of the posterior fossa (such as vermial dysplasia) and dysgenesis of the corpus callosum, and better identified the cause of ventricular enlargement. In a study by Levine and colleagues, in fetuses with sonographically suspected CNS anomalies, fetal MRI identified additional unsuspected CNS anomalies in 55% of cases. Importantly, the additional information provided by MRI may affect patient counseling, particularly with regard to fetal outcome. It is important to note that a normal fetal MRI examination does not exclude the possibility of an anomaly. In addition, there are some circumstances in which fetal MRI may not be as sensitive as sonography in detecting certain anomalies. For instance, small neural tube defects/meningoencephaloceles may go undetected on fetal MRI.

Fetal MRI may be performed with several imaging protocols. On a 1.5-T system, fast multiplanar spin echo T2W and gradient-echo T1W sequences may be obtained. Fetal immobilization can be obtained by maternal premedication with flunitrazepam given orally 1 hour before MRI examination. However, multiplanar imaging with the HASTE (half-Fourier single-shot turbo spin echo) sequence has been quite successful. Given the rapidity of imaging using the HASTE sequence, fetal immobilization by maternal premedication is not necessary. Because the risk to the fetus from MRI is unknown, imaging should not be performed in the first trimester.

Notes

Index of Cases

255

Index of Terms